LISTEN TO YOUR BODY

ELLEN MICHAUD, LILA L. ANASTAS
and the editors of PREVENTION Magazine

MJF BOOKS

NEW YORK

Notice: This book is intended as a reference volume only, not as a medical manual. If you suspect that you have a medical problem, we urge you to seek competent medical help. Keep in mind that nutritional needs vary from person to person, depending on age, sex, health status and total diet. The foods discussed and recipes given here are designed to help you make informed decisions about your diet and health. They are not intended as a substitute for any treatment prescribed by your doctor.

Published by MJF Books
Fine Communications
Two Lincoln Square
60 West 66th Street
New York, NY 10023

Copyright © 1988 by Rodale Press, Inc.
Prevention is a registered trademark of Rodale Press, Inc.

Library of Congress Catalog Card Number 94-75372
ISBN 1-56731-038-9

Published by arrangement with Rodale Press, Inc.
Manufactured in the United States of America

MJF Books and the MJF colophon are trademarks of Fine Creative Media. Inc.

10 9 8 7 6 5 4 3 2 1

Editor: Debora Tkac

Research Coordinator: Jan Eickmeier

Research and Fact-checking: Susan Nastasee, associate research chief; Holly Clemson, assistant research chief; Sue Ann Alleger, senior research editor; Ann Gossy, Alice Harris, Jill Jurgensen, Sally Novack, research associates; JoAnn Williams, researcher

Editorial/Production Coordinator: Jane Sherman

Copy Editor: Linda Harris

Office Personnel: Roberta Mulliner, Kelly Trumbauer

Book Design: Lynn Foulk, Jane Knutila

Cover Design: Acey Lee

Executive Editor, Prevention®*Magazine Health Books:* William Gottlieb

Group Vice President, Health: Mark Bricklin

The authors are indebted to many people for helping to make this book accurate and complete. Although each chapter has been reviewed for accuracy by an expert in the field, the authors assume all responsibility for the information in this book, including judgments, evaluations and opinions.

PROFESSIONAL BOARD OF REVIEW

H. Randall Hicks, M.D., clinical instructor of psychiatry, University of California at San Diego School of Medicine, San Diego, California.

Richard E. Honicky, M.D., associate professor, Department of Pediatrics and Human Development, Michigan State University, East Lansing, Michigan.

Marvin H. Klapman, M.D., dermatologist, Kaiser Permanente Medical Center, Los Angeles, California.

Samuel Klein, M.D., M.S., assistant professor, Division of Gastroenterology, Division of Human Nutrition, University of Texas Medical Branch at Galveston, Texas.

Merrill Knopf, M.D., diplomate, American Board of Ophthalmology, practicing in Long Beach, California.

Robert S. Kunkel, M.D., head, headache section, Department of Internal Medicine, Cleveland Clinic Foundation, Cleveland, Ohio.

Robert G. Loudon, MB, ChB, professor of medicine, University of Cincinnati College of Medicine, and director, Pulmonary Disease Division, University of Cincinnati College of Medicine, Cincinnati, Ohio.

Ronald A. Lutz, M.D., chairman, Department of Emergency Medicine, Lehigh Valley Hospital Center, Allentown, Pennsylvania, and clinical associate professor of Emergency Medicine, Hahnemann University Medical School, Philadelphia, Pennsylvania.

Richard J. Macchia, M.D., acting chairman, Department of Urology, State University of New York Health Science Center at Brooklyn, New York.

William Norcross, M.D., associate clinical professor of Community and Family Medicine, University of California at San Diego School of Medicine, San Diego, California.

John Phillips, M.D., Lassen professor of cardiovascular medicine, and Chief, Cardiology Section, Tulane University Medical Center, New Orleans, Louisiana.

Lawrence Pottenger, M.D., Ph.D., associate professor of orthopedic surgery, University of Chicago, Chicago, Illinois.

E. Stanley Rodier, M.D., dermatologist practicing in La Jolla, California.

Anne Rosenberg, M.D., assistant professor of surgery, Jefferson Medical College, Philadelphia, Pennsylvania.

Lyon Rowe, M.D., chief of dermatology, Kaiser Permanente Medical Center, Los Angeles, and associate clinical professor of dermatology, University of California at Los Angeles, California.

Cherilyn Sheets, D.D.S., spokesperson for the Academy of General Dentistry, practicing in Inglewood and Newport, California.

Michael R. Spence, M.D., chairman, Department of Obstetrics and Gynecology, Hahnemann University Medical School, Philadelphia, Pennsylvania.

Nagagopal Venna, M.D., assistant professor of neurology, Boston University School of Medicine, Boston, Massachusetts.

Stephen Weinberg, D.P.M., director of podiatry, Columbus Hospital's Running and Sports Medicine Clinic, Chicago, Illinois.

Contents

Notice

This book is intended as a reference volume only, not as a medical guide or manual for self-treatment. If you suspect that you have a medical problem, please seek competent medical care. The information here is designed to help you make informed decisions about your health. It is not intended as a substitute for any treatment prescribed by your doctor.

Acknowledgments

This book was a team effort from front to back. In particular, we'd like to thank the physicians and researchers we interviewed, all of whom were as committed to putting practical health information into your hands as we were; our editor Debora Tkac, who shepherded the book to its conclusion and was always ready to make it better; our research coordinator Jan Eickmeier, who checked, checked and checked again to make sure that the stacks of journals, reports, books and interviews we gathered were accurate; and our families, who heard more at the dinner table about stomachs, rashes and bunions than any of them ever wanted to.

Introduction

It would be nice if none of us ever got sick. Or hurt. Or even slightly sniffly. And we do our best to prevent it, don't we? We eat our fruits and vegetables, lay off hot dogs and munch only whole grain snacks. We swear we'll never look at those long, snowy loaves of French bread again. Or the high-fat cheeses that go with them. And we take 35-minute walks through our neighborhoods four times a week to seal the bargain. Well, maybe three times a week.

What we're doing, of course, is trying to practice good preventive care. And for the most part we succeed. But we live amid a stew of microorganisms determined to give us everything from sore throats, wheezes and sneezes to sore bottoms, aching joints and queasy stomachs.

That's why *Listen to Your Body* was written. Whenever your body is under attack and sending out messages of pain, swelling, sneezing, aching, nausea or whatever, *Listen to Your Body* can translate. With the flip of a page it can tell you what those messages mean, what causes them and what medical experts suggest you do about them.

Take discolored urine, for example. Normal urine usually ranges from crystal clear to dark yellow. But let's say one morning you get up and go to the bathroom, then notice that the urine in your toilet bowl is red. "My God!" you think. "I must be bleeding inside!"

You don't panic. Instead you head straight for the bookshelf in your living room, take down your copy of *Listen to Your Body* and turn to chapter 18, Urinary Tract. You flip through the alphabetically ordered symptoms to Urine, Discolored and find out about a one-minute test —made from materials usually found in your kitchen—to tell whether or not there's blood in your urine.

What's in this homemade blood detector? Baking soda. You sprinkle it into the toilet bowl, and if the red goes away, then returns when you add a few drops of vinegar, you can be sure that it was last night's beets—and not this morning's blood—that tie-dyed your urine red. If your urine *doesn't* change color the way *Listen to Your Body* describes, the book's medical experts suggest you see a doctor. Pronto.

Listen to Your Body is meant to be an easy-to-use source of medical information that can help you avoid running to your doctor for every little thing. But it is not intended to replace your doctor. In fact, you shouldn't even use the over-the-counter drugs or preparations mentioned by *our* experts without checking with *yours*: your family doctor. Your own personal physician is the only one who can evaluate a particular symptom in the context of your body as a whole.

But this book will help. Each chapter outlines symptoms that affect a specific body part or system, including their common causes and possible treatments. And, to further increase your awareness, at the end of each chapter there is a brief discussion of common conditions that may be responsible for some of the messages your body is sending. All of this adds up to information you need to decide how quickly you should see your doctor, to intelligently discuss your symptoms and to ask questions that will reveal treatment options and alternatives.

Listen to Your Body is the book that puts you in charge of your own health care. After all, as the title says, it's *your* body.

Chapter 1

Abdomen and Digestive System

SEE YOUR DOCTOR IMMEDIATELY IF:

- *You have pain in the upper abdomen that lasts longer than five minutes and is not relieved by taking an antacid*
- *You have pain in the abdomen that is accompanied by vomiting and fever*
- *You have severe pain in the abdomen that doesn't go away*
- *You have a sudden pain and a bulging lump in your lower abdomen*
- *You feel a throbbing in the abdomen that doesn't go away*
- *Your abdomen is board-hard and you feel feverish and ill*
- *You're vomiting bright red blood*
- *You're vomiting dark material that resembles coffee grounds*
- *You've been vomiting uncontrollably*
- *You begin vomiting following a head injury*
- *You haven't had a bowel movement for more than two weeks*
- *You have diarrhea for more than 48 hours*
- *You have discharge from the rectum*
- *You have black or maroon-colored stools or severe rectal bleeding*

The digestive system creeps into conversations in the oddest ways. You haven't the "stomach" for this. You can't "digest" that. You don't have the "guts" to do *anything*. But your stomach becomes a lot more than small talk when it starts talking back to you.

That "rumbly in the tummy" that Winnie-the-Pooh once described can leave you mighty bewildered when you're trying to find out what's really going on in there. That's because what's in there is a lot more than your stomach.

The abdominal area contains the liver, gallbladder and pancreas. And while these organs can signal distress through the abdomen, it's the

1

organs in the digestive tract, like the intestine, small bowel and colon, that most often are the cause of abdominal upsets.

The digestive tract is a complex system that is primarily responsible for the digestion and absorption of food. The chain of command begins in the mouth, where food is broken down by the mechanical action of the teeth and the chemical action of the saliva. This food passes through the 10- to 12-inch-long esophagus (or "gullet," as Grandma called it) on its route to the stomach, where it's stored and broken down into small particles.

The broken-down food then snakes through the 20-foot-long small intestine, the main site where it is further digested and absorbed into the bloodstream. The next stop is the 5-foot-long large intestine, where more fluid is absorbed, compacting what's left for the final journey through the rectum and anus.

For most of us, the digestive tract is an unappreciated conveyor belt to which we give little thought—until something goes wrong. In this chapter, you will find a "belly-full" of ailments that overuse and abuse can cause.

SYMPTOM: **Belching**

COMMON CAUSES: When you swallow too much air, gases in the stomach are forced back up the esophagus and out of the mouth. The result: You burp. It's normal and common behavior. Even excessive belching may not be due to an abnormality.

Some air is unavoidably swallowed as you eat and drink. But larger-than-average amounts may be gulped when you're anxious or you eat too quickly, chew gum, smoke or drink carbonated beverages— especially if you drink them with a straw.

Belching, however, isn't always a problem of aerodynamics. Excess belching can be attributed to such digestive upsets as indigestion (see Symptom: Indigestion) or an ulcer (see Common Abdominal and Digestive System Conditions).

BEST RESPONSE: If swallowing too much air is the cause of your belching (and chances are it is), a few changes in some of your personal habits will help alleviate the problem. Experts recommend the following tips, all of which will help you take in less air.

Eat slowly and, if you're the fidgety type, stay calm and relaxed at mealtimes. Chew your food completely—with your mouth closed—before swallowing. Avoid chewing gum, carbonated beverages (they contain air or gas), drinking out of cans or bottles and drinking through a straw. Don't smoke before eating or between courses. Foods with a high air content also should be avoided. These include, but are not limited to, beer, ice cream, soufflés, whipped cream and omelets.

To help alleviate a problem that already exists, digestive disease experts recommend over-the-counter antacids containing simethicone, such as Mylanta II, Maalox and Di-gel, which act by breaking up the "big bubbles" in your stomach.

ACCOMPANYING SYMPTOMS: If fatty foods seem to make you belch, and you also feel pain in your upper right abdomen, you could have gallbladder trouble (see Common Abdominal and Digestive System Conditions).

If your belching is more severe when you're lying down or bending over, and you're also experiencing flatulence, you could have a hiatal hernia (see Common Abdominal and Digestive System Conditions).

SYMPTOM: **Bloating.** *See* Symptom: Swelling

SYMPTOM: **Bulge, Abdominal.** *See also* Symptom: Lump, Abdominal

COMMON CAUSES: A bulge in the abdomen is most often the sign of a hernia, which is a protrusion of soft tissue (often a portion of the intestine) through a weak muscle wall. The muscle wall can tire for a number of reasons; strain and a congenital weakness are most often to blame.

The bulge of a hernia usually appears gradually—over a period of several weeks—although hernias have been known to show up suddenly. Hernias are, for the most part, not serious, although complications can occur.

Hernias can appear anywhere in the abdominal area, and the location usually determines the type of hernia. A bulge or lump near the groin, for example, is called an inguinal hernia; one near the navel is called a periumbilical hernia. Although rare, an incisional hernia can be the result of surgery or a wound.

BEST RESPONSE: If you suspect you have a hernia, you should see your physician to confirm the diagnosis. Most often, say doctors, hernias can be repaired through a routine surgical procedure in which the protruding tissue is pushed back into place.

ACCOMPANYING SYMPTOMS: If you have an abdominal bulge and are experiencing pain, nausea and vomiting, you could have an obstructed hernia. This can occur when the protrusion is a length of intestine that obstructs passage of intestinal contents through the digestive route. A hernia that becomes large, red and painful is strangulated, meaning that the blood supply is being cut off to the portion of intestine causing the bulge. Both conditions require immediate medical attention.

SYMPTOM: **Colic**

COMMON CAUSES: Those who've ever had a child don't need an explanation of what colic is all about—they've lived it. But colic isn't the exclusive domain of infants. Several types of colic occur in adults. If it occurs in the biliary tract—the tube that connects the liver and gallbladder to the intestine—it's called biliary colic and refers to severe come-and-go pain (see Symptom: Pain, Abdominal, Recurring) that can last for a few minutes to a few hours.

In adults, the most common cause of biliary colic is a sudden blockage of one of the bile ducts, usually by a gallstone. Symptoms can be made worse by fatty foods that stimulate the excretion of bile.

But adult colic also can be caused by a kidney stone blocking the ureter, the tube through which urine passes from the kidney to the bladder. Or it can signal an intestinal obstruction or gastroenteritis (see Common Abdominal and Digestive System Conditions).

When parents speak of colic, however, they're referring to a complex set of symptoms that affects 20 percent of all newborns to one degree or another. It usually starts a few weeks after birth and can last from three to six months, even though it's frequently referred to as the "three-month colic." (Colic that starts after two months of age is probably not colic at all, but an allergy or food intolerance.)

Colic can be frightening to new parents as they try to comfort a screaming baby who turns red in the face, clenches the fists, draws up the legs, arches the back and pushes out a little belly that is frequently distended by gas. But colic in babies is not as bad as it sounds or looks. Despite their obvious distress, they eat well and gain weight, and the flatulence is due more to swallowing air during crying than anything else.

But what causes the symptoms that start your baby crying to begin with? Nobody really knows. Too much food at a single feeding may cause painful contractions as food is forced through the digestive system, say some scientists, while too few stomach enzymes may make it difficult to digest carbohydrates and butterfats, say others. Too little of a particular hormone may lead to intestinal spasms, some doctors suggest, or an underdeveloped central nervous system may cause the infant's brain to erroneously signal pain, say others.

BEST RESPONSE: If you're an adult and you have symptoms of colic, you should see your doctor, who can give you an examination and provide the best treatment.

If your baby has colic, keep him or her clean, well fed, well burped and well cuddled. Feeding the infant a little warm water and applying a warm (not hot!) water bottle to the abdomen may also provide some degree of comfort. And check with your doctor or pediatrician. Only a physician can tell one kind of pain from another—including colic.

To help a colicky child get to sleep, you can try rocking or walking your baby in a "front-pack" carrier (it keeps him or her "up close and personal"), driving the baby to sleep in the car, administering a belly-massage with your fingertips, putting the child in an automatic wind-up swing and reducing outside stimulation by keeping the child's room warm, dim and activity free.

To minimize the symptoms of colic, doctors suggest, you might try keeping your baby in a sitting position during feeding and burping to aid the movement of food and the passage of gas. You may also want to eliminate potentially allergenic foods from the child's diet, including butterfat, carbohydrates and cow's milk. If you're nursing, you might want to eliminate milk, eggs and other troublesome foods from *your* diet, although you should check with your doctor before trying this approach.

This is by no means the complete list of colic quenchers. There are probably as many other tips as there are parents (and grandparents) who've been through it. It's most important to keep in mind that a colicky baby is not an unhealthy baby, and although there is no "cure," the storm will pass.

In the meantime, experts recommend that the best thing for parents is to take a break from a colicky baby for short periods of time to relieve parental tension (although you might find it difficult getting the babysitter to come back the second time). And, if all else fails, wrap your child in a thin blanket, put him or her to bed, shut the door and turn up the radio.

As for drugs, their role in the treatment of colic is controversial. Antispasmodic and sedative drugs (such as phenobarbital) are occasionally prescribed by some doctors.

ACCOMPANYING SYMPTOMS: If your colicky baby also suffers from diarrhea, constipation, excessive vomiting, signs of allergies such as skin rashes, or troubled breathing, call your doctor. It's likely that the trouble is more than colic.

SYMPTOM: **Constipation**

COMMON CAUSES: It's not necessary to move the bowels *every* day. For some, regularity means three times a week. For others, it can be three times a day. True constipation, then, is a change from *your* normal pattern.

Doctors say that constipation *in the absence of other symptoms* is usually not a serious symptom. Nevertheless, it's one of the most common digestive complaints, and it is associated with a number of diseases.

Constipation may be the result of a low-fiber diet and/or not drinking enough fluids, which enhance movement through the bowel. Interruptions in normal routine—dieting, stress, inactivity, travel or illness, for example—can also cause constipation. And it tends to become more of a problem with age.

Chronically postponing your answer to nature's call can cause a loss of normal bowel reflexes. The result? Constipation. This is why those with hemorrhoids or an anal fissure often complain of constipation: The pain of a bowel movement may cause the person to frequently delay defecation.

Medications can also cause the problem. Antihistamines and decongestants can make the stool drier, causing more difficult bowel movements.

Other drugs slow down movement in the intestinal tract. These troublemakers are antacids containing calcium carbonate, amphetamines, diet pills, painkillers, many cough preparations made with codeine, phenothiazine tranquilizers, tricyclic antidepressants (Sinequan, Elavil), atropine, cholesterol-lowering drugs (Questran), and certain anticancer drugs (Oncovin).

Ironically, however, possibly the most troublesome drugs of all are the ones marketed to alleviate constipation—laxatives. Excessive use of some laxatives can result in chronic constipation. The reason for this is not clear, but it may be due to thinning of the muscular wall of the colon. Without adequate muscle tone, the colon can no longer contract as it should, and you're left with painful spasms that can be soothed but not cured.

Constipation is very common during pregnancy and is often a problem for some women premenstrually. A rectocele, which occurs when part of the rectum presses up into the floor of the vagina, can also cause constipation. A rectocele is caused by stretched and weakened muscles resulting from multiple pregnancies, age or a congenital problem.

People who are bedridden or who suffer from such neurological abnormalities as multiple sclerosis, Parkinson's disease or spinal cord injuries are prone to constipation. Constipation is a major problem for children who are born with megacolon, an abnormally large colon that lacks the nerve cells necessary for normal movement in the intestinal tract. The condition can also occur later in life.

Also, a diet dependent on only one food group—for example, eating only dairy foods or eating just green vegetables—can be constipating.

BEST RESPONSE: The most effective constipation remedy is diet, most specifically a high-fiber diet, say doctors and nutritionists.

"You can increase fiber in your diet by eating whole grain breads and cereals—a bran-type cereal for breakfast is especially good—and increasing the amount of raw fruits and vegetables that you eat," says Jacqueline Sooter-Bochenek, a registered dietitian and director of clinical nutrition at the University of California at San Diego Medical Center. "Eating prunes and drinking prune juice will also stimulate bowel action and help regularity. Just as important, you should drink at least one quart of liquid every day."

In many cases, these simple dietary changes are all that will be necessary, she says. However, if constipation remains a problem, you can add two teaspoons of unprocessed bran to a meal by sprinkling it over food.

The nutritionist cautions, however, that bran should be added gradually to the diet, since too much too soon may result in diarrhea or increased flatulence. She also cautions that you keep within these guidelines. Since bran may bind with certain minerals, such as zinc and calcium, it may cause nutritional deficiencies. Also, she recommends that you vary your diet so that you're eating foods from all food groups.

Finally, another constipation fighter is exercise, say doctors. Exercise helps keep the body working more efficiently. They also recommend establishing a regular time schedule for bowel movements-- it's what regularity is all about.

If, after trying all these measures, you are still constipated, you should try a laxative, say doctors. But, they warn, laxatives are for occasional use only. And you should use a brand that is least abusive to your system. According to the experts, here's how the major forms of laxatives stack up.

Bulk-forming agents, such as psyllium preparations (Metamucil, Effer-Syllium, Konsyl), calcium polycarbophil (Mitrolan) and plantago (Siblin granules), are your best bet. They are the safest laxatives you can take because they encourage your own system to do the work by absorbing water and expanding. The added bulk stimulates contractions, while the absorbed water softens the stool, making it easier to pass. These agents may take a while to work—from one to three days. Until recently, several of these products were high in sodium, but that's no longer true. They must be taken with at least eight ounces of water or other fluid to prevent a possible blockage of the gastrointestinal tract.

Lubricants, such as liquid paraffin and mineral oil, act by coating the stool, allowing it easy passage. But they definitely have their drawbacks. For example, they sometimes cause rectal leakage. More important, when taken over a long period, mineral oil can deplete the body of the fat-soluble vitamins A, D, E and K by blocking their absorption.

Stool softeners, such as Colace, are often prescribed after a heart attack or rectal surgery, when straining should be avoided. They use the chemical docusate sodium sulfosuccinate (DSS), which doesn't interfere with the absorption of nutrients from the intestinal tract but has been reported to enhance the absorption of mineral oil and shouldn't be used along with it.

Osmotic or saline (salt) laxatives, such as magnesium hydroxide (milk of magnesia), magnesium sulfate (Epsom salts) and sodium sulfate, absorb and pull water into the feces for fast (in two to six hours) and often liquid relief. The problem here is the threat to patients with heart or kidney failure, due to excessive absorption of sodium or magnesium. If you're on a salt-restricted diet, you should use sodium-containing laxatives only under the guidance of your doctor. Glycerin suppositories are classified in this category and are generally safe.

Chemical stimulants, such as senna (Senokot, Fletcher's Castoria), phenolphthalein (Ex-Lax, Correctol, Feen-A-Mint), danthron (Dorbane), bisacodyl (Dulcolax) and castor oil, are the strongest and most abused laxatives. All of these chemicals work fast—usually in less than eight hours. Unfortunately, they may also produce painful cramps, diarrhea, dehydration and, when taken regularly, depletion of certain minerals from the body.

Doctors have advised against stimulant laxatives in general but have come down especially hard on the phenolphthalein ones. They're the most toxic of all the products that you could use for constipation, says Jacques Thiroloix, M.D., author of *Constipation: Its Causes and Cures*. Phenolphthalein acts by irritating the colon wall.

The other chemical stimulants, however, aren't much better. Bisacodyl can cause rectal burning. Senna is excreted in the breast milk of lactating women and can cause diarrhea in the infant. Castor oil is potentially damaging to the lining of the small intestine.

ACCOMPANYING SYMPTOMS: If your constipation is accompanied by abdominal pain, you could be suffering from appendicitis, diverticulosis, irritable bowel syndrome or intestinal obstruction (see Common Abdominal and Digestive System Conditions). You should see your doctor for a diagnosis.

If you're constipated and also have a fever and repeatedly vomit foul-smelling liquid, you could be suffering from ileus, which is an obstruction of the intestines. This condition can be caused by abdominal surgery or a perforated ulcer and requires medical attention.

Constipation can be a sign of colorectal cancer. If your problem is accompanied by any suspicious signs, see your doctor.

SYMPTOM: **Diarrhea, in Adults**

COMMON CAUSES: Diarrhea can be caused by literally hundreds of diseases, and some of them are serious. For the most part, though, diarrhea is mild and short-lived.

Diarrhea results when one of a number of viruses infects the bowel, making it weep fluid. This extra fluid in the bowel causes runny stools, often accompanied by cramping abdominal pain.

Gastroenteritis, lactose intolerance and malabsorption syndrome (see Common Abdominal and Digestive System Conditions) and intestinal flu are common causes of diarrhea. Food poisoning (see Common Abdominal and Digestive System Conditions) can also cause intestinal turmoil, and you can consider the diagnosis sealed if others who ate the same food also come down with the same symptom.

Traveler's diarrhea, aptly known as "Montezuma's revenge," is a variation of gastroenteritis that results in persistent diarrhea for three to five days—more than enough time to ruin a vacation. It's caused by bacteria, viruses or protozoa that are known to invade raw food and water in developing nations.

Sorbitol, a common sweetener found in many diet products (including ice cream) is suspected of causing diarrhea if ingested in large amounts. "The amount that will cause a problem varies from one person to another," says Steven Brozinsky, M.D., a gastroenterologist and assistant clinical professor at the University of California at San Diego Medical Center. "Sorbitol is a sugar that's not absorbed by the small intestine, so it gets into the large intestine intact. This draws fluid into the large intestine and causes the diarrhea."

Many drugs, whether prescription or over-the-counter, have the potential to cause diarrhea. Antibiotics, in particular, are associated with diarrhea, says Dr. Brozinsky. Antibiotic-induced diarrhea can begin as early as one day after starting the drug but can occur up to a month following treatment.

But diarrhea isn't always caused by some outside invader. Anxiety and a case of "nerves" can cause such inner turmoil in some people that they end up with diarrhea.

BEST RESPONSE: Most cases of diarrhea due to intestinal invaders should go away by themselves, says David A. Lieberman, M.D., a gastro-enterologist and assistant professor of medicine at Oregon Health Sciences University in Portland. "Most cases of diarrhea clear up in one to four days. If it doesn't, you should see your doctor.

"Unless a person has severe fluid loss, my philosophy is to do nothing for diarrhea," says Dr. Lieberman. "That's because diarrhea is usually a response to an infection, and the body's trying the best it can to rid itself of that infection. Generally speaking, then, you don't want to do anything to slow down the gut."

Dr. Lieberman suggests that if you have diarrhea, you should rest and eat lightly. "Milk and milk products should be avoided because you may be temporarily deficient in lactase, an important enzyme. On the other hand, chicken soup is good when you're recovering. It has a little salt in it, which is readily absorbed and will help replenish what's been lost. Carbonated beverages and crackers will help replace lost electrolytes, which are important in the balance of body chemistry."

If you've come down with a case of Montezuma's revenge, effective relief can be found by taking an adsorbent medication (like Pepto-Bismol), an antimotility agent (Lomotil or Imodium) or an antibiotic. You should check with your doctor before taking these, because Pepto-Bismol may react with other medications, antimotility agents may slow down recovery and different antibiotics are required to zap different organisms.

Prevention, however, is your best bet. Before embarking on a vacation in a high-risk area, see your doctor, who may want to give you a medication to prevent or treat diarrhea. You can guard against it ever happening by avoiding tap water, ice, raw fish and seafood, raw vegetables, fruits that you haven't peeled yourself, undercooked meat and unpasteurized milk and dairy products. Generally safe foods are those that have been adequately cooked and are served hot, bottled carbonated beverages, hot coffee or tea, beer, wine and boiled and bottled water (check to make sure that the seal is intact).

If your diarrhea is caused by antibiotic therapy, you should contact your physician. Often the only treatment necessary is stopping the antibiotic, although occasionally your doctor will need to prescribe additional medication.

ACCOMPANYING SYMPTOMS: If your diarrhea is accompanied by bouts of cramping, abdominal pain and constipation, you may be suffering from irritable bowel syndrome or diverticulosis (see Common Abdominal and Digestive System Conditions).

If periodic diarrhea is accompanied by cramps, abdominal pain and a general sense of feeling ill, you could have Crohn's disease (see Common Abdominal and Digestive System Conditions). You should see your doctor for all of these problems.

If you've had stomach surgery and your diarrhea and abdominal discomfort are accompanied by palpitations, dizziness, nausea and vomiting, you could be suffering from "dumping syndrome"—too-rapid movement of food and fluid through the digestive tract. The usual treatment is changing your diet to include more fruits, frequent small feedings of dry, high-protein foods and lying down after meals.

Diarrhea that alternates with constipation and lasts for more than seven to ten days can be a sign of colorectal cancer. You should have the problem checked out by a physician.

SYMPTOM: **Diarrhea, in Children**

COMMON CAUSES: Diarrhea in infants and young children can be serious, doctors say, because it can quickly cause dehydration. It can be triggered not only by the germs that cause diarrhea in older individuals but also by cold germs and other germs that don't affect older children and grown-ups at all. Usually the stools are loose and more frequent, and they have a different odor and color—most commonly they turn green.

Parents often blame diarrhea on teething. While it may be a factor, teething doesn't create the problem. But diet might. The risk of diarrhea in infants receiving formula is 6 times greater than in infants receiving breast milk, researchers say, and 2½ times greater than in infants receiving cow's milk. And one study indicates that whole milk is less likely to cause the problem than low-fat milk.

Another study found that infants and toddlers newly enrolled in day-care centers had a tendency to come down with diarrhea. The researchers also found that children and staffers who washed their hands infrequently increased the risk of causing the problem.

When an otherwise normally developed young child has diarrhea for more than three weeks, and the doctor is not able to identify a specific cause for the condition, physicians usually label the problem chronic nonspecific diarrhea of childhood (CNDC). The youngster is typically 6 to 30 months old and has three to six loose stools with mucus daily.

CNDC is probably not a single disorder, doctors say, but a mixed bag of two or more intestinal problems. These include a reaction to new foods or drugs, an enzyme deficiency, genetic predisposition, a form of irritable bowel syndrome (see Common Abdominal and Digestive System Conditions), an inadequate diet or excessive water intake typically recommended for children who suffer from diarrhea.

In addition, drinking apple juice seems to trigger many cases of CNDC. "Kids tend to like apple juice and drink a lot of it," says Richard M. Katz, M.D., pediatric gastroenterologist at Children's Hospital and Health Center in San Diego, and assistant professor at the University of California at San Diego Medical Center. "The problem is that the fructose, or sugar, is not easily absorbed and can cause diarrhea."

BEST RESPONSE: In 90 to 95 percent of cases, infant diarrhea will clear up by itself in three to five days, says Dr. Katz.

Smaller, more frequent feedings every 2 to 3 hours are advised for a child who has suddenly started having diarrhea. Continue breastfeeding if that's what you've been doing, since breast milk is well tolerated and contains antibodies to some of the germs that cause the illness, he says. If you've been bottle feeding, cut the formula concentration in half. In 24 to 36 hours, the baby should be improved and back to regular feedings. If not, the child should be seen by a doctor. In some stubborn cases of infant diarrhea, hospitalization may be necessary, and physicians may prescribe intravenous fluids and antibiotics to clear up the problem.

For children on solid foods, many doctors recommend that one day of liquids (but no apple juice) can be followed by the BRAT diet—bananas, rice cereal, applesauce and toast. "The major problem with the BRAT diet is that it's low in calories and protein, and we're finding now that children do better if some chicken or turkey is added to the BRAT diet," says Dr. Katz. "After two or three days, a normal diet can gradually be resumed."

If your child suffers from CNDC, you can restrict apple juice and see if this helps control the problem, says Dr. Katz. "Actually, CNDC is more of a bother to the family than it is to the child. In spite of the unexplained diarrhea, toddlers with this problem are healthy, and it's just a question of waiting until they outgrow the problem. In the meantime, I sometimes recommend that certain juices or milk products be restricted—if these make the problem worse. Otherwise, nothing needs to be done." Ninety percent of children with CNDC are free of diarrhea by 36 to 39 months of age, doctors say.

ACCOMPANYING SYMPTOMS: Diarrhea in babies should be considered severe if *any* of the following symptoms are present: if the baby has watery stools, pus or blood in the stools, vomiting, fever of 101°F or more, lacks vitality or has sunken eyes with gray circles under them. In such cases, you should see your doctor immediately.

SYMPTOM: **Flatulence**

COMMON CAUSES: Passing gas is almost never a sign of a serious health problem. It's usually caused by something you swallowed— either air or, more likely, food.

When you swallow too much air at mealtime, gases can build up in the lower intestine that are then forced through the bowel for release. (If they lodge in the upper intestine, they're released through the esophagus. See Symptom: Belching.) Some foods are also gas producing: dairy products, wheat products, beans, legumes, broccoli, onions, cauliflower, cabbage, apples and radishes. So, too, is sorbitol, a sugar substitute used in many diet drinks and diet foods.

By far, however, the most common cause of persistent flatulence is dairy products, or, to be more specific, the inability to properly digest dairy products. The condition even has a name—lactose intolerance (see Common Abdominal and Digestive System Conditions).

Flatulence, however, can also be a symptom of gallbladder disorders and irritable bowel syndrome (see Common Abdominal and Digestive System Conditions).

But before you decide that your passing of gas is, in fact, a bona fide problem, you might want to consider the research findings of David Altman, M.D., of the Division of Gastroenterology at the University of California at San Francisco School of Medicine. Dr. Altman actually went to the trouble to find out what the daily norm is for passing gas. He came up with the number 14—if you pass gas up to 14 times a day, you can consider it just a part of everyday life.

BEST RESPONSE: If you really want to know what is causing your excess flatulence—air or food—modern science can give you an answer. You can actually have your intestinal gas analyzed. If the analysis indicates the presence of oxygen and nitrogen, swallowed air is the problem, and dietary change will not help. (But a few life-style changes will. See Best Response under Symptom: Belching.)

On the other hand, if large quantities of hydrogen and carbon dioxide are found, it means that ingested substances are reaching bacteria in the intestine, and change in diet is the right prescription.

For all practical purposes, however, going to such extremes is not necessary. If excessive flatulence is your problem, it's best to assume that it *is* diet related. And finding the offending food or foods is the only way to quell the condition.

You can begin by keeping a list of all the foods you eat for a few days and noting when you have gas problems, says Theodore Bayless, M.D., director of the Meyerhoff Digestive Disease Center at Johns Hopkins University School of Medicine in Baltimore. It usually takes at least two to four hours for a meal to reach the lower part of the colon. This is about the time you can expect your gas problems to begin. If you can pare the offending food down to one or two items, such as beans or onions, the solution is as simple as eliminating them from your diet. If wheat flour is the source of your discomfort, the gassiness may not begin for six or eight hours. You could try switching to foods made with rice or gluten-free flour to avoid it.

If you notice that you have excess gas problems after ingesting milk or dairy products, you could have lactose intolerance. "There are different degrees of lactose intolerance," says Dr. Bayless. "Some people have to drink a quart of milk at one sitting before they are bothered. Others can be bothered by half a glass.

"You should suspect the problem if you generally feel fine but have bouts of abdominal bloating and distress, gas or even diarrhea after you consume dairy products," says Dr. Bayless.

There are a number of tests that your physician can order to detect if you have lactose intolerance, but you can, on your own, try the "lactose challenge," says Dr. Bayless. It goes like this:

Skip all lactose-containing foods (dairy foods) for several days, then drink two glasses of skim milk on an empty stomach. "If you feel pain or bloating in your abdomen within the next several hours, chances are you're lactose intolerant," says Dr. Bayless. Avoid all lactose-containing products for the next several days. If your digestive distress is gone, you can consider the diagnosis sealed.

To keep the problem under control, Dr. Bayless says you'll have to learn to take in only the amount of lactose that your body can handle. Eight out of ten people who are bothered by a glass of milk can tolerate yogurt, for example. Some dairy products may be more agreeable than others—buttermilk and sweet acidophilus milk, as well as some of the hard cheeses, are less likely to "backfire"—and lactose-reduced milk and cheese are now available in many markets. You can even buy capsules of the missing enzyme at your local drugstore and add them to regular milk. And, according to a study published in the *American Journal of Clinical Nutrition,* there's a 47 percent reduction in lactose malabsorption when breakfast cereal, egg and banana are taken with milk.

As for getting the flatulence itself under control, researchers at Loma Linda University School of Medicine in California found that activated charcoal, available in capsule form, cuts down on the amount of gas formed after eating gas-producing foods. However, it should not be used on a daily basis, because charcoal absorbs vitamins along with any bad substances.

Also, over-the-counter antiflatulents containing simethicone, such as Mylanta II, Maalox and Di-gel, may offer relief and reduce belching.

ACCOMPANYING SYMPTOMS: If you react to milk and/or hard cheeses with flatulence plus itching, sneezing, wheezing, hives or coughing, you are probably allergic to dairy products and should see a doctor for testing.

SYMPTOM: **Gurgles, Grumbles and Rumbles**

COMMON CAUSES: Everyone has had that classic moment—sitting in church, being interviewed for a job. The moment is quiet. Suddenly, from the depths of your bowels come gurgles, grumbles and rumbles. You wish for noise, *loud* noise. All you get are stares.

What is it that makes the abdomen growl at such inopportune moments?

One obvious answer is hunger. If you delay a meal too long, your gut rebels by growling. "Rumbling can also be a sign that peristalsis— the muscle contractions that help push food through your system—is doing its job of moving air and fluid through the intestines," says Theodore Bayless, M.D. So what it really means is that you're healthy, not sick.

The only time gurgling would be a significant symptom—and this is *not* the usual case—is when it is accompanied by severe pain or when severe pain is followed by a lot of stomach noise, says Dr. Bayless. It could be a sign that you're suffering from a partial bowel narrowing.

BEST RESPONSE: Turn on some music, start talking, or, if you're really embarrassed by it all, leave the room. If you're guilty of missing a meal or two, have a snack. Or simply disregard the noise; it'll go away. If you suspect something serious, see your doctor.

SYMPTOM: **Heartburn.** *See also* Symptom: Indigestion

COMMON CAUSES: Heartburn is that burning sensation you experience under your breastbone after you've eaten something you liked that didn't like you. Sometimes the fiery feeling is mistaken for a heart attack (see myocardial infarction under Common Circulatory, Heart and Lung Conditions in chapter 5). Or worse, a heart attack may be labeled as heartburn.

Heartburn is the result of esophageal reflux, which is the failure of the lower esophageal sphincter (the muscle at the end of the esophagus), explains Gordon McHardy, M.D., professor emeritus of medicine at Louisiana State University Medical Center in New Orleans. Normally this muscle relaxes to let food into the stomach, then immediately contracts to close off the esophagus from the stomach contents. But if the muscle weakens—a common result of pregnancy and, sometimes, obesity —acid and bile from the stomach can back up into the unprotected esophagus and irritate it, causing a burning sensation in the chest.

"The burning sensation can often turn into actual pain, and the pain can mimic that of a heart attack by radiating into the neck and left shoulder," says Dr. McHardy. "In fact, most people who experience such severe heartburn for the first time go to a hospital emergency room or to their physician."

Many foods can trigger heartburn. Peppermint, spearmint, fatty foods and chocolate are among the most menacing. Citrus juice, tomato products, coffee (even decaffeinated coffee), tea, colas and alcohol can also aggravate or initiate heartburn.

Certain drugs also have been indicted. Progesterone in oral contraceptives, nicotine in cigarettes, the tranquilizer Valium, antibiotics such as tetracycline, asthma medications such as aminophylline, and certain heart medications are just a few examples. The acidity in vitamin C (ascorbic acid) tablets can cause the problem, too.

But heartburn can also be disease related. The major symptom of a gastric ulcer (see ulcers under Common Abdominal and Digestive System Conditions) is a burning, gnawing pain, usually felt throughout the upper part of the abdomen and sometimes in the lower chest. It usually occurs just after eating and can last from half an hour to three hours. The problem can come and go, with weeks of intermittent pain alternating with short pain-free periods.

A duodenal ulcer (see ulcers under Common Abdominal and Digestive System Conditions) produces a similar gnawing pain, usually confined to a small area in the upper middle abdomen but sometimes radiating throughout. The pain is often temporarily relieved by eating, but then returns several hours later and lasts for a couple of hours. It's often worst at night. In fact, nighttime aggravation is such a telltale sign that if you're being awakened by pain in the wee small hours, take it as a clue that you may have a duodenal ulcer.

BEST RESPONSE: The first reaction to an attack of heartburn is usually to take an antacid tablet (such as Rolaids) and lie down. But it's the *wrong* reaction. The best way to get immediate relief from heartburn is to take a liquid antacid (such as Mylanta) and sit up, says Barbara Bachman, M.D., of the University of South Florida in Tampa.

Sitting up helps reduce the pressure against the lower esophageal sphincter muscle, she explains. And while antacid tablets may be more convenient, liquid preparations have the edge because they coat more of the surface of the esophagus and stomach, providing more soothing relief.

Antacids contain at least one of four neutralizing ingredients—sodium bicarbonate, calcium carbonate, magnesium hydroxide and aluminum hydroxide—each of which can have its own set of side effects. For this reason, warns Dr. Bachman, antacids should be used only for occasional bouts of heartburn. Long-term use should be monitored by a physician.

Antacids containing calcium carbonate (such as Tums and Alka-Mints) and aluminum hydroxide (such as AlternaGel) can cause constipation. Sodium-containing products, obviously, can load up your system with sodium. Those on salt-restricted diets should choose low-sodium antacids and eat less sodium in their diet. And any antacid can interact with certain antibiotics, heart medications and other drugs, so if you are under treatment for any medical condition, you should check with your doctor before self-prescribing antacids.

To minimize attacks, avoid the foods or drugs that aggravate them. This can be done by keeping a food diary and noting which food or foods bring on an attack. If you're obese, losing weight may also help to relieve pressure on the weakened sphincter muscle.

In addition, you should eat small, frequent meals instead of infrequent, heavy ones, eat your last meal of the day several hours before bedtime, rinse your esophagus frequently by slowly sipping water throughout the day and avoid lying down after meals.

If heartburn is a frequent problem at night, say doctors, raise the head of your bed four to six inches. This will elevate your upper body without "folding you in half," which can aggravate the condition. Also, avoid using extra pillows for the same reason.

Heartburn should not be ignored. If left untreated, chronic heartburn can lead to more serious medical problems, warns Myron Goldberg, M.D., a New York City gastroenterologist and author of *The Inside Tract: The Complete Guide to Digestive Disorders.*

"The constant backflow of acid can cause ulcers in the esophagus, because the delicate tissues there are susceptible to damage by stomach acid and even bile," he notes. "This can lead to scarring of the esophagus and eventual narrowing, which can make swallowing food difficult or even impossible."

SYMPTOM: **Hiccups**

COMMON CAUSES: Hiccups are caused by the collision of two sudden and involuntary contractions within the diaphragm. Occasional and brief episodes of hiccups are never cause for concern. Even stubborn cases are innocent in nature, although occasionally they can indicate a serious disorder.

You can get hiccups if you eat too much or too fast, if you eat something that doesn't agree with you or, classically, if you've had a few too many. And men are more prone to hiccups than women.

Babies are notorious hiccupers in their early months, but again, it's usually no cause for concern. Hiccups are also a common complaint during pregnancy. Exercising too soon after a big meal, swallowing food "the wrong way," indigestion and nervousness are also among their benign causes. Sometimes an emotional upset can cause an attack. Hiccups can also plague those who have had recent surgery.

Prolonged and recurring hiccups can accompany a variety of diseases, although it's more than likely that other symptoms will have already warned you that there is something amiss. These conditions include pneumonia (see Common Circulatory, Heart and Lung Conditions in chapter 5); pancreatitis (see Common Abdominal and Digestive System Conditions); bladder irritation; uremia, in which urination is less than normal, poisoning the body; diaphragmatic pleurisy, an inflammation of the membrane that covers the diaphragm; disorders of the stomach, esophagus and bowel; and liver problems.

BEST RESPONSE: Most hiccup remedies are based on the scientific principle that high blood levels of carbon dioxide inhibit hiccups, while low levels aggravate them. But doctors will tell you there's no sure cure for the problem. In fact, any know-it-all on the block will tell you his or her solution is best!

Classic remedies for mild attacks include holding your breath for as long as possible, drinking a glass of water while holding your breath, drinking a glass of water rapidly, and swallowing three times with your mouth closed while holding your breath.

If none of these methods seems to do the trick, you might want to try one or more of these not-so-classic remedies culled from experts and those who swear they work.

Hold a paper—*not* plastic—bag tightly over your nose and mouth and breathe in and out for a minute or two. You will be rebreathing your own carbon dioxide, and this should relax the involuntary contractions.

Grasp the end of your tongue with your fingers and *gently* pull it out of your mouth as far as it will go without producing discomfort. Keep it extended for a minute or two.

Bend over as far as possible and drink a glass of water from the far rim of the glass. You'll be drinking from the glass backward.

Dissolve a teaspoon of sugar on your tongue. Or close your eyes and gently press on your eyeballs. And, if all else fails, someone might sneak up from behind and yell "Boo!" in your ear.

When it comes to infants, there's really nothing you need to do for hiccups aside from making sure that stomach bubbles have been brought up, say pediatricians. You can also try giving the child a drink of *warm* water.

A normal attack of hiccups should subside within 30 minutes, says Joel Wacker, M.D., assistant professor of medicine at the University of Wisconsin School of Medicine in Madison. "If you're plagued by persistent and long hiccups, you should see your doctor, who will check for a medical cause," says Dr. Wacker. Sometimes a sedative or a tranquilizer is necessary for serious cases, he says. This is especially true if the cause is emotional.

SYMPTOM: **Incontinence**

COMMON CAUSES: Incontinence—loss of bowel control—affects 16 to 25 percent of all elderly persons living in institutions. Its causes range from a complication of constipation to serious neuromuscular disease.

Any disease that causes severe diarrhea (see Symptom: Diarrhea) can result in urgency and accidents. You can also have the problem if you suffer from diabetes mellitus (see Common Whole Body Conditions in chapter 19), multiple sclerosis or dementia (see Common Neurological System Conditions in chapter 12), a spinal cord injury or deformity, psychosis, or hepatic encephalopathy, which is a neuropsychiatric disorder due to liver disease.

It can also be a complication of anorectal surgery for such conditions as hemorrhoids, anal fissure, anorectal fistula and anorectal abscess (see Common Abdominal and Digestive System Conditions), and rectal prolapse, a protrusion of the rectum through the anus. And a serious tear during childbirth can also cause loss of bowel control.

BEST RESPONSE: Treatment of bowel incontinence depends on the cause of the problem and the degree of severity, doctors say. Exercises to strengthen the sphincter muscle—the muscle surrounding the anus that controls its opening and closing—can be effective in mild cases.

In more serious cases, doctors recommend deliberately promoting constipation by prescribing a low-fiber diet and drugs (such as Lomotil or Imodium) to slow movement through the intestines, then giving enemas every one to three days.

Biofeedback conditioning is a fairly new treatment that may be useful in people with diabetes or those with congenital spinal deformities.

Biofeedback is based on the premise that patients who can feel some rectal distension can be trained to tighten the contractions of their external anal sphincter in response to that feeling. In this way they can retain a stool.

This is how the biofeedback works: A three-balloon device that's attached to polyethylene tubes is inserted into the rectum. As air is pumped into the balloon and the rectum is distended, you'll be asked to contract the sphincter muscle. This simulates normal bowel action. Pressure measurements are made on a machine and shown to you so that you become aware of how muscular contractions match up with normal readings. As you learn to respond better to your own body signals, there is gradual weaning from the biofeedback equipment. Sometimes the whole process takes less than three sessions.

Some studies have shown that this procedure can substantially reduce the frequency of incontinence in 70 to 83 percent of patients. Because of the low number of sessions required and the apparent safety, as well as the appeal and success of biofeedback, it is considered the most promising therapy.

In severe cases of incontinence, such as patients who have to constantly wear a perineal pad (adult diaper), or for those who have a tear in the sphincter muscle, surgery may be the only solution.

SYMPTOM: **Indigestion.** *See also* Symptom: Heartburn

COMMON CAUSES: Indigestion is actually a cluster of symptoms that spell general discomfort in the abdomen, explains Theodore Bayless, M.D. These can include pain, nausea, bloating, gas, belching and an acidic taste in the mouth. So if you've recently been eating or drinking and feel a bit rocky in the stomach, chances are you've got indigestion.

Indigestion is almost always related to food and drink. Rich, unpalatable and fatty foods can cause it. So can gas-causing foods such as beans, cabbage, onions, radishes and cucumbers. Wine, coffee, tea and carbonated beverages are also among the accused. And indulging in either too much food or too much drink can bring it on. Those who smoke heavily or are stressed or overworked can suffer from indigestion after meals.

Sometimes, however, indigestion can be a side effect of a medical condition. It's a common complaint in constipation, and during pregnancy and menopause.

BEST RESPONSE: The fastest route to relief is an antacid, available over the counter or through prescription, says Dr. Bayless. He warns, however, that if you take such medications, be careful not to exceed the recommended dosage (for more on antacids see Best Response under Symptom: Heartburn).

The problem with indigestion, however, is that if you have it once, you'll probably have it again. So your best bet is to take measures to keep the episodes to a minimum.

This can be done by making mealtime a relaxing, not harried, occasion, says Dr. Bayless. This means avoiding emotional issues and personal confrontations at meals. Also, eat slowly and chew completely. And avoid wearing clothing that is too tight. This can aggravate any discomfort that you might feel.

Some doctors feel that a leisurely walk after meals will enhance digestion—and thus eliminate indigestion—by decreasing the time necessary to empty the stomach. Others say that relaxing for half an hour after a heavy meal is beneficial. You might want to try both to find out what's best for you.

ACCOMPANYING SYMPTOMS: If your bouts of indigestion are getting more frequent and severe, it could be a sign of any number of abdomen-related illnesses, including appendicitis, gallstones, gallbladder disease, ulcers or cirrhosis (see Common Abdominal and Digestive System Conditions), and reflux esophagitis, an inflammation of the esophagus resulting from the backup of acid and pepsin from the stomach. In addition, if you notice a long-term, gradual loss of appetite, it could be a sign of a tumor of the stomach or large intestine. See your doctor, who will probably give you a physical examination and may recommend a gastroscopy, a procedure that gives physicians a look at the inside of the stomach.

SYMPTOM: **Itching, Anal**

COMMON CAUSES: If this problem plagues you, be assured that you're not alone. It's quite an ordinary affliction and one that can bother some of its victims for years.

There are a number of factors that encourage anal itching to develop, doctors say. Poor personal hygiene, such as bathing incorrectly or not bathing enough, can cause the problem, especially in those with irregularly furrowed and/or hairy skin. Scratching, vigorous rubbing with a towel or using harsh, dry toilet paper can damage the skin of the anal area, also causing the problem. Moisture collecting in the area as a result of sweat, discharge or wearing tight, nonporous clothing can aggravate the problem, too.

In some people, the use of steroids, antibiotics or local anesthetic agents can result in decreased skin resistance to fungi and yeasts, causing anal itching.

Certain diseases or conditions can also cause itching. The most common are anorectal fistula, hemorrhoids and proctitis (see Common

Abdominal and Digestive System Conditions) or worms (see Symptom: Stools, Worms in).

These are the common causes of anal itching. Unfortunately, about half of those who suffer from chronic, recurring itching around the anus have what doctors call idiopathic pruritis ani. "Idiopathic" means that your doctor doesn't know what's causing the itch, but has ruled out known disease as a suspect.

BEST RESPONSE: See your physician to make sure that no diseases are causing your itching, doctors advise. If no problem is found, you can begin at-home treatment by keeping the anal area scrupulously clean. The use of soap, particularly rubbing with a bar of soap, should be avoided, doctors say, because it only adds to the irritation. But the area can be cleansed after each bowel movement with premoistened tissues such as those used for cleaning a baby's bottom. Do not rub the area excessively with harsh toilet paper or bath towels and avoid wearing synthetic materials, tights, panty hose, tight jeans or jockey shorts. Instead, wear loose clothing made from natural fabrics like cotton.

Most, if not all, local medications should be avoided, doctors say, because topical anesthetic agents and antibiotics are often allergenic— they can aggravate the itch.

Topical steroids are not recommended for chronic itching. But in the case of a sudden flare-up, 1 percent hydrocortisone cream may be applied sparingly two or three times a day for no longer than one week. Aluminum acetate lotion—available at drugstores as Burow's solution— can be used as a simple astringent to soothe the inflamed tissues. Otherwise, pills or creams should be used only on the advice of a doctor.

SYMPTOM: **Lump, Abdominal.** *See also* Symptom: Bulge, Abdominal

COMMON CAUSES: A lump in the abdomen can be a sign of a benign kidney cyst. Or it can be a symptom of intestinal cancer. A lump is also part of the package of symptoms in a number of digestive-related conditions, including diverticulitis and Crohn's disease (see Common Abdominal and Digestive System Conditions).

A lump in a child's abdomen may be a first sign of Wilms's tumor, a major childhood cancer originating in the kidney.

BEST RESPONSE: Any lump in the abdomen that lasts more than a week should be checked by a physician. Doctors say you should pay close attention to any other symptoms you may be experiencing and describe them *all* when you see your doctor. It can help in finding the source of your problem.

SYMPTOM: **Lump, Anal**

COMMON CAUSES: You have this symptom if you have the sensation that "something" is in the anus or if you reach down and can actually feel the "something."

The "something" probably is hemorrhoids (see Common Abdominal and Digestive System Conditions) or skin tags, which are the empty remains of a hemorrhoidal vein that was once swollen or held a clot.

Other causes include an anorectal abscess (see Common Abdominal and Digestive System Conditions) or a rectal prolapse, a protrusion of the rectum through the anus. In children, a prolapse can be a sign of celiac disease, which is a malabsorption syndrome disease (see Common Abdominal and Digestive System Conditions), or cystic fibrosis, a rare, inherited disease that affects the pancreas.

A tumor, although rare, can also be responsible for a lump.

BEST RESPONSE: "Having your problem diagnosed by a doctor is top priority," says David Lieberman, M.D. "Treatment is very different, depending on whether you're suffering from hemorrhoids or a tumor, so an initial medical evaluation is crucial."

Hemorrhoids are treated with a high-fiber diet, increased fluids (six to eight glasses a day), bulk-forming agents such as Metamucil or stool softeners such as Colace, no straining at stool and gentle cleansing after bowel movements with premoistened cleansing pads. Doctors may also recommend medication, warm compresses and sitz baths, in which you soak your bottom in warm water.

Sometimes, in severe cases, hemorrhoids may need to be removed through surgery or laser therapy.

"The treatment for rectal prolapse depends on the cause of the prolapse," says Richard M. Katz, M.D. "Sometimes it's a harmless problem caused by straining during a bowel movement. This can be triggered by severe constipation or diarrhea, and the prolapse will improve once these conditions are under control.

"In some cases, when the prolapse persists, a simple surgical procedure is necessary," says Dr. Katz. Surgery is frequently the treatment for anorectal abscess and tumor.

SYMPTOM: **Nausea**

COMMON CAUSES: That queasy sensation known as nausea is Mother Nature's way of keeping unwanted and potentially dangerous food out of an already "sick" stomach.

The causes of nausea are numerous and can be as abstract as a reaction to an emotional upset or as telltale as a sign of early pregnancy. More often than not, it is a sign of a worse indignity yet to come—vomiting.

Nausea can occur—with or without vomiting—in conditions such as Meniere's disease (see Common Ear Conditions in chapter 6), migraine headaches (see Symptom: Headache, Migraine in chapter 12), menopause, ovarian cysts, painful menstrual periods and motion sickness. It can also be an individual reaction to a strong medication.

In addition, nausea can be brought on by virtually anything that affects the gastrointestinal system, including appendicitis, cirrhosis of the liver, diverticulitis, gallstones and gallbladder disease, gastritis, gastroenteritis, hepatitis, peritonitis, ulcerative colitis and ulcers (see Common Abdominal and Digestive System Conditions).

BEST RESPONSE: "Nausea in the absence of vomiting will generally go away within a few hours," says Joel Wacker, M.D. You can help get rid of the queasy feeling by slowly sipping fluids—water, flat soft drinks and fruit juices (except orange juice) are best, says Dr. Wacker. Chewing on dry crackers can also be helpful. Avoid carbonated beverages, which are gas producing, and milk, which may be difficult to digest.

If you suspect medication is causing your problem, discuss it with your doctor, who may be able to change your prescription or lower your dosage. If you're frequently plagued with spoil-all-the-fun motion sickness—

whether it's caused by car, plane or boat—you can prevent it from happening again by taking an over-the-counter motion sickness medication, such as Bonine or Dramamine, *before* your next venture. Dr. Wacker warns that if you take the medication when the symptom hits, it's already too late.

Also, there is a topical prescription medication called a scopolamine patch that is taped behind the ear and can be effective against nausea for several hours.

Since it's best to avoid all drugs during pregnancy, there are some self-help measures you can take to control your "morning sickness." (This term, by the way, is a misnomer, since the condition can occur at any time of the day.)

Eat small, frequent meals to keep food in your stomach, since nausea is most bothersome on an empty stomach, suggest obstetricians. In the same vein, avoid eating heavy and full meals. Always be kind to your stomach by drinking fluids slowly and sparingly. Some obstetricians suggest keeping dry crackers on your nightstand. If you wake up feeling queasy, you can eat them before getting out of bed. After eating, you should lie down for 20 minutes.

Also keep in mind that for the majority of the pregnant population, morning sickness is only temporary. It usually subsides within a few weeks.

For the most part, though, avoiding nausea can be difficult, especially if it's disease related or an emotional reaction. "Some people have a higher sensitivity to their inner workings," says Dr. Wacker. "There's really not much you can do about such reactions except to know that you may be one of those people who gets nauseated easily."

ACCOMPANYING SYMPTOMS: If your nausea causes vomiting that persists for five or six hours, and you're also experiencing abdominal pain and fever, call your doctor. You're probably suffering from one of any number of gastrointestinal ailments that require immediate attention.

SYMPTOM: **Pain, Abdominal, Burning.** *See* Symptom: Heartburn

SYMPTOM: **Pain, Abdominal, Recurring**

COMMON CAUSES: This is a kind of come-and-go pain that comes and goes over a long period of time. There are numerous digestive problems related to such pain, but by far the most likely cause is irritable bowel syndrome (see Common Abdominal and Digestive System Conditions).

IBS, as it is called, is actually a collection of digestive-oriented symptoms characterized by episodes of persistent or spasmodic pain, usually concentrated on one side of the lower abdomen, that are often relieved by a bowel movement. It's usually accompanied by constipation or diarrhea or a combination of the two. Gas, bloating and nausea are also common side effects. It's common in both adults and children, and, although a specific cause has not been identified, psychological or stressful factors often accompany or aggravate the condition, says Stephen Hanauer, M.D., a gastroenterologist at the University of Chicago Medical Center.

"The good news about IBS is that the symptoms rarely get worse and there is no danger of medical complications," says Dr. Hanauer. "The bad news, however, is that the discomfort can go on for years."

IBS, however, is usually the diagnosis only if organic disease can be ruled out. Gallbladder disease (see Common Abdominal and Digestive System Conditions), for example, is characterized by recurring pain. Attacks usually occur after consuming a fatty meal. Pain is generally felt in the upper abdomen and lasts at least 20 minutes and often up to two to four hours.

An ulcer (see Common Abdominal and Digestive System Conditions) is also characterized by recurring pain, usually in the upper part of the abdomen. The pain can occur immediately following a meal or up to several hours later, and it can last for up to three hours. The "hunger pains" of a duodenal ulcer are usually felt in a small spot in the upper middle abdomen and occur several hours after a meal.

Other diseases characterized by recurring pain include diverticulitis, colitis and ulcerative colitis, Crohn's disease and pancreatitis (see Common Abdominal and Digestive System Conditions), endometriosis (see Common Reproductive System Conditions in chapter 14), and cancers of the stomach, large intestine and pancreas.

BEST RESPONSE: Pain is impossible to diagnose on your own, so your best bet is to see your doctor, who will listen to your symptoms (make sure you pay attention to and can describe all of them) and possibly run a battery of tests to determine the origin of your discomfort. If there is no sign of a specific disease, you may be suffering from irritable bowel syndrome.

"There's no one treatment for all persons who suffer from irritable bowel syndrome," says Dr. Hanauer. "A lot depends on the individual case—what the person's symptoms are, what aggravates them and what relieves them."

Diet can often be a modifying factor in IBS. "If pain accompanies diarrhea, I have patients avoid irritants such as alcohol, caffeine and highly spiced food," says Dr. Hanauer. "They should also reduce raw roughage in favor of cooked, canned or peeled fruits and vegetables. I also suggest avoiding highly concentrated fruit juices or irritants such as orange juice."

If the pain is accompanied by constipation, Dr. Hanauer recommends a more liberal intake of roughage. "These patients should increase their consumption of fruits and vegetables or add bran fiber to their diet," he says. Bran acts as a natural laxative. If constipation persists, he recommends a mild bulk laxative, such as Metamucil.

For *all* IBS sufferers, Dr. Hanauer suggests regular eating habits, including regularly scheduled meals. If milk is found to cause gas, bloating or diarrhea, it should be avoided or treated with enzymes. "You should also stop smoking, since cigarettes produce intestinal spasm, and at least learn to recognize and try to minimize those situations that aggravate the stress that creates the problem," he says. As for drugs, Dr. Hanauer says, "some patients benefit from antispasmodic drugs with or without a sedative. Some find antidepressants helpful. Antidiarrhea medication may be necessary for those who cannot get rid of the problem through natural means."

Since stress is an important factor in IBS, some have found stress-management courses, biofeedback or psychotherapy to be helpful.

ACCOMPANYING SYMPTOMS: If you begin noticing changes in your normal IBS symptoms, especially rectal bleeding or unexplained weight loss, you should make an appointment to see your doctor, says Dr. Hanauer.

"IBS can go on for years without indicating there is something more seriously wrong," says Dr. Hanauer. "However, a change in symptoms calls for a complete workup to find if there's a new source of the problem."

SYMPTOM: **Pain, Anal**

COMMON CAUSES: Hemorrhoids (see Common Abdominal and Digestive System Conditions) are notorious pain causers, although the pain is generally most intense while trying to pass a stool.

Anal fissure and anorectal abscess (see Common Abdominal and Digestive System Conditions) and trauma are other common causes of chronic pain. "Fissures can cause so much pain that people hold in their bowel content until it becomes hard and difficult to move," says David Lieberman, M.D.

For some, though, pain occurs only during defecation. "Hard stools cause straining and irritation, which in turn cause the sphincter muscle to go into spasm," says Herand Abcarian, M.D., former secretary of the American Society of Colon and Rectal Surgeons.

BEST RESPONSE: If you suffer from anal pain, you should see your physician for proper diagnosis, recommends Dr. Lieberman. A change in your diet most likely will be in order.

Hemorrhoids are treated with a high-fiber diet, increased fluids (six to eight glasses a day), bulk-forming agents such as Metamucil or stool softeners such as Colace, no straining at stool and gentle cleansing after bowel movements with premoistened cleansing pads. Doctors may also recommend medication, warm compresses and sitz baths, in which you soak your bottom in warm water.

Dietary changes will also help relieve the pain caused by excessively hard stools, says Dr. Abcarian. "A high-fiber diet—unprocessed bran is preferred—plus fruits and vegetables and lots of water will help soften the stools. You can also take one tablespoon of a bulking agent three times a day. Once the stools are soft and mushy, the pain should lessen."

For anal fissures, over-the-counter pain relievers such as acetaminophen (Tylenol) may be helpful, says Dr. Lieberman. Also, taking a sitz bath, using over-the-counter anesthetic ointments such as benzocaine or pramoxine hydrochloride and taking stool softeners will help soothe the ache. Anorectal abscess often requires surgery to open the abscess and drain the pus.

ACCOMPANYING SYMPTOMS: If you engage in anal intercourse and have painful bowel movements accompanied by ineffectual straining at stool, see your doctor. You're at high risk for infection and could have proctitis (see Common Abdominal and Digestive System Conditions) or a sexually transmitted disease (see Common Reproductive System Conditions in chapter 14).

SYMPTOM: **Regurgitation**

COMMON CAUSES: Regurgitation, the backup of undigested food, acid or water into the mouth, is usually the result of a weakness in the valve between the esophagus and stomach.

Regurgitation is different from vomiting, although the sensation may be similar. In vomiting, a coordinated series of events, including nausea and muscular contractions of the diaphragm, results in the expulsion of stomach contents. In regurgitation, on the other hand, contents from the stomach or esophagus back up into the mouth effortlessly, without nausea or muscular contractions.

In adults, many disorders that affect the esophagus may cause regurgitation. These include hiatal hernia (see Common Abdominal and Digestive System Conditions), ulcer of the esophagus and esophagitis, an inflammation of the lining of the esophagus.

In infants, regurgitation, or "spitting up," is a common, harmless condition. Babies tend to have a weak esophageal valve, and overfilling their small stomachs can cause them to spit up.

BEST RESPONSE: A liquid antacid such as Mylanta can help adults bothered by regurgitation, say doctors (for more information on antacids, see Best Response under Symptom: Heartburn). You should, however, discuss the problem with your doctor.

The same advice does not apply to infants. They will eventually outgrow the problem as the esophagus gets stronger.

ACCOMPANYING SYMPTOMS: If you're regurgitating food and also have difficulty swallowing, you could have Zenker's diverticulum, an unnatural pouch that develops along the wall of the esophagus. Treatment for this somewhat rare condition ranges from no treatment at all to surgery, depending on the size of the pouch.

If swallowing food is difficult and causes you to regurgitate, you could be suffering from achalasia, a condition caused by failure of the muscles of the esophagus to relax. Treatment can range from a low-bulk diet for mild cases to corrective surgery for severe cases.

SYMPTOM: **Stools, Black**

COMMON CAUSES: A normal bowel movement is brown, soft and formed. Very black, tarry stools—usually liquid or semiliquid—are a sign of bleeding taking place high in the intestinal tract.

Black stools, however, can also be caused by such harmless things as taking certain pills or eating certain foods. Iron pills, bismuth (found in some over-the-counter antacids) and charcoal can cause dark stools. Eating foods such as licorice, chocolate sandwich cookies such as Oreos and Hydrox, grapes, raisins and cranberries can also cause stools to turn a very dark color. So before jumping to the conclusion that your dark stools are due to internal bleeding, try to remember what you ate over the past day or two.

The serious causes of black, tarry stools include bleeding from an ulcer and gastritis (see Common Abdominal and Digestive System Conditions), esophageal varices, which are dilated veins in the esophagus, or tumors of the stomach or intestines.

Blood in the stool can also be a complication of drug therapy. This can result in gastric erosion—a worn spot in your stomach—or ulcers, and the most common culprit is aspirin, which is taken frequently by arthritics. Nonsteroidal anti-inflammatory agents such as Motrin can also cause bleeding.

BEST RESPONSE: If you overdosed on Oreos or other "suspicious" foods within the last 18 to 24 hours, there may be no need to fear, but you should see your doctor as soon as possible to be sure. Even if you suspect the cause is related to medication, you should leave it up to your doctor to make the diagnosis.

If you suffer from ulcers or some other intestinal problem, you should routinely check your stools for any change in color and report it to your doctor.

ACCOMPANYING SYMPTOMS: If you live in the southern United States and notice black stools, along with great hunger, weakness, fatigue, pallor, shortness of breath on exertion and palpitations, you could be suffering from hookworm. The hookworm larva penetrates the body through the soles of the feet, and then moves to the small intestine and attaches itself to the intestinal wall, where it feeds on its victim. Anemia frequently results. The eggs of the hookworm are excreted in the stool. If you think you have this problem, you should see a doctor, since medication can be prescribed to kill the hookworm and treat the anemia.

SYMPTOM: **Stools, Bloody or Red**

COMMON CAUSES: This is the rectal symptom that most frequently sends people to their doctor. And with just cause—it can be a very serious symptom. In most cases, however, it's not.

In fact, it often turns out that bloody-looking stools aren't bloody at all. They only look that way because of something you ate or drank. In babies, for example, undigested beets or tomatoes can make the stools red. And if you've been drinking cherry-flavored drinks such as Kool-Aid and Hawaiian Punch or eating breakfast cereals that are reddish in color, you may also end up with red-looking stools. Drugs that have red dyes in them can also be the cause. And one physician reported to the British medical journal *Lancet* that cherry-flavored medicines for children can cause stools that closely resemble the bloody stools of serious disorders.

If what you see is actually blood, the cause could be hemorrhoids, anal fissure or proctitis (see Common Abdominal and Digestive System Conditions), polyps, which are benign growths in the rectum, or colorectal cancer.

BEST RESPONSE: Even if you think that your red stools are due to something you ate or a drug you're taking, doctors say you should have it checked out by your physician, since the diagnosis is often too close to call.

"It's good that this is a symptom that worries people enough to see their doctor, because only a doctor can sort out what the true cause of the bleeding could be," says David Lieberman, M.D. "Although hemorrhoids are most likely to be the cause, the symptoms of this condition are the same as those produced by other disorders, including cancer."

When you see your doctor, he or she may examine your abdomen, perform a rectal examination and test your stool for blood. If the doctor suspects cancer or a polyp, he or she may use a device called a sigmoidoscope to look inside the rectum and lower colon. A sigmoidoscopic examination enables doctors to detect colorectal cancer in its early stages, even before it shows up on x-rays. Because doctors can detect problems at extremely early stages, they are able to head off many complications that could be potentially life-threatening.

SYMPTOM: **Stools, Hard.** *See* Symptom: Constipation

SYMPTOM: **Stools, Pale**

COMMON CAUSES: You can have pale stools if your diet consists mostly of milk. But pale or yellowish-gray stools that are greasy-looking, soft and bulky and have a strong odor are most likely due to poor digestion or malabsorption. This can result from a number of conditions, such as Crohn's disease and malabsorption syndrome (see Common Abdominal and Digestive System Conditions), and pancreatic disease, like cystic fibrosis.

BEST RESPONSE: If you're persistently passing pale-colored stools—especially if you're not feeling well or are experiencing any other symptom—you should see your doctor. It may be a sign of disease or a complication of an existing disease.

SYMPTOM: **Stools, Worms in**

COMMON CAUSES: Worms in stools are usually easy enough to detect; they often are quite visible.

Pinworms are the most common variety. They look like small white threads that wiggle and can be seen both in the bowel movement and around the anus. They occur most often in children and are spread by touching the worms or eggs with the hands and then touching the mouth. They also cause itching, especially at night.

Roundworms can also be found in the stool, although this is rare. Roundworms, which look like earthworms with tapered ends, are harder to detect than pinworms or may not be seen at all. They are caused by eating beef or pork that has not been properly cooked.

BEST RESPONSE: If you think you've found a worm in a stool, save the specimen to show your doctor. Proper identification will allow your doctor to select a drug that will kill the parasite.

"Pinworms are very common and are easily treated with one dose of a prescription medication called mebendazole (Vermox)," says Richard M. Katz, M.D. Since they can be spread easily, everyone in the family should be treated at the same time. Also, wash all sheets and undergarments at the same time."

SYMPTOM: **Straining at Stool**

COMMON CAUSES: Don't confuse this with constipation. The official name here is rectal tenesmus, meaning ineffectual straining at stool. You feel an urgent need to go to the bathroom, but often achieve no result.

The problem is frequently caused simply by ignoring nature's call. However, if straining at stool is a routine complaint, you might have a medical problem.

"Any condition that expands the rectum and gives it a sense of fullness can cause tenesmus," says David Lieberman, M.D. It could be caused by an inflammation such as proctitis, large internal hemorrhoids or an impacted stool (see Common Abdominal and Digestive System

Conditions), rectal polyps or tumors. It can sometimes be a problem for those with ulcerative colitis (see Common Abdominal and Digestive System Conditions). In women, straining can be caused by a droopy bladder or rectum.

BEST RESPONSE: Set aside a regular time to move your bowels and stick to that routine. If you can't move your bowels easily and you find yourself straining, doctors say you should leave the bathroom until the urge returns.

Straining can aggravate hemorrhoids or hernias and can adversely affect blood pressure and heartbeat, says Dr. Lieberman. Therefore, you should take measures to prevent it from happening. A high-fiber diet, drinking more fluids (including juices) and getting regular exercise are all helpful in promoting regularity.

He also suggests taking a tip from our long-ago ancestors, who moved their bowels in a more natural stance—squatting. You can do this by placing a few books in front of the toilet and resting your feet on them, thus raising your knees.

If none of these measures helps, it's time to see your doctor. "If straining is being caused by disease, then the disease needs to be treated before the symptom can be alleviated," says Dr. Lieberman.

SYMPTOM: **Swelling**

COMMON CAUSES: Swelling or bloating in the abdomen can have several causes: It may mean you're retaining water due to your menstrual cycle or possibly that fluid is accumulating in your abdomen or that gas or air is trapped in your stomach. (Of course, it's also part of the process of pregnancy.)

The cyclical bloating that precedes a menstrual period—usually two to ten days before—is common and no cause for concern. It's part of the package in a condition now known as premenstrual syndrome, or PMS (see Common Reproductive System Conditions in chapter 14). Such bloating does have a physiological basis, however. Research indicates that a shortage of progesterone, the hormone that, among other things, keeps water from accumulating in the body, may spur many PMS symptoms.

Bloating that stems from a digestive problem is actually a secondary symptom; it's caused by gas or air in the intestinal tract. It's often been associated with gastroenteritis and irritable bowel syndrome (see Common Abdominal and Digestive System Conditions).

Among the less common—but by no means rare—causes of fullness and swelling is the formation of "bezoars" in the stomach or small intestine. This is the ultimate "knot in the stomach" and, in 55 percent of the cases, the knot is composed of hair, wool strands or carpet fibers (this occurs most frequently in girls who have the nervous habit of chewing on their hair).

Bezoars also can be composed of densely entangled fruit and/or vegetable fibers or other materials. In fact, one medical journal reported the unusual case of a psychiatric patient who had a bezoar composed of 290 shoestrings. (Maybe he took "living on a shoestring" literally.) The cordlike mass ran from the esophagus through the colon. Bezoars can also occur after certain types of gastrointestinal surgery. The danger of bezoars is that they can cause obstruction or long-term interference with normal digestion and absorption of nutrients.

Distended abdomens are common in children with hypothyroidism; cystic fibrosis, a rare hereditary disease that affects the pancreas; or megacolon, an unusually large colon.

BEST RESPONSE: If fluid retention is common prior to your menstrual period, try to cut down your intake of salty foods such as processed meats, cheese and highly seasoned foods.

Diuretics ("water pills") are sometimes prescribed, although these should be taken sparingly because of their potential side effects. You should take them only under a doctor's supervision. After all, premenstrual water retention is only a temporary condition.

Fullness created by gas or air can be alleviated only by finding the cause of your belching or flatulence—sometimes a food that can be eliminated from your diet.

Only a physician with the aid of diagnostic tests can tell you if you have a bezoar in your stomach or small intestine. According to doctors, treatment for this condition includes clear-liquid diets, use of organic solvents and enzymes to dissolve the "knot" and, in emergencies, surgical removal of the mass. Complete passage of stomach bezoars can take as long as ten months.

ACCOMPANYING SYMPTOMS: A swollen abdomen accompanied by puffy ankles and shortness of breath (especially at night) may be a result of heart failure (see Common Circulatory, Heart and Lung Conditions in chapter 5).

If your stomach is bloated and you notice that you are also passing less urine than usual, you could be suffering from glomerulonephritis (see Common Urinary Tract Conditions in chapter 18).

Diarrhea, abdominal pain and swelling may be present in celiac disease (see Common Abdominal and Digestive System Conditions) and sprue, common malabsorption syndrome diseases. Swelling in the abdomen accompanied by severe abdominal pain and fever may mean peritonitis (see Common Abdominal and Digestive System Conditions).

All of these conditions require care by a physician.

SYMPTOM: **Tenderness**

COMMON CAUSES: Abdominal tenderness—soreness that is felt when pressure is applied—can be the result of something as innocuous as overdoing it in aerobics class or something as serious as appendicitis (see Common Abdominal and Digestive System Conditions).

Tenderness that is not accompanied by other symptoms and lasts only a short period of time—say a few days—is usually no cause for alarm, say doctors. It can be caused by overdoing it, and you may not even realize you've overdone it. A bout with the flu or a cold, for example, can cause a tender abdomen just from the "exercise" of coughing or vomiting so much.

A number of digestive problems are characterized by a sore and tender stomach, although they are almost always accompanied by other symptoms. However, the location of the tenderness is often a clue to what ails you.

If you're tender just below the ribs on the right side, the problem could be hepatitis (see Common Abdominal and Digestive System Conditions). Tenderness in the pit of the stomach can indicate pancreatitis (see Common Abdominal and Digestive System Conditions). Tenderness in the lower half of the abdomen can be the result of appendicitis or ulcerative colitis (see Common Abdominal and Digestive System

Conditions). And tenderness in the left side of the abdomen could be diverticulosis (see Common Abdominal and Digestive System Conditions).

BEST RESPONSE: Tenderness caused by strain or overdoing it requires no attention; it will simply go away by itself. But if you suspect that your tenderness is disease oriented, don't attempt to make a diagnosis on your own. Pay close attention to *all* your symptoms and see your physician, who can examine you and give you any of a series of tests to determine the cause of your discomfort.

SYMPTOM: **Vomiting**

COMMON CAUSES: You may not appreciate it at the time, but vomiting is often a *helpful* symptom. It rids your body of unwanted poisons—whether it's food that's spoiled or inedible for some other reason or food that is contaminated or poisoned (see food poisoning under Common Abdominal and Digestive System Conditions). Often if someone swallows a substance that could be or is poisonous, doctors give medicine to *force* vomiting.

Overeating, overdrinking and emotional upsets are classic examples of situations when getting sick is your ticket to feeling better. The experience is usually short-lived. Sometimes, however, you feel the misery is never going to come to an end. This is when you can suspect the cause is more than something you ate.

Gastritis and gastroenteritis (see Common Abdominal and Digestive System Conditions) are common ailments characterized by vomiting. But you may suffer from other symptoms, too, such as pain and diarrhea.

Vomiting may also be a dominant (but not necessarily the only) symptom in more serious conditions such as appendicitis, gallbladder disease, hepatitis, pancreatitis, peritonitis and ulcers (see Common Abdominal and Digestive System Conditions); heart attack (see myocardial infarction under Common Circulatory, Heart and Lung Conditions in chapter 5); allergic reactions to insect and spider bites and poisonous snake bites (see Symptom: Bites and Stings in chapter 15); heat exhaustion (see Common Whole Body Conditions in chapter 19); kidney failure (see Common Urinary Tract Conditions in chapter 18); bowel obstruction; diabetic coma; withdrawal from drugs; or shock due to injuries. And, of course, anything that causes nausea (see Symptom: Nausea) also can lead to vomiting.

In the gynecological department, vomiting can be a companion to morning sickness, a condition that occurs in the early weeks of pregnancy, and it is a symptom of toxemia, which occurs in the last three months and is not considered normal. Vomiting may also be a problem for women who suffer from painful menstrual periods.

Vomiting is also a frequent accompaniment to such neurological problems as stroke (see Common Neurological System Conditions in chapter 12); migraine headache (see Symptom: Headache, Migraine in chapter 12); acute glaucoma (see Common Eye Conditions in chapter 7); brain injuries and brain tumors.

Vomiting in babies often can be brought on by appendicitis or intestinal obstructions (see Common Abdominal and Digestive System Conditions); pneumonia (see Common Circulatory, Heart and Lung Conditions in chapter 5); the syndrome associated with colic (see Symptom: Colic); allergies; car sickness; viral infections; poisoning; or Meckel's diverticulum, a congenital sac found in a portion of the small intestine.

BEST RESPONSE: Routine treatment for those suffering from food poisoning is to let the vomiting take its course, say doctors. In the meantime, clear liquids are all that should be taken by mouth. When your nausea is gone and your stomach is ready to tolerate it, gradually reintroduce food to your diet, beginning with soft foods. Also, heat can be applied to the stomach with a heating pad or hot water bottle.

Although food poisoning from contaminated or spoiled food is not life-threatening, it is wise to see your doctor just the same. There are some foods, such as certain species of berries and mushrooms, that are potentially fatal.

For vomiting associated with intestinal upsets, avoid solid foods until vomiting ceases, advise doctors. However, make sure you replace lost fluids by frequently sipping liquids. This is a guard against dehydration. Plain water, carbonated beverages (shake them up to eliminate the fizz), tea, juice or bouillon are good to sip. Regular food should be reintroduced to the diet gradually.

In the case of a child, give small sips (about one teaspoon) of liquid (no orange juice) every 10 to 20 minutes, say doctors. Gradually increase the amount if the child keeps this down. Slowly work back to a regular diet once the stomach is settled.

Any vomiting that is severe or lasts longer than a day or two needs medical attention, because it increases the danger of dehydration and electrolyte imbalance due to loss of water and salts. This is especially true in infants, the elderly or those who are chronically ill.

ACCOMPANYING SYMPTOM: If someone is unconscious and vomiting, there is a danger of inhalation of vomit. The person should be made to lie forward with the head turned to one side to prevent choking.

Common Abdominal and Digestive System Conditions

Anal fissure.   A small crack or tear that occurs in the mucous membrane of the rectum or in the skin around the anus, an anal fissure causes severe pain, especially during bowel movements.

The usual cause is passage of an unusually large stool, childbirth, trauma, diarrhea or injury caused by a medical procedure.

Fissures may not heal if left untreated, because each time the bowels move, the crack is reopened. Conservative treatment includes a high-fiber diet, stool softeners, local anesthetic ointments and sitz baths, in which you soak your bottom in warm water. When conservative measures are ineffective, surgery may be required.

Anorectal abscess.   This is an infection in the area of the anus and rectum caused by bacteria. It is characterized by rectal pain, swelling and warmth. Often there will also be pus. The problem is more common in men and is often a problem in those who suffer from Crohn's disease.

An abscess of this type is treated by surgically opening it and allowing the pus to drain.

Anorectal fistula.   An anorectal fistula is an abnormal tubelike tract that goes from the rectum to an opening in the skin near the anus. It causes a discharge and sometimes a sore bottom. Anal fistulas usually result from recurrent abscesses around the anus or are associated with Crohn's disease. Some fistulas can be treated medically; others may require surgery.

Appendicitis. The appendix is a short, wormlike, dead-end tube located near where the large and small intestines join—in the lower right area of the abdomen. Your appendix really serves no useful purpose, which is fortunate, since a "sick" appendix generally requires surgical removal.

An inflamed appendix—appendicitis—may result when an obstruction, such as intestinal worms or a piece of fecal matter, plugs up the organ, making drainage impossible.

The classic symptoms of appendicitis include pain or tenderness, usually in the lower right area of the abdomen, nausea, vomiting and low-grade fever. In children, the fever is usually quite high. The pain of appendicitis is usually unrelenting and can be aggravated by motion.

If performed early, removal of the appendix is a relatively simple procedure. If the organ ruptures, however, it can cause the infection to spread in the abdomen, resulting in peritonitis, a much more serious and life-threatening condition.

Celiac disease. *See* Malabsorption syndrome

Cirrhosis. This disease, in which damage in the liver is replaced by scar tissue, causes serious malfunction of the vital organ responsible for detoxifying body poisons, metabolizing nutrients and producing important proteins for normal body functions.

It's a serious, life-threatening disease because we have only one liver and, like the heart, it's an organ we can't do without.

Alcohol abuse is the major, although not the only, cause of this disease. Not all alcoholics get it; only 10 to 15 percent of confirmed alcoholics contract the disease. Cirrhosis also can be caused by various forms of hepatitis and can result from excessive use of drugs, prolonged exposure to environmental toxins and rare inherited forms of liver disease.

Although cirrhosis is generally considered to be a disease of middle-aged men, women are now suffering in greater numbers. Twenty years ago, according to one study, men with alcoholic cirrhosis outnumbered women with the condition five to one. In the past ten years, the male-to-female ratio has fallen to about two to one.

Mild cirrhosis may not have any symptoms, although enlargement and contraction of the liver is one of the early signs. Those with more advanced alcoholic cirrhosis have a massive amount of fluid in the abdominal cavity, causing swelling from the ribs to the groin. Small, red spider marks may appear on the face, arms and upper trunk, and large veins appear on the abdomen. Jaundice and mental confusion set in.

An extremely serious complication of cirrhosis is esophageal varices, which are swellings of the veins in the esophagus that can rupture and bleed.

When cirrhosis is due to alcoholic poisoning, progression of the disease can be halted if drinking is stopped. But the damage that is already present can't be reversed. Treatment is aimed at preventing further damage. A well-balanced diet, usually with low salt intake, is often recommended. In severe cases, diuretics ("water pills") and sometimes steroid therapy are used.

Crohn's disease. Sometimes referred to as regional ileitis or regional enteritis, Crohn's disease is an inflammatory condition that can attack any portion of the intestinal tract, although it most often affects the ileum, which is the bottom portion of the small intestine.

Some of the symptoms and complications of Crohn's disease are similar to those of ulcerative colitis—diarrhea, abdominal pain and rectal bleeding—and the two are often grouped together under the name inflammatory bowel disease.

Crohn's disease can begin slowly or develop suddenly, with symptoms such as diarrhea, abdominal pain, fever and sometimes decreased appetite, loss of weight and stunted growth. More than half of the patients with Crohn's disease have diarrhea and abdominal pain. Persons with Crohn's disease may also develop kidney problems, gallstones, arthritis and/or ankylosing spondylitis, a form of arthritis.

The cause of Crohn's disease is not known. Diagnosis is made with the aid of an upper and sometimes a lower gastrointestinal x-ray series, as well as internal examinations of the colon. Treatment may include dietary changes and steroid and antibiotic therapy. To compensate for nutritional losses, extra vitamins and minerals—including zinc and vitamin C—are sometimes recommended. When medical therapy is not effective, surgical removal of the diseased intestine may be necessary.

Diverticulosis/diverticulitis.   In diverticulosis, small pouches form in weakened muscle walls of the large intestine or colon. It is found in about a third of the population of industrialized countries after middle age—it's one of the most common colon problems in people over 40 years of age.

Diverticulosis can be symptomless, but it may have symptoms similar to those of irritable bowel syndrome—pain or tenderness, bloating and alternating diarrhea and constipation. Diagnosis is made by barium x-ray.

Diverticulitis is a complication of diverticulosis and results when the pouches break, spilling the contents of the bowel into surrounding tissues. The symptoms of diverticulitis are severe pain in the abdomen, fever, nausea and vomiting. Less than 15 percent of people with diverticulosis get diverticulitis, however.

Treatment of diverticulitis varies depending on the severity of symptoms. Often bed rest at home and antibiotics are all that's necessary. Sometimes hospitalization and even surgery are required.

A possible preventive and treatment for diverticulosis may be simple and inexpensive: a high-fiber diet. "With a high-fiber diet we can relieve, quite dramatically, over 90 percent of the symptoms of diverticular disease," claims Neil Painter, M.D., a British physician who helped revolutionize treatment for diverticular disease. "Already the widespread adoption of this diet in England, for example, has reduced, quite remarkably, the need for surgery."

You can put fiber back into your life by adding up to two tablespoons of bran a day to your meals as well as increasing whole grain products, fruits and vegetables. You should, however, avoid such indigestible roughage as nuts, corn, popcorn, strawberries, raspberries, figs, grapes with seeds, poppy seeds and caraway seeds. The seeds can get caught in the pouches, causing inflammation.

Food poisoning.   True food poisoning is caused by eating food containing poisons or toxins produced by bacteria growing in the food. Staphylococcal food poisoning is the most common type in the United States.

Although staphylococcal poisons do not harm the body directly, they produce poisonous substances in the body, causing disease symptoms such as vomiting, pain or cramping, weakness, diarrhea and dizziness. The symptoms usually come on quickly, between one and four hours after eating the contaminated substance.

This type of infection can be passed on easily—food handling is the most notorious way—and it's most easily spread through food that is not refrigerated. Food-borne infections (like salmonellosis) are caused by eating food containing organisms that grow or multiply once they're inside your body. The symptoms of salmonella poisoning—pain, vomiting and diarrhea—can take several days to appear.

Gallbladder disease.   The gallbladder is a pear-shaped organ that is located below the liver and serves as a storage place for bile. When trouble hits the gallbladder, it usually comes in the form of gallstones, which are lumps of solid material usually composed of either cholesterol or bile. They can range in size from smaller than a pinhead to three inches across.

Between the ages of 20 and 60, women are three times more likely to have gallstones than men. By the age of 60, almost 30 percent of all men and women have them. You're a likely candidate if you're overweight and eat a lot of dairy products and animal fats, if you're a woman who's been pregnant or if you're over age 60.

Almost half of the people with gallstones have no symptoms. When a symptom does occur, it's likely to be severe, steady pain in the upper abdomen that lasts at least 20 minutes and up to four hours. You may also feel pain between the shoulder blades or in the right shoulder. Nausea and vomiting are common.

As the gallstones move out of the gallbladder, they can lodge in a channel called the cystic duct. If gallstones block the duct for a prolonged period, the gallbladder can become inflamed, resulting in cholecystitis. Other ducts can be blocked, causing pancreatitis or common bile duct obstruction. These complications can cause severe abdominal pain with a high fever and sometimes jaundice.

Gallstones can be identified by x-ray or ultrasound examination. Surgery is usually recommended for gallstones that cause symptoms. Some gallstones can be dissolved with drugs taken by mouth, but there are significant side effects and, when the drugs are discontinued, stones reappear. A new technique—endoscopic retrograde cholangiopancrea-tography, or ERCP—can remove gallstones without surgery. An endoscope, a flexible tube, is passed through the mouth and the digestive tract until it reaches the opening of the bile duct. After identifying the stone, the doctor can open up the muscle at the end of the bile duct and remove the stone through a procedure called sphincterotomy. In this procedure the patient is given "twilight sleep" rather than a general anesthetic.

Diet may play a role in gallstone formation. In one study, vegetarian women—who tend to eat less saturated fat and no meat and have a high intake of fiber—had half the incidence of gallstones. Young women seem to be at higher risk if they take oral contraceptives. Many doctors recommend low-fat diets for preventing gallbladder attacks, but one recent study reported in the *American Journal of Gastroenterology* suggested no significant therapeutic advantage to following such a diet.

Gastritis. One of the most common stomach disorders, acute gastritis is an inflammation of the lining of the stomach. It can be caused by too much alcohol, food poisoning or a bacterial infection. In some people, it can be caused by certain drugs, such as aspirin and other antiarthri-tic medicines.

Many people may not have symptoms, but abdominal pain and tenderness, loss of appetite, nausea and vomiting may be present.

The usual treatment for gastritis is to eat nothing for a full day. Small amounts of liquids should be drunk frequently to prevent dehydration. After 24 hours, small amounts of bland foods may be eaten. Your doctor may prescribe an antacid or, if nausea and vomiting are severe, may administer an injection of an antiemetic, an antinau-sea drug.

Some people suffer from chronic gastritis. Although this occurs frequently with aging, it may also be associated with other disorders, such as a vitamin B_{12} deficiency or chronic stomach ulcers.

However, some cases of chronic gastritis may be caused by an invasion of bacteria that wiggle into the lining of your stomach and establish a permanent residence. One way to get rid of them is simple: two tablespoons of bismuth subsalicylate—sold over the counter as our old friend Pepto-Bismol—four times a day for two to three weeks will zap most of the little critters into oblivion, say researchers at Baylor College of Medicine. However, since Pepto-Bismol is a relative of aspirin, and aspirin can cause bleeding, you should check with your physician before taking it.

Gastroenteritis.   This is an inflammation of the lining of the intestines. It can be brought on by food poisoning, too much alcohol or a bacterial or viral infection. Allergies to certain foods can also result in gastroenteritis. However, emotional upsets, such as fear, anger and anxiety, also have been linked to this disease.

The illness comes on suddenly and can range from a mild single episode of vomiting and loose stools to more severe symptoms, including bloating, stomach cramps, diarrhea, repeated episodes of vomiting, fever and weakness.

Treatment usually includes bed rest. No food should be eaten until all vomiting has ceased and the nausea clears. Then food should be reintroduced gradually. Clear liquids should be taken frequently to prevent dehydration. Because of the threat of dehydration and chemical imbalance due to loss of water, treatment by a physician is advised.

Hemorrhoids.   Also known as piles, hemorrhoids are small distended veins in the rectum and anus. They're similar to varicose veins of the legs in that in both cases the veins take on odd shapes because their supporting walls are weak.

Common causes include obesity, prolonged sitting or standing, heavy lifting and constipation. The single most common cause of hemorrhoids in women is pregnancy. Hemorrhoids can develop inside the rectum (internal) or in the anus (external).

A large percentage of the population suffers from hemorrhoids, and the usual symptom is bright red blood seen on the toilet tissue or on the stool. Minor bleeding is usually the first clue to either kind of hemorrhoids, although external hemorrhoids are usually the only kind that cause pain.

If the hemorrhoids protrude only slightly, they are classified as first degree. Second-degree hemorrhoids protrude and descend into the anal canal during straining but return to their place when straining stops. Third-degree hemorrhoids protrude with less effort, and gentle pushing with the finger is required to get the protrusion back in place.

Fourth-degree hemorrhoids are prolapsed so much that they persistently protrude through the anus and can't be reduced.

Hemorrhoids can sometimes develop complications. If they form blood clots that stop blood flow, they are called thrombosed hemorrhoids. They can also become irritated, ulcerated or infected.

Treatment for hemorrhoids is routine—a high-fiber diet, stool softeners, bulk-forming agents and sitz baths, in which you soak your bottom in warm water to relieve discomfort. In addition, straining should be avoided, and the hemorrhoids that protrude should be gently pushed back into the rectum.

If these measures aren't effective, the doctor may inject a special shrinking agent into an internal hemorrhoid or destroy the hemorrhoid by cryosurgery, a procedure in which the affected tissue is frozen. Ligation, or placing a tight rubber band over the base of each hemorrhoid, is an outpatient procedure. The traditional treatment of hemorrhoids—which gets rid of them once and for all—is cutting them out in a surgical procedure that requires a hospital stay.

A brand-new treatment for hemorrhoids is infrared probe coagulation. In this procedure, a ray of infrared heat is applied to a hemorrhoid. The blood coagulates—thickens into an unmoving clot—and the damaged blood vessel collapses. Because the procedure is very precise, healthy tissue is not destroyed, as is the case with banding or injection therapy. The result is less pain. Laser surgery is also being used for severe cases.

Hepatitis.   An inflammation of the liver, hepatitis can come on slowly or quickly, at first mimicking flulike symptoms—slight fever, headache, aching muscles, weakness, nausea and loss of appetite. A more distinguishing symptom is tenderness and a feeling of deep pain or pressure just below the ribs on the right side—the site of the enlarged and infected organ.

Other symptoms can include hives or general body itching; jaundice; loose, clay-colored stools and dark urine. Recovery from hepatitis is slow, and patients with the disease often complain of fatigue for a long time.

There are three kinds of viral hepatitis. Hepatitis A, or infectious hepatitis, is a viral infection spread by fecal contamination of food, clothing, toys, eating utensils and other objects. You don't actually have to be able to see the offending substance for it to be present. It's the prime reason that food handlers (and you, for that matter) are asked to wash their hands after using the bathroom. It usually takes four to six weeks for the symptoms to develop after the initial contact. Mainly a disease of the young, hepatitis A doesn't cause lasting liver damage, and complete recovery is expected.

Hepatitis B, formerly known as serum hepatitis, was once thought to be spread only by blood transfer, such as through transfusion, contaminated needles shared by drug addicts or even acupuncture, ear piercing and tattooing. But the virus is now known to be present in other body fluids, such as tears, semen and saliva, meaning the disease can be spread by sexual contact.

With hepatitis B, there's a long time between exposure to the virus and development of symptoms—anywhere from 40 days to six months, with an average of two months. It's during this incubation period, when there are no symptoms, that hepatitis B is most contagious. Anyone who suspects that he or she may have had contact with the disease can be immunized against it. Although most people who develop type B hepatitis recover completely, some will go on to have chronic liver inflammation and/or be infectious to others for years.

The third type of hepatitis—non-A, non-B—is usually spread by blood transfusions or contaminated needles. There is as yet no method for screening blood for this kind of infection. This form can also result in chronic hepatitis and can even progress to more serious cirrhosis of the liver. The incubation period for this particular type of hepatitis is between one and ten weeks.

Treatment for all forms of hepatitis includes rest, a well-balanced, nutritious diet and monitoring by a physician. To prevent spread of the infection, contaminated bowel movements should never be touched, and the toilet should be cleaned frequently with a disinfectant. Frequent hand washing is essential.

Also, during the most active stage of the disease, doctors advise that you treat your liver tenderly. That means avoiding liver irritants such as alcohol and certain drugs, including birth control pills, tranquilizers, certain tetracyclines and other antibiotics, antidepressants and high-dosage acetaminophen (Tylenol).

Hiatal hernia. In this condition, a small portion of the stomach slips through an opening (hiatus) in the diaphragm, allowing the stomach to "ride up" into the chest. This may be associated with an increased backup of stomach acids into the esophagus, which can cause belching, heartburn and general discomfort.

Although found in all ages and both sexes, a hiatal hernia is generally a disorder of the middle-aged. It can be present at birth, but most often it results from tremendous pressure on the diaphragm, which can be caused by such things as injury.

Not everyone with a hiatal hernia suffers discomforting symptoms, however. Those who do usually respond well to antacids, weight reduction and small but more frequent meals. For those in whom strain due to constipation is the cause, a high-fiber diet is often advised.

Impacted stool. This condition results when a large, firm mass of stool forms in the rectum. It's caused by not completely emptying the bowels. The problem occurs most commonly in elderly, bedridden people or those with painful rectal diseases. Occasionally the problem occurs in children, especially those with emotional problems or an undiagnosed megacolon, an abnormally large colon that lacks the nerve cells to pass bowel movements.

Diagnosis is made by rectal examination, and treatment can be as simple as manual removal and/or an enema. The impaction must be removed by a physician, and patients sometimes require general anesthesia while the procedure is being done.

Intestinal obstruction. This is a partial or complete blockage of the intestines and can be caused by a hernia near the area of the groin (known as an inguinal hernia), adhesions resulting from surgery, a twisting or kinking of the bowels (known as volvulus), cancer of the colon and even swallowing an indigestible object, such as a large button.

A partial obstruction can cause diarrhea; a complete blockage causes constipation. An obstruction in the small intestine causes vomiting and cramping pains in the middle of the abdomen. If the problem is in the large intestine, there may be no vomiting.

Hospitalization is required for intestinal obstruction, and x-rays are often taken to determine the origin of the obstruction. Treatment includes administering intravenous fluids and electrolytes. Also, a method called decompression is used, in which a tube is inserted into the intestine to remove trapped fluids and gases. Although decompression sometimes results in removal of the obstruction, surgery is often required.

Irritable bowel syndrome.   Also known as IBS, irritable colon, spastic colon or mucous colitis, this very common intestinal problem affects 10 to 20 percent of the population and is responsible for more than half of all disorders of the digestive system.

For unknown reasons, twice as many women as men fall victim to it, and symptoms usually start before age 25. IBS is believed to be due to abnormalities in gastrointestinal motility. One of the more common abnormalities occurs when certain muscles in the bowel contract too quickly, while others contract too slowly. Abdominal pain, bloating, constipation, diarrhea or alternating constipation and diarrhea are the classic symptoms.

Since these same symptoms are also present in a number of other intestinal conditions, an examination by a doctor is needed to confirm the diagnosis. IBS, incidentally, usually turns out to be the diagnosis only after no other cause is found.

No one knows for sure what causes IBS, although stress influences the symptoms. Because stress is a factor, many sufferers have reported improvement with psychotherapy, hypnosis, biofeedback and other stress-management techniques. Medically, antispasmodic drugs and some-times antidepressants are prescribed.

A change in diet is routinely advised. Doctors suggest avoiding gas-producing foods or any foods that may trigger an attack. For those with constipation, high-fiber foods—whole grains, fruits and vegetables— are ordered. A tablespoon or two of bran added to food is particularly helpful.

Lactose intolerance.   In order to digest milk and dairy products, which are rich in *lactose,* your body needs an intestinal enzyme called *lactase.* If you have reduced levels of this enzyme, as many adults do, the undigested milk sugar will sit in your large intestine and cause gas, bloating, pain and diarrhea.

Almost all babies are born with sufficient quantities of lactase to digest milk. (Although it's rare, a baby can be born with too little lactase, in which case lactose-free formula must be given.) Normally, lactase levels decline during childhood, and by adulthood many people have such a deficiency that they are unable to tolerate products containing lactose.

Those who suffer from other common and not-so-common digestive disorders may also have problems digesting lactose. These conditions include inflammatory bowel disease (Crohn's disease or ulcerative colitis) and malabsorption syndrome. A recent intestinal infection can also create the problem. In addition, those who have had intestinal surgery, have used antibiotics, are immune deficient or have been in cancer therapy may also be affected by lactose intolerance.

There is no cure for this condition. The best ways to control the disease are to buy capsules of the missing enzyme at your local drugstore and use them in your milk, or to buy milk and milk products to which the enzyme is already added; avoid dairy products altogether; or find your own tolerance level by keeping a diary of what you eat and how your intestine responds to it.

Malabsorption syndrome. This is actually an umbrella term for a group of diseases that interfere with the absorption of nutrients from the intestinal wall into the body. The causes are numerous; enzyme deficiencies, intestinal ailments, changes in intestinal bacteria, drugs or laxatives and intestinal surgery are among them.

Celiac disease is the most notable form of malabsorption syndrome. It is characterized by the body's inability to tolerate gluten, a protein found in wheat and other grains. The intolerance leads to abnormal changes in the lining of the small intestine and impairs absorption of nutrients. The disease usually begins in a child after six months of age, although it may begin or even reappear in adulthood.

Children with the disease have pale, foul-smelling, bulky stools and suffer painful abdominal bloating. They fail to grow and have iron deficiency anemia. Adults with celiac disease often show the same digestive symptoms.

Treatment of the disease is aimed at eliminating gluten from the diet. Substitute grains are corn, rice and buckwheat. Following a strict gluten-free diet is a great challenge, since there are many foods and products—including beer and communion wafers—that contain gluten.

Nutritional supplements such as zinc, iron and B vitamins are usually necessary to help replace lost nutrients.

Pancreatitis. The pancreas has many functions. Two of the most important are producing insulin needed to regulate sugar in the bloodstream and producing digestive enzymes needed to help take nutrients into the body. When the pancreas becomes inflamed, the pancreatic juices run amok, causing the enzymes to actually digest pancreatic tissue. The pancreas appears to be digesting itself.

Pancreatitis can be brought on by alcoholism, drugs, gallstones, a perforated ulcer, hyperparathyroidism or a virus. The major symptom is tenderness and severe pain in the midabdomen. Pancreatitis often requires hospitalization and must be diagnosed through medical testing. Blood tests and/or ultrasound and computerized axial tomography are generally the routine followed. Painkilling drugs, fasting and intravenous fluids generally lead to improvement.

Pancreatitis can become a chronic condition. This can cause the organ to become inefficient, so that pancreatic enzymes must be administered. It can also cause such great pain that narcotics are sometimes required.

Peritonitis. The peritoneum is a two-layered membrane that lines the abdominal cavity and also covers the stomach, intestines and other abdominal organs. Peritonitis is the inflammation of this membrane, and it is always a complication of another disease. It can be caused by problems such as a ruptured appendix or gallbladder, a perforated ulcer, a tearing wound to the abdomen, alcoholic cirrhosis or pelvic inflammatory disease.

Peritonitis usually causes severe abdominal pain. The abdomen will also feel tender and rigid. Nausea, vomiting and fever are other symptoms. Peritonitis is a serious disorder that may require removal or repair of the offending organ. Intravenous antibiotic therapy is a necessary part of treatment.

Proctitis. This is an inflammation of the rectum and anus that can occur in those with ulcerative colitis, hemorrhoids or anal fissures. It's also being seen in increasing numbers of homosexual men because of frequent anal sex.

The usual symptoms are pain, discharge and straining at stool with no results. Healing occurs through treating the disease (or stopping the sex act) that's causing the inflammation, but symptoms can sometimes be relieved by resting and taking sitz baths, in which you soak your bottom in warm water.

Ulcerative colitis.   This is a serious and chronic inflammation of the colon that causes repeated attacks of diarrhea, abdominal pain and rectal bleeding. The cause is unknown; there is no evidence that emotional factors cause the disease.

Chronic ulcerative colitis can lead to colon cancer. When the disease is severe or when there is evidence of precancer or a cancerous lesion, surgical removal of the colon is necessary.

Ulcerative colitis usually attacks young adults, with three-quarters of the cases developing before age 40. Diagnosis is made by direct examination of the diseased area. A low-fiber diet is usually suggested, and treatment often includes steroid drugs.

You should know, however, that drug dependence has become so prevalent among those with inflammatory bowel disease (IBD)—the term used to refer to both ulcerative colitis and Crohn's disease—that doctors now label it a medical complication of the condition. The problem is exacerbated by the fact that people with IBD frequently consult with a number of specialists, each of whom may write a different prescription. To avoid setting yourself up for a drug problem, experts advise that you have all your medications prescribed and coordinated by one doctor.

Ulcers.   Ulcers are sores or "raw spots" created by an imbalance between stomach acids and the gastrointestinal tract's natural defenses. An ulcer that appears on the lining of the stomach is known as a gastric ulcer; one that appears on the small intestine, or duodenum, is known as a duodenal ulcer.

An ulcer is characterized by a burning, gnawing pain around the breastbone. Flare-ups can last from 30 minutes to three hours, and the pain may be troublesome for weeks and then go away, only to reappear later.

Why some people get ulcers and others don't remains unknown, although certain life-style factors—mainly smoking, stress, alcohol and caffeine—may play a role. Recently, however, doctors have begun to realize that a type of bacterium found in roughly 25 percent of all adults may cause the problem. According to Barry Marshall, M.D., an Australian researcher, these bacteria cause a stomach inflammation that thins the stomach's protective layer of mucus and leaves it open to the ravages of digestive acids. The acids then begin to digest the stomach instead of the food in it, and the resulting injury is an ulcer.

Ulcers are diagnosed only after a series of tests, which usually consist of a set of x-rays that show your upper digestive tract or an endoscopic exam, in which a thin, flexible tube is inserted into the stomach, allowing the doctor to view the stomach wall.

Most ulcers can be treated, but tend to recur after therapy is stopped. Your doctor might order you to give up cigarettes, coffee, alcohol and aspirin, all of which can irritate a sensitive ulcer. But the mainstays of modern ulcer treatment are antacids such as Maalox TC and the drugs cimetidine (Tagamet), ranitidine (Zantac) and sucralfate (Carafate).

If your ulcer is caused by bacteria, you're in luck—Pepto-Bismol can kill the bugs and cure your ulcer. If your ulcer is from other causes, however, you can still frequently prevent it from recurring by taking antacids; medications that block acid secretion, like cimetidine or ranitidine; or other substances, like sucralfate, that coat the ulcer and enhance the protective barrier lining the stomach and intestine.

Sometimes, however, surgery is required. Also, ulcers can get worse, causing bleeding, obstruction or perforation of the stomach or intestine. These complications require immediate medical care.

Chapter 2
Back and Spine

SEE YOUR DOCTOR IMMEDIATELY IF:

- *You have pain in any part of the spine as a result of an accident or other trauma*
- *You suffer a sudden, severe attack of back pain accompanied by shortness of breath, pain in the chest or abdomen and/or a throbbing lump in the abdomen*
- *Your backache is so severe it wakes you at night*
- *Your backache is accompanied by pain, numbness, tingling or weakness in the extremities or loss of bowel or bladder control*
- *Your back pain is accompanied by chills and fever*
- *You have pain in your lower or middle back that spreads to the abdomen or groin and is accompanied by cloudy or bloody urine and/or fever greater than 101°F*
- *You're over 60 years old and/or have recently been bedridden and suffer persistent sharp pain in one place on your spine*
- *You have a stiff neck accompanied by such symptoms as headache, nausea and vomiting, and you cannot tolerate bright light*
- *You suspect a severe injury to the spine. But don't move! Instead, have someone call your local emergency number for assistance*

The trouble with backs is that we take them for granted—until they stop working.

The backbone—that hollow column that extends from the brain to the bottom of the buttocks—protectively houses the spinal cord, which is a major part of the central nervous system. When you consider that this spinal column—our pillar of strength—is made up of 33 oddly shaped bones (called vertebrae) linked by ligaments and separated by thin discs—well, that's not steel and concrete. It's no wonder that years of excess weight, strain and twisting can take their toll! Our backs rebel.

Caring for your backbone should be a lifetime commitment. And practicing proper posture, using your back correctly (by stooping, instead of bending, to pick up a baby, for example), eating calcium-rich foods and keeping fit are part of it.

Every year millions of American backs transmit distress signals that send their owners to emergency rooms and doctors' offices. Why? Rodney Dangerfield might put it this way—backs get no respect. Give yours some.

SYMPTOM: **Curvature**

COMMON CAUSES: This is a symptom you may not even notice until your 10- to 15-year-old child (usually your daughter) comes home from school with a note saying that he or she has "flunked" the routine screening examination for scoliosis (see Common Back and Spinal Conditions).

You begin to recollect. That's why your daughter's hemline or waistband has been looking uneven, or one of your son's pant legs has been riding higher than the other. Or that's why your child's hip or shoulder blade is more prominent on one side. It's the reason for that slight hump you've noticed on one shoulder. And it explains that habit of tilting his or her head to one side. You think ahead. You think the worst—surgery, body casts, years of pain and deformity. You panic. But relax. Failing that test doesn't mean things are all that bad.

Gilbert Simon, M.D., coauthor of *The Parent's Pediatric Companion,* points out that out of 25,000 boys and girls in their first year of high school, only 7 percent were found to have some sideways curvature. All of these children went on to have back x-rays to confirm the diagnosis. With this test, 27 percent were found to have no curve at all (a curve was probably detected initially because the children weren't standing up straight when the nurse was checking them). Of those who did have spinal curves, only 6 percent had curvature severe enough to require bracing. The vast majority of curves were mild enough to require no treatment. So, suggests Dr. Simon, the odds are in your child's favor that his or her spinal curvature—even if confirmed by an x-ray—will be the mild kind and is not a signal for panic and distress.

BEST RESPONSE: The purpose of school screening exams for scoliosis is to detect mild cases so they can be followed through the teen years.

If your child has flunked the test, he or she should be seen by a physician (preferably an orthopedic surgeon) on a regular basis, since severe scoliosis, left untreated, can get worse and could cause deformity. The doctor may recommend physical therapy or a spinal brace or, in a few cases, scoliosis surgery may be necessary.

Warning to parents: There is increased concern that repeated x-rays of teenage girls can increase the risk of breast cancer. Because of this fact, researchers at the Food and Drug Administration's Center for Devices and Radiological Health have recommended protective measures that can dramatically reduce radiation doses without interfering with a doctor's getting the information needed to determine the severity of a child's curvature.

SYMPTOM: **Hunchback**

COMMON CAUSES: It's medically known as kyphosis, and it's commonly called by a variety of names—hunchback, humpback, dowager's hump. It's not uncommon to see it in adolescents (age 12 to 15 years) —round shoulders and a stoop are the characteristic signs. Adolescent stoop is usually not a serious problem; it usually is corrected when growth stops.

Hunching that begins in older adults, however, should be considered a serious sign. The main cause of hunchback is osteoporosis (see Common Bone, Joint and Muscle Conditions in chapter 3), which literally means "brittle bones." Its most likely victims are women past menopause.

At the University of California at San Diego School of Medicine, there's a diverse group of doctors and scientists who meet regularly to investigate the disease. J. William Hollingsworth, M.D., an internist and professor there, is a spokesman for the Osteoporosis Study Group. "Osteoporosis is a very common problem for older women—by age 80, half of all women will have broken vertebrae as a result of the disease," says Dr. Hollingsworth. "The tip-off in diagnosis is the humpback, but there's also loss of height, chronic back pain and immobility."

Another cause, although rarely found today, is tuberculosis of the spine, an infection that can cause a sharp bend in the upper part of the back. This is the disease the Hunchback of Notre Dame was supposed to have had.

BEST RESPONSE: Mothers of round-shouldered children frequently chide their youngsters to "stand up straight!" But this may not be enough, say doctors. Exercise is necessary to strengthen back muscles. Swimming is particularly good. A flat, firm mattress is also helpful.

For women with osteoporosis, Dr. Hollingsworth recommends calcium—1,500 milligrams daily. But his best advice is prevention. He recommends that women become aware of the risk factors for the disease and eat calcium-rich foods or take supplements of calcium, the mineral most important in bone strength. If you're a white or Asian woman who is frail and has a family history of osteoporosis, you are most at risk.

"I would recommend regular exercise—walking is best—and an intake of 1,500 milligrams of supplemental calcium a day in addition to a well-balanced diet," says Dr. Hollingsworth. "I would also suggest that you strongly consider estrogen and progesterone replacement therapy at the time of menopause and continue this treatment for the rest of your life."

ACCOMPANYING SYMPTOMS: If adolescent kyphosis is accompanied by backache or appears to be getting worse, a doctor should be consulted. It could be more than a posture problem.

SYMPTOM: **Inability to Straighten Up**

COMMON CAUSES: This is the way some—but by no means all—back pain stories start out: You bend down to pick up something and you're unable to straighten up again. It can be scary (to put it mildly).

The reason you can't unkink is spasm, a contraction of muscle fibers so severe that you're unable to straighten up. It can be caused by any of the conditions that cause lower back pain (see Symptom: Pain, Lower Back). You can also have trouble straightening up if you've fractured a vertebra.

BEST RESPONSE: If your back pain starts in the dramatic fashion described above, no one needs to tell you that absolute bed rest is the first order of business. (You won't feel like doing anything but going to bed anyway.) When you're able to move again, usually in a few days, you can consult a physician to find out the cause of your discomfort.

If, however, you've recently fallen or been injured and experience this symptom, you should see your doctor right away.

ACCOMPANYING SYMPTOMS: If you can't straighten up and also experience pain, numbness, tingling or weakness, you could have a slipped or ruptured disc (see Common Back and Spinal Conditions). You should see your doctor.

SYMPTOM: **Numbness**

COMMON CAUSES: Numbness in any part of the body can be a very disturbing symptom. The back is no exception. One of the cardinal signs of a slipped or ruptured disc (see Common Back and Spinal Conditions) is numbness in the lower back and legs. You'll also experience abnormal sensitivity—even a light touch is painful—tingling or sensations like "pins and needles." These are all signs that an intervertebral disc is impinging on a nerve.

If you've suffered a serious fall or a crushing injury or have been in a car accident, you may have a fracture of the spine (see Common Back and Spinal Conditions) with damage to the spinal cord. Along with severe back pain, you will have numbness or feel "dead" below the site of injury. Depending on the amount of damage to the spinal cord, this numbness may herald some form of paralysis or may be a temporary problem.

BEST RESPONSE: Numbness associated with lower back pain requires investigation by a physician to diagnose the problem and prevent permanent nerve damage. If you've suffered any type of sudden back injury, it should be treated as a suspected fracture until proven otherwise. That means don't move. Moving or transporting a person with such a problem is best left to professionals who are trained to handle these emergencies.

SYMPTOM: **Pain, Base of Spine**

COMMON CAUSES: This pain is usually felt over the sacroiliac joint, which is located low down in the back where, in most people, there is a dimple. Pain in this area is common after giving birth. And golfers often complain of pain here because of injury to the ligaments while hitting a drive. Stomach sleepers may also complain about it. Most sacroiliac pain is caused by spraining the ligaments.

BEST RESPONSE: Pain in this area should be treated like other types of lower back pain—initial rest followed by gentle activities (see Best Response under Symptom: Pain, Lower Back). Sacroiliac pain may last a long while.

SYMPTOM: **Pain, Lower Back**

COMMON CAUSES: Eight out of ten Americans experience lower back pain at some time in their lives. If you asked a physician about the causes of such pain, he or she might counter with, "How much time do you have?"

Certainly, if you have had the flu (see influenza under Common Whole Body Conditions in chapter 19), you know that lower back pain can make you almost as miserable as the fever and other symptoms. And before the rash of shingles (see Common Skin Conditions in chapter 15) shows itself, a person can suffer pain in the middle to lower back.

For women, periodic or persistent lower back pain can go with the package of side effects that may accompany normal menstruation or pregnancy. But it could also signal problems such as endometriosis or pelvic inflammatory disease (see Common Reproductive System Conditions in chapter 14). It is less likely, but your pain could indicate a fracture somewhere in your back or even a tumor of the spine (see Common Back and Spinal Conditions).

But the most likely suspects in lower back pain, says Robert Boyd, M.D., assistant clinical professor of orthopedic surgery at Harvard Medical School and director of the Problem Back Clinic at Massachusetts

General Hospital in Boston, are a slipped or ruptured disc (see Common Back and Spinal Conditions), degenerative disc disease or a strain.

In spite of all the publicity it receives, only about 5 percent of back problems belong in the slipped or ruptured disc category. If you have this problem, pain starts in the lower back and radiates down the leg, often extending below the knee, causing numbness and weakness.

"Most back pains written off as disc problems are really muscle problems," says Willibald Nagler, M.D., New York Hospital-Cornell University Medical Center's physiatrist-in-chief (a physiatrist is an M.D. specializing in physical medicine and rehabilitation). "Most people with back problems have back and hamstring muscles too tight for toe touching, and abdominal muscles too weak for sit-ups."

Because the back and hamstring muscles support the entire structure of the back, they must be strong but flexible in order to allow you to bend over, sit or twist without straining your back. In addition, excess baggage—especially around the waist—can cause back pain because the weight stresses soft back tissue and compresses discs.

Degenerative disc disease is part of the inevitable aging process and can often begin in your thirties. Discs begin to shrink and narrow, resulting in periodic bouts of pain brought on by nothing more strenuous than bending over to pick something up off the floor.

A strain can be caused by a sudden injury, emotional stress, bad posture or the cumulative effects of wear and tear. Back strain usually lasts only a few days, but if allowed to build up, the pain can become a persistent ache.

BEST RESPONSE: A visit to your gynecologist will solve the mystery of whether your back pain is due to a gynecological problem. If you're pregnant, lower back pain may be alleviated by wearing low-heeled shoes. In addition, a maternity belt is on the market that relieves back pressure and helps women to remain active during pregnancy. The belt consists of two sections that support the abdomen and lower back without compression while allowing good circulation. Fully adjustable, the belt is available in four sizes (for more information, write Reenie Enterprises, P.O. Box 2816, Prescott, AZ 86302).

Most people, however, don't fit into the category of back pain caused by pregnancy. Their condition is due to a back problem. What can you do about the pain, which at times can be excruciating?

When severe back pain hits, the usual recommendation is bed rest. But for how long? Two days is usually enough to get you back on your feet, according to Richard Deyo, M.D., of the University of Texas Health Science Center in San Antonio.

Dr. Deyo studied over 200 people with lower back pain and advised half to remain in bed for seven days and the other half to stay there for two days. Both groups also were told to apply heat to the painful area, do back exercises and avoid heavy lifting. When he compared the two groups several weeks later, Dr. Deyo found they didn't differ in the number of days their activities were actually limited or in the degree of self-rated improvement.

Of course, the way you rest in bed is also important. You should lie on your back with several pillows tucked under your knees to keep your pelvis flat against the mattress. You can alternate this position by lying on your side in the fetal position (knees bent at a right angle to your body) with small pillows under your waist and between your knees. You should avoid lying on your stomach, since this position is hard on the back. If you must lie this way, put pillows under your stomach to support your lower back.

To get out of bed, roll onto one side and use your arms to push your trunk upright. The mattress? It doesn't seem to matter so much anymore—anything that gives good support and feels comfortable to you is fine. (If you're uncertain what that means, see Best Response under Symptom: Stiffness for suggestions on selecting a mattress and pillow.) Heat (warm baths or showers, a heating pad or hot water bottle) or cold (an ice pack) can relieve aching muscles.

Heat increases blood flow and can be soothing. Cold reduces blood flow and deadens nerve perception, which is why cold is often recommended in the first 48 hours following injury—sometimes alternated with heat. Finally, some physicians recommend a back brace for temporary support and pain relief in the early days of recuperation.

At some time during this acute period of back pain, you've probably seen a doctor, who has examined you and may have put you through a number of tests (the CAT—computerized axial tomography—scan has overtaken spinal tap as the most popular diagnostic test). If tests suggest you have a slipped or ruptured disc, some doctors may recommend chymopapain injections into the disc or back surgery to relieve the pain. Many doctors, however, feel that chymopapain can be dangerous and that surgery may also not be in your best interests. According to Edward

A. Abraham, M.D., author of *Freedom from Back Pain,* one-third of all disc operations, whether successful or not, require some form of follow-up surgery.

After the acute attack of back pain has subsided—in Dr. Abraham's experience, 70 percent of attacks will pass within ten days to three weeks —it's time to identify and solve the problems and behaviors that led to the pain. The easiest way to do this is to take your back to school. There are now more than 5,000 outpatient back clinics in the United States. Almost every major hospital and university has one, and although none are free, many are covered by insurance. Most require a doctor's recommendation to enroll. At these back schools, good posture and proper body mechanics are stressed. In addition to attending back school, you might consider some other measures to prevent future back problems.

Any kind of pounding of your feet, for example, can show up as backpain, especially if your muscles are weak or you're older. That's why joggers end up with more injuries than walkers, swimmers or bicyclists. One study showed that switching to lightweight, flexible-soled shoes fitted with simple shock-absorbing viscoelastic cushions produced surprisingly rapid and significant pain relief in about 80 percent of the 382 back sufferers tested.

You should also avoid prolonged sitting. Take a stand-up break every hour and select a chair that helps you to sit comfortably erect. Avoid slouching when sitting by inserting a small pillow, two or three inches thick, behind your back.

Yoga is a good way to relax muscles. And biofeedback and progressive relaxation training can help you relax deeply even while you're active.

Doctors recommend that you should also learn to lift properly. Bend at the knees rather than the waist, and squat close to the object you want to pick up. Keep your back straight and abdominal muscles tense as you take hold of the object and draw it to your chest. Rise slowly by straightening your legs. Never try to move weights that are too heavy.

SYMPTOM: **Pain, Middle Back**

COMMON CAUSES: Pain between the shoulder blades and the end of the ribs (just above the waist) is not uncommon. Everyone feels it at one time or another. Did you overdo it in the garden? Are you a mother with a new baby to carry around all day (and night)? If so, your problem is probably nothing more than tender muscles and ligaments.

Occasional middle back pain can also be part of the package if you suffer from scoliosis (see Common Back and Spinal Conditions). Pain and stiffness in this area can be caused by several types of arthritis of the spine (see Common Back and Spinal Conditions). Ultimately, it may interfere with the ability to expand the chest or stand up straight.

In many cases, pain in the middle back indicates trouble in front of the spine. When you consider the organs that are located within the ribs—the lungs, heart, pancreas, gallbladder and kidneys, as well as major vessels—you may have a greater appreciation for the difficult job that a doctor has in diagnosing and fixing the problem that's causing your pain. Injury to or disease of the kidney, for example, frequently shows up as pain in the middle to lower area of the back. And if you are in the early stages of pneumonia (see Common Circulatory, Heart and Lung Conditions in chapter 5) or you have an ulcer (see Common Abdominal and Digestive System Conditions in chapter 1), you may feel pain in the back area.

BEST RESPONSE: If your pain is due to overdoing it, gentle massage or stroking may be particularly helpful. You don't need to be an expert to do massage—there are seminars in many cities that teach therapeutic massage, done either by you or a partner. Or, if you prefer, a licensed massage therapist can be located through local medical practitioners or health clubs. In addition to massage, many of the self-help measures explained under Best Response for Symptom: Pain, Lower Back, and Symptom: Pain, Neck and Upper Back can be useful here.

If, however, you cannot associate your ache to the pains and strains of everyday living, you should see your doctor, who can examine you to find out the cause of your problem.

ACCOMPANYING SYMPTOMS: If you have intense pain between the shoulder blades and pain in the upper right side of the abdomen that tends to peak and fade, and this pain is accompanied by nausea and vomiting, you could have gallstones (see gallbladder disease under Common Abdominal and Digestive System Conditions in chapter 1) and should see your physician.

SYMPTOM: **Pain, Neck and Upper Back**

COMMON CAUSES: Is someone or something giving you a pain in the neck? Do the cares of the world always seem to rest on *your* shoulders?

If everyday upsets and frustrations are causing your muscles to tense up, then neck and shoulder pain can result. But other factors besides stress can contribute to the problem.

"One major cause of neck and shoulder pain is a round-shouldered posture," according to Susan L. Fish, a registered physical therapist in New York City. "It throws your head forward and leaves you looking down. But you tend to want to see where you're going, so you arch your head back. Holding your head up in that forward-jutting position puts a tremendous amount of stress on the muscles in the back of the neck and upper shoulders. And a muscle that's in a constant state of contraction can become a painful muscle.

"Part of the problem is habit," Fish says. "Part is genetic. Part is just generally poor posture, from the feet all the way up. For instance, large-busted women may get round-shouldered because of the weight of their breasts. In postmenopausal women, osteoporosis can contribute to it. And fatigue can cause you to be round-shouldered because people who don't get enough sleep just can't hold themselves up straight."

Slouching in an easy chair is another problem. "If you let yourself scoot down in your chair and slouch in your lower back, you're going to go into that round-shouldered posture," she says.

Carrying the equivalent of the weight of bricks in your shoulder bag or briefcase can also make your body tilt sideways, though you may not realize it. The result? Muscle tension.

Still another modern-day problem is holding a telephone between your ear and shoulder while you stir the soup or take notes. This keeps the shoulder muscles in a constant state of tension, and neck and shoulder pain can result.

Sleeping habits, as well as the choice of pillow and mattress, can also contribute to neck and shoulder pain (see Symptom: Stiffness).

Specific conditions or diseases, such as temporomandibular joint syndrome, or TMJ (see Common Facial, Jaw and Mouth Conditions in chapter 8), arthritis of the spine or a slipped or ruptured disc (see Common Back and Spinal Conditions) in the neck region also can cause pain in the neck and shoulders.

Finally, there is the pain caused by a whiplash injury (see Common Back and Spinal Conditions) as a result of the neck being snapped back, then forward like a whip. Most frequently this occurs when a person is sitting in a car and the car is hit from behind. But it can occur from *any* accident where the neck is snapped back and then forward, says Steven R. Garfin, M.D., associate professor of orthopedics and rehabilitation at the University of California at San Diego School of Medicine. He says it's the ligaments, muscles and joint capsules that bear the brunt of a whiplash injury.

"Occasionally a patient suffers this type of injury but has no pain," says Dr. Garfin. "Usually, though, neck pain lasts six weeks or less, but it's not uncommon for the discomfort to go on for six months or, occasionally, even for years. The pain, however, is rarely permanent and surgery is rarely necessary."

BEST RESPONSE: To help relax muscles, doctors say you can let a hot shower run on the back of your neck, or you can ask a friend to give you a massage by running his or her hands smoothly from the nape of your neck across your shoulders, stroking toward your heart.

To prevent pain from recurring, make an effort to stand up straight. And when you sit, you should perch right on the base of your buttocks with a support at your lower back. That way, you can't slouch!

If you work at a computer, you should make sure the screen is at eye level. The same goes for typists—use a book stand to copy from rather than laying the material flat on the desk. Lighten up on the baggage you carry around or, when carrying heavy items, divide the weight evenly between both arms. In the case of a shoulder bag, switch sides occasionally or don't carry one at all. If you've been ringing up pain with your telephone habits, you should get a phone rest—or give your phone a rest.

The usual treatment for whiplash injury is a cervical collar. "The majority of whiplash injuries are healed with a collar, rest and anti-inflammatory medication," says Dr. Garfin. "Sometimes physical therapy and isometric exercises are useful."

ACCOMPANYING SYMPTOMS: If your neck pain is accompanied by numbness or tingling in the arms and/or your head and neck are in an unnatural position, you could have a slipped or ruptured disc (see Common Back and Spinal Conditions) in the neck or a broken neck. A broken neck is a medical emergency.

SYMPTOM: **Pain, Shooting, in Legs**

COMMON CAUSES: Some folks know this as sciatica. The pain, which starts in the back and then shoots down the legs, can also cause tingling or "pins and needles" in the leg. It can even cause abnormal sensitivity, where even a light touch is painful. You may also feel a weakening of the buttock and calf muscles. Coughing, sneezing or straining can make it worse.

Sciatica occurs when the sciatic nerve or a portion of it is being compressed in some fashion. *True* sciatica is a structural problem. It is caused by a slipped or ruptured disc (see Common Back and Spinal Conditions) that impinges on the sciatic nerve or by spinal stenosis, a narrowing of the spinal canal that leaves inadequate room for nerves.

Spinal stenosis most commonly affects people older than 50. Spondylolisthesis, a defect in which the vertebrae slip out of alignment, or a tumor or fracture of the spine (see Common Back and Spinal Conditions) can also cause the problem.

If you're experiencing shooting pain down the back of your legs, however, it probably is not true sciatica. More than 90 percent of the people who suffer sciatica-like pain have some other problems, says Edward A. Abraham, M.D. Pain shooting down the legs is often due to tissue swelling somewhere along the course of the sciatic nerve, and this is believed to cause temporary irritation of the nerve.

"Often a person's occupation or personal habits can be the problem," says Dr. Abraham. "Anyone who sits for a long time, such as a truck driver, or repeats certain motions for a number of years, such as a bricklayer or mechanic, can suffer from this type of pain. I've treated several male patients who kept big wallets in their back pockets and whose jobs kept them sitting most of the day. The wallet put pressure on the sciatic nerve as it came through the buttock, and the result was pain down the leg. Once they removed the wallet, the pain went away."

BEST RESPONSE: If you have one minor, isolated episode of shooting pain, you probably don't need medical attention, say doctors. But if your pain goes on for several days, you need to see a physician, who is likely to recommend rest and other conservative treatment.

If the problem takes care of itself in a week or ten days, then no further treatment is necessary. If the pain is unrelenting, then it makes sense to see a specialist—an orthopedic surgeon, a physiatrist, a neurologist or a neurosurgeon—for further evaluation. A physical examination and various tests such as x-ray, CAT (computerized axial tomography) scan or spinal tap may be in order. In the small percentage of cases where physical defects are found, such as a slipped or ruptured disc or spinal stenosis, surgery may be necessary.

But in *most* cases, there is no "miracle cure," and you may have to change your life-style or at least change the way you do some things—like sitting less and exercising more. Dr. Abraham feels yoga, stretching exercises and swimming are best. Or, the cure may be as simple as removing your wallet from your back pocket!

SYMPTOM: **Pain, Tailbone**

COMMON CAUSES: We are talking coccyx (the scientific term for tailbone) here, and anyone who has suffered the often severe pain that a coccyx problem can cause knows the precise location.

If someone has given you a swift kick in the rear or you've taken a heavy fall and landed on your derriere, you could feel pain here—and the pain could be due to a cracked bone. (Only an x-ray can say for sure.) After giving birth, women can also suffer from coccyx pain.

Still another cause for pain could be a slipped or ruptured disc (see Common Back and Spinal Conditions) higher up in the back, which presses on nerves in this region. A pilonidal cyst, an infolding of skin in which hair continues to grow, can cause pain or tenderness in the area around the coccyx and is aggravated by sitting or riding in an automobile.

These are the usual explanations for tailbone pain. Now for a bit of the unusual—something you might want to think about if your teenager is the one complaining about the pain.

Doctors from the department of pediatrics at Cleveland's Case Western Reserve University reported two such cases in the journal *Pediatrics*. Two teenage girls, who wore tight jeans with heavy reinforced seams, complained of pain in the area of the tailbone. Examination revealed no other findings. The doctor's prescription was to avoid wearing the jeans and to sit in a more erect position on the hard school seats. Following this recommendation, the pain and tenderness soon disappeared.

BEST RESPONSE: Doctors say that most people with pain in the tailbone find that carrying a soft pillow with them is the only way to travel. Whether the practice of carrying and sitting on the pillow—or the passage of time—is the healer is open to question. Sooner or later, the pillow stays home.

Painkillers and sitz baths, in which you immerse your bottom in warm water, also help to soothe the hurt. But the important thing is that little can be done in terms of treatment. It's a simple case of letting time heal the wounds.

Slipped discs and pilonidal cysts should be treated by a doctor.

SYMPTOM: **Posture, Poor**

COMMON CAUSES: When your back's against the wall (literally), your head, shoulders, buttocks, lower legs and the backs of your heels should all be touching the wall's surface. If you fail this simple test, your posture leaves something to be desired. And poor posture leads to back pain.

But there are other possible causes: A spinal deformity such as that caused by osteoporosis (see Common Bone, Joint and Muscle Conditions in chapter 3), scoliosis or arthritis of the spine (see Common Back and Spinal Conditions); fatigue; emotional problems or periods of rapid growth. If you're pregnant or overweight, a swayback will develop to compensate for your protruding abdomen.

BEST RESPONSE: Standing tall can increase your height an inch or two and can reduce the stresses on the front of the spine that cause stooped-forward postures, suggests David Fardon, M.D., author of *Osteoporosis*.

"Imagine a wire coming down from the sky, attached to the top of your head, that pulls you upward," he explains. "Now adjust your posture to go with the upward pull. Tilt your pelvis forward and suck your stomach in, and you will feel your lower back flatten and become longer. Imagine that you have a third eye in the front of your neck. To clear the way for that eye to see, you must pull your head and shoulders back and tuck in your chin, so your neck will become straighter and longer. Those are the postures of standing tall; make them a habit."

SYMPTOM: **Spasms**

COMMON CAUSE: When a ligament or vertebral joint is injured, the surrounding muscles will go into painful spasm. With spasm the fibers can't get adequate blood supply or dispose of waste. The result: more pain and a vicious cycle of more pain, more spasm and so on. Spasms can come in alternating waves of contraction and release (clonic spasm) or may be persistent and steady (tonic spasm).

BEST RESPONSE: Some doctors suggest that you should immediately go to the emergency room or see your physician when you're suffering from muscle spasm. But in a survey published in *Backache Relief,* participants said they avoid seeing a physician during this very acute stage—the effort of getting out of bed and waiting to see the physician more than offsets the value of any treatment. A physician can be consulted *after* several days of bed rest and supportive treatment (see Best Response under Symptom: Pain, Lower Back).

SYMPTOM: **Stiffness**

COMMON CAUSES: Stiffness in the spine or neck, especially on awakening, is frequently the result of nothing more serious than bad sleeping habits, a draft or a poor choice of pillow and/or mattress. It commonly occurs as you get older.

Stiffness is also a companion to back pain that occurs after you've lifted a heavy object, fallen, stayed in an awkward or cramped position for some time or done some unaccustomed exercise. It commonly accompanies neck pain (see Symptom: Pain, Neck and Upper Back). As the pain goes, so goes the stiffness.

Stiffness can be more of an ongoing problem if you suffer from arthritis of the spine (see Common Back and Spinal Conditions) or kyphosis (see Symptom: Hunchback).

Stiffness can also be a symptom of a wryneck (see Common Back and Spinal Conditions). Besides having pain and difficulty moving, the posture of the head is different—the angle of the jaw pulls toward one shoulder and the forehead and eyes go in the other direction. This is due to the tightening of a specific muscle. "A wryneck can be caused by a virus or a ruptured cervical disc, or can be due to a fracture or muscle and ligament damage," according to Steven R. Garfin, M.D. "Emotional stress also plays a role. Sometimes babies are born with this condition and the cause is unclear."

BEST RESPONSE: The first thing you should do is investigate your sleeping habits to see if they could be contributing to morning stiffness, recommend doctors.

First, the mattress. A good mattress will hold your spine as close as possible to a position you would assume while standing with good posture. Body weight should be distributed evenly so that no one part of the body is pressured more than another. A high-quality, firm mattress supported by a box spring that was designed to go with it is best for most people.

As important as the mattress is, the pillow you use may be even more crucial, according to Lionel A. Walpin, M.D., medical director of the Walpin Physical Medicine and Pain Institute in Los Angeles. A back sleeper should use a pillow that's thin and soft, but not so thin and soft that it forces you to scrunch up your neck and shoulders to keep the pillow in place. A side sleeper with narrow shoulders should also use a thin pillow. But a side sleeper with broad shoulders should choose a thicker model. With the proper pillow, you shouldn't need to place your arm or hand under the pillow, which can cause pinched nerves in the elbow or wrist.

Also, try to avoid sleeping in drafts, since neck and shoulder muscles tend to contract in a cold environment. Besides eliminating drafts, wearing a turtleneck shirt may help because it keeps the upper body warm.

To alleviate the ache that stiffness brings on, you can apply the same self-help measures that are useful for pain in the lower back (see Best Response under Symptom: Pain, Lower Back).

For wryneck, Dr. Garfin explains that treatment can vary from "nothing, to collars, physical therapy, anti-inflammatory drugs, muscle relaxants, traction or surgery. For babies who suffer from wryneck, physical therapy is the usual treatment, although sometimes surgery is necessary."

Common Back and Spinal Conditions

Arthritis of the spine. The most common type of arthritis that affects the back is osteoarthritis (degenerative arthritis). What happens is that the surfaces of the back joints slowly wear out and cause stiffness.

Mild cases of osteoarthritis are often initially without symptoms, and you can have the problem without knowing it. When pain does surface and an x-ray confirms the diagnosis, the doctor may recommend aspirin or anti-inflammatory drugs to relieve pain, along with gentle exercise, maintenance of normal weight and even wearing a back brace.

A less common form of arthritis is rheumatoid arthritis, which involves the lining of the joint, or synovium, which secretes the fluid that lubricates the joints. What happens in the spine is that the lining of the joint thickens and the joint is actually destroyed. Treatment for this condition is variable and complex. Anyone suffering from rheumatoid arthritis should be under the care of a physician.

Fracture of the spine. Since the vertebrae, which make up the spinal column, are made of bone, they can break just like any other bone in the body. What makes a broken vertebra a serious injury is the fact that the spinal cord threads through each bone and can easily be cut or damaged by the jagged ends of a broken vertebra.

A fracture of the neck or back may occur with little damage to the cord at the time of injury and, with proper handling, the person may recover completely. But if such a person is improperly handled, the broken bone may pinch or shear off the spinal cord at the point of injury—with permanent paralysis or death as the result.

So what should you do if you suspect that injury has caused a broken back? Medical aid should be sought immediately, but the patient should be moved only by a person who is trained in such techniques.

Incomplete fractures of the vertebrae can occur if you suffer from osteoporosis, a condition that causes loss of bone mass. An incomplete fracture is one in which the break doesn't extend through the whole circumference of the bone. Treatment of incomplete and complete fractures varies with the severity of the injury.

Scoliosis.   This is a sideways curvature of the spine that causes the rib cage to lose its symmetry. It can be caused by weakness or paralysis of the spinal muscles or a developmental abnormality of the spine, or it can be associated with a disorder such as dwarfism.

Scoliosis is more common in girls than in boys, and in many cases the cause isn't known. A mild curvature becomes noticeable in the adolescent years and needs to be followed at this time. Severe scoliosis, if left untreated, can be painful and deforming and may even interfere with the working of the heart and lungs.

Treatment of scoliosis begins with physical therapy, and sometimes a spinal brace must be worn. Surgery is only necessary in more serious cases.

Slipped or ruptured disc.   The discs, which are made of cartilage and serve as cushions between the vertebrae, can rupture and press directly against an adjacent nerve root as it emerges from the spinal cord. This is not the most common cause of back pain, but it can cause the most agony and has the potential for disability.

Disc trouble most often turns up in men in their thirties and forties, although people at almost any age (past the teen years) can be affected.

Since cartilage can't be seen on an x-ray, a special test called a myelogram is frequently used to diagnose the problem. In this test, a needle is inserted into the sheath around the spinal cord, releasing a dye that can be seen on an x-ray. Unfortunately, myelography has serious drawbacks, one of which is severe headache following the procedure. For this reason, the CAT (computerized axial tomography) scan has become more popular with doctors—and patients.

At one time the treatment of choice for a slipped disc was almost always surgery. Later came injections of chymopapain, a papaya derivative, to shrink the disc. Now it is felt by many doctors that conservative therapy may be the best approach. Sometimes, local application of ice or heat, aspirin, and stretching and other exercises can be useful.

Tumors of the spine.   Not all tumors mean cancer. Benign tumors can occur in the spine and can cause pain, but they won't spread. They can usually be removed by surgery. Cancer that starts in the bone is uncommon.

However, many other types of cancer that begin elsewhere in the body can either cause "referred" pain to the back or can eventually spread to the back itself.

Whiplash injury.   This problem most commonly occurs as a result of rear-end automobile collisions in which a person's neck snaps back, then forward. Whiplash can also occur when you land on your feet or buttocks after a fall or accident.

The injury causes torn muscles and ligaments in the lower level of the neck vertebrae. Pain can vary from mild to very severe, with pain sometimes radiating to the hands, causing tingling and numbness.

Treatment usually involves wearing a neck collar for several weeks, and sometimes traction is used. Heat helps relieve pain and muscle spasm. Pain relievers and muscle relaxants also are frequently prescribed.

Wryneck.   Officially called spasmodic torticollis, this is a spasm of the neck muscles that causes rotation and tilting of the head. It can occur at any age (sometimes babies are born with wryneck), but most frequently occurs between the ages of 20 and 50. It can begin either suddenly or (more likely) gradually. Both sexes are equally affected.

The condition varies from mild or occasional episodes to a condition that lasts a lifetime and is difficult to treat. If the wryneck is caused by a physical problem, treatment is usually effective. Sometimes, however, emotional problems bring on the spasm and, in this case, psychiatric treatment may be necessary.

Chapter 3
Bones, Joints and Muscles

SEE YOUR DOCTOR IMMEDIATELY IF:
- *You experience unexplained numbness or tingling in your hands or feet*
- *Your skin turns red around a swollen joint*
- *A lump in your bone begins to grow*
- *You develop a muscle weakness that spreads through your hands, feet, arms, legs, abdomen and chest*

When an arm, leg, hip or shoulder aches, swells, clicks or collapses, it's hard to figure out whether you've got a problem with a bone, a joint or a muscle. That's because they're all related. Like a bunch of nosy aunts, uncles and cousins, they're tied together with a telephone-line network of tendons, ligaments and nerves that not only seem to talk back and forth to one another but also tend to shoot symptoms from one end of your body to the other the way Great Aunt Stella zips the latest family gossip to your mother.

That's why if you go to your doctor complaining of knee pain, you shouldn't be surprised if he or she presses on your hip and asks, "Here?" It's not that the doctor hasn't heard you or is getting senile. It's because doctors know that the knee bone's connected to the thigh bone in more than one particular way. And the site of your pain and the site of your problem may be as far apart as you and your Great Aunt Stella.

If you have bone, joint or muscle problems, the information in this chapter may help you figure out what's going on and where—and maybe what to do about it.

SYMPTOM: **Cramps**

COMMON CAUSES: Muscle cramps are the painful contraction of a muscle anywhere in your body. They're usually caused by exercising an untrained muscle too hard or by demanding that extra mile from a trained one. In pregnant women, doctors suspect, muscle cramps may be caused by a calcium deficiency.

Cramps can tie you into knots at any time, of course, but nighttime cramps are known to awaken roughly 15 percent of all healthy adults at some time or another. And the incidence of nighttime cramps seems to increase as you get older.

Not getting enough water, magnesium or salt can aggravate muscle cramps, as can thyroid disease (see Common Whole Body Conditions in chapter 19), or even uremia, a condition in which urination is less than normal, poisoning the body. Cramps that occur when you first start to exercise are usually due to an imbalance of such minerals as calcium, sodium or potassium. Cramps that come on after you've exercised for a little while are most frequently caused by inadequate blood supply to the muscle. This does not mean that you have poor circulation. During exercise, your muscles have an increased need for blood, and cramps mean that your body is not meeting the increased demand.

BEST RESPONSE: Stretch the muscle, doctors suggest. If it's your calf that's tying itself into a painful knot, you can, for example, grab your toes and the ball of your foot, then pull toward your kneecap. Or simply stand with your foot flat against the floor and press down as hard as you can.

Better yet, stand about two feet away from a wall, with your feet pointing toward it. Place your palms against the wall in front of your shoulders and lean into the wall with your legs and knees stiff and your feet flat on the floor. If you can touch the wall with your nose, you're doing it right. When you slowly do this several times, you'll feel your legs loosen up, says Lawrence Pottenger, M.D., Ph.D., associate professor of orthopedic surgery at the University of Chicago. If nighttime cramping is a problem, says Dr. Pottenger, do this stretching exercise before you go to bed. Keeping your muscles stretched and limber will help prevent muscle cramping from recurring, says Dr. Pottenger.

Pregnant women may need to supplement their diet with either calcium or magnesium to relieve cramping. One and a half to two grams a day of calcium carbonate or calcium gluconate has been the traditional therapy for pregnant women with leg cramps, doctors report, but a recent study indicates that magnesium may also be helpful.

At Brigham Young University in Provo, Utah, researchers found that 266 milligrams a day of supplemental magnesium reduced cramping in all their groups of pregnant women. The women were followed during the final two months of their pregnancy. The groups with the most cramps—women over age 27 who already had at least one child—were helped the most by the magnesium. Their cramps were reduced by 57 percent.

SYMPTOM: **Joint, Swelling around**

COMMON CAUSES: A swollen joint usually means there's extra fluid in the area, says Lawrence Pottenger, M.D. And it's frequently your body's reaction to injury. "Usually that kind of swelling goes away at night," he adds, so if swelling is still present after you've been to bed, it might be triggered by something more serious.

Some forms of arthritis (see Common Bone, Joint and Muscle Conditions) and rheumatic fever (see Common Whole Body Conditions in chapter 19) are common causes of swelling.

BEST RESPONSE: Any swelling that cannot be explained by such things as a bump, bruise or injury should be seen by a doctor. Swollen, painful joints can be a symptom of many diseases, and treatment depends on the cause.

If you have infectious arthritis, for example, you may need to have the fluid drawn out of the swollen joint and a splint or cast put on. You may also need long-term treatment with antibiotics. The same thing goes for rheumatic fever. Long-term treatment with antibiotics is frequently necessary, doctors say, and your physician will probably send you to bed with a bottle of aspirin to reduce any inflammation around your joints.

And don't ignore swollen joints even if you've already been diagnosed as having one condition or another. Several of the more serious causes of swollen joints can coexist (infectious arthritis with osteoarthritis for example), and swelling may be the only tip-off that your body has been invaded by a new villain.

Once you have been to your doctor and you know what's causing the problem, there are general treatments that you can follow to reduce the swelling.

"If you have swelling anywhere from your hips to your toes, lie down with your ankles higher than your heart," Dr. Pottenger says. Use a recliner, he suggests, or toss a couple of pillows on the sofa and lie down with your feet propped on top. Just sitting down with your feet on a footstool is not effective.

Ibuprofen (Advil or Nuprin) taken two to four times a day will also help to get rid of the swelling, says Dr. Pottenger.

ACCOMPANYING SYMPTOMS: See your doctor if you lose your appetite, have a swollen joint and feel as though you've run out of steam. You may have hepatitis (see Common Abdominal and Digestive System Conditions in chapter 1) and need medication.

SYMPTOM: **Joints, Crackling**

COMMON CAUSE: The kind of crackling sound your joints make when you "snap" your knuckles or "pop" your ankles is caused by the sudden opening of a vacuumlike space within the joint. It is natural and it is not an indication that there is anything wrong.

BEST RESPONSE: It may sound like your joints are falling apart, but they're not. You don't need to do a thing.

SYMPTOM: **Knee, Collapsing**

COMMON CAUSE: "A collapsing knee is actually a pain reflex," says Lawrence Pottenger, M.D. "It's the same as if you stepped on a tack or a sharp stone. Your spinal cord will automatically flex the muscles behind your knee, relax the muscles in front and withdraw your foot—even before your head perceives the need."

But what triggers the pain? "Instant pain that causes the knee to collapse usually means that it's a mechanical thing," explains Dr. Pottenger, rather than a symptom of disease. Usually it's a past injury that has come back to haunt you in the form of damaged cartilage in your knee.

Small pieces of cartilage—no bigger than a grain of rice—were probably torn off at the time of the injury and have been floating around inside the fluid that surrounds the joint. Since knee cartilage derives its nourishment from that fluid, the "rice-bodies," as they are sometimes called, kept on growing. "In some people they'll grow to a fair size," says Dr. Pottenger. "Then they'll get caught in the joint and cause pain.

"The pain is so sudden that your leg reacts faster than your brain," he adds. But as your knee collapses and you begin to fall, "you become so interested in the fact that you're falling that you don't even recognize the pain."

BEST RESPONSE: Check with your doctor, advises Dr. Pottenger. "In most cases, you'll require arthroscopy to remove whatever's getting caught in the knee."

Arthroscopy is an outpatient surgical procedure in which a pencil-thin telescopic instrument is inserted into the knee joint through a quarter-inch incision. A thin fiber through which light can travel illuminates the inside of your knee, allowing the doctor to actually see what's inside. Any torn cartilage, bone chips or scar tissue that are caught in the joint can be siphoned out using microsurgical instruments introduced through minuscule neighboring incisions. The procedure is so quick and simple that athletes can get back to exercise one to two weeks after surgery.

SYMPTOM: **Legs, Restless**

COMMON CAUSE: Did you ever have a weird feeling deep inside your legs that produced an irresistible urge to move them, especially right before bedtime? That's what "restless legs" are.

"What I think is involved in this is a dull, poorly localized pain," says Lawrence Pottenger, M.D. "Nobody really knows what causes it, although in children people call it growing pains. There's cramping at night, too."

BEST RESPONSE: Don't resist the irresistible. Get up and walk around. Avoiding food that contains caffeine, particularly at supper and before bed, may also help the problem, since caffeine is known to make even the strongest man shake when he's had too much.

SYMPTOM: **Lumps**

COMMON CAUSES: "Anytime you have a lump around a joint, you have to worry about cancer," says Lawrence Pottenger, M.D., although it's more likely you have gout or a form of arthritis (see Common Bone, Joint and Muscle Conditions) called osteoarthritis.

In gout, lumps around joints are actually a collection of uric acid crystals. In osteoarthritis, they may be formed by an overgrowth of bone. In fact, lumps are so characteristic of arthritis that scientists are beginning to wonder if the ends of bones near arthritic joints may be more like dense fluid than solid bone.

Imagine one end of a warm candle, Dr. Pottenger suggests. Then think about pushing it against a wall. The candle almost seems to curl back upon itself and bulge out at the end. That's the way some researchers feel arthritic bone works. New bone forming on the outside of the bone—a condition specific to arthritis—curls back and forms a lump.

If the lump is behind your knee, however, it's more likely to be a collection of fluid called a Baker's cyst. "The cyst feels like a little cherry or a little knot," says Dr. Pottenger. It generally occurs in people who manufacture a lot of joint fluid. The fluid builds up in the knee and tends to bulge out like a balloon on a tire at the weakest point.

A lump around your wrist or on top of your foot joints, however, is likely to be a swelling under the skin called a ganglion. Generally no bigger than a pea, a ganglion actually has nothing to do with your bone or muscles. It is nothing more than the accumulation of a harmless jellylike substance.

BEST RESPONSE: Any lump should be evaluated by your doctor. In the case of a Baker's cyst or ganglion, for example, your physician may very well choose to leave it alone. And there's not much you can do to eliminate lumps due to osteoarthritis.

But there are several drugs your physician can prescribe to melt away the uric acid crystals of gout, says Dr. Pottenger. And frequently a diet low in purine—a substance found in such foods as anchovies, asparagus, consommé, gravies, heart, herring, kidney, liver, meat extracts, mincemeat, mushrooms, mussels, sardines and sweetbreads—can help prevent a recurrence, since uric acid is a by-product of the way your body digests purine.

Drinking lots of water may also help by keeping the uric acid dissolved in your bloodstream instead of collected into lumps around your joints.

Occasionally, however, gouty lumps need to be surgically removed— especially if they interfere with nerves and blood vessels or actually begin to destroy skin, tendons or ligaments.

SYMPTOM: **Pain**

COMMON CAUSES: Pain in a bone, joint or muscle can be caused by anything from overexercising to cancer. But because bones, joints and muscles work so closely together, it's hard to tell which one is the site of your pain. And the site of the pain is not always the source of the problem.

"Pain can be extremely difficult to localize," explains Lawrence Pottenger, M.D., "because it's often referred from one area to another down the distribution of a nerve.

"People with hip problems, for example, will complain of pain just a little above the knee. But an examination of the knee will be absolutely normal. Then when you twist and internally rotate the hip or touch the hip in any way, you'll find that this movement extenuates the pain down around the knee." The problem is in the hip—even if it's the knee that hurts.

The same thing happens with tendons, says Dr. Pottenger. Tendons are cords or bands of strong, white, fibrous tissue that hold muscle to bone. If you were a marionette, tendons would be your strings. When a muscle shortens, for example, it pulls on the tendon, which yanks your bone into the place you want it. If a tendon becomes inflamed—from that extra mile on your evening walk, perhaps, or the lawn mower you lifted out of the car—it's hard to tell from the pain exactly where the injury is.

If the tendon around your ankle becomes inflamed, for example, you might say, "My whole leg hurts," or "The upper part of my leg hurts." Then, according to Dr. Pottenger, "what I will do—and what a smart patient would do—is press around on the different areas of your hip and leg until you find a particular area of tenderness. Whereas pain is poorly localized, tenderness—which means it hurts when you press it—is very well localized to the anatomic structures. The tenderness usually points exactly to the source of your pain."

Once the source of your pain is pinpointed, ten to one you'll find it's caused by an inflammation of the joints, tendons or bursae—those little fluid-filled sacs that act as internal cushions between skin, bone, joint and tendon. And that means arthritis, tendinitis or bursitis (see Common Bone, Joint and Muscle Conditions).

BEST RESPONSE: "Tendinitis—what we now call soft-tissue rheumatism—is often very hard to get rid of," says Dr. Pottenger. That's because it's usually due to being overweight and/or weak muscles. So just going about your everyday activities—putting away the dishes, making the bed or bathing the dog—can strain your tendons and cause a flare-up. The same thing is true of your bursae.

Ice packs and an anti-inflammatory medication such as aspirin or a nonsteroidal anti-inflammatory drug like naproxen (Anaprox) or ibuprofen (Advil or Nuprin) may be necessary during the first three days of an attack, but once the worst of your pain is over, ice or heat—hot showers, compresses or heat lamps, for example—can usually control your pain. Rest and physical therapy, plus a firm bandage or sling around the affected area, should do the rest.

If your pain continues, however, your doctor may suggest a shot of anesthetic or an anti-inflammatory drug right to the center of your pain—the tendon or bursa that's causing all the trouble.

Occasionally, chronic bursitis can develop, and your doctor may recommend injecting the offending bursa with corticosteroids.

Chronic tendinitis can frequently be treated with exercise aimed at keeping the surrounding muscles strong, says Dr. Pottenger. You should exercise to the point of pain but not beyond. For problems with the knee or hip, exercising on a stationary bicycle is a good bet. By adjusting how hard you pedal and how far, you can safely increase the amount of exercise you do. And for problems just about anywhere in your body, swimming is a good exercise.

For the pain of tendinitis, nonsteroidal anti-inflammatory drugs such as naproxen or ibuprofen may make exercising easier. If your pain is not getting any better, or if you have swelling, heat and/or redness at the site of the pain, you should see your doctor.

Exercise is also a key component in relieving and preventing chronic pain in arthritis, says Dr. Pottenger. That's because exercise strengthens the muscles surrounding the affected joints and prevents them from literally "fading away" into nothingness—or at least the medical equivalent.

It also prevents your joints from stiffening up and may, in some cases, make the difference between living a normal life and living the life of an invalid. A study of arthritis sufferers by the Upjohn Company indicated that, unfortunately, less than half of those surveyed exercised to keep their joints flexible. Generally, doctors advise, you should exercise twice daily, ten minutes at a stretch.

Loosen up your joints in the morning with a warm shower, says Emmanuel Rudd, M.D., a clinical associate professor of medicine at Cornell University Medical College in Ithaca, New York. Then lie down—on your bed if it's firm or on the floor if it's not—and contract the muscles in your buttocks ten times. Hold each contraction for a count of five. Then contract the muscles in your upper thighs ten times, again holding each contraction for a count of five. If you're wondering how on earth you contract an upper thigh muscle, Dr. Rudd explains that it's done by pushing the back of your knee down to the bed or floor.

The third exercise is just as easy. Keeping your knee absolutely straight, raise your leg slowly off the bed until it is halfway up. Then slowly lower your leg. Repeat the exercise ten times with each leg.

And don't neglect hip exercises if you have osteoarthritis in your hips, says Dr. Rudd. Lying on your bed, stretch your legs straight out and point your big toes first at each other and then at the walls on either side of you. "You're guided by your feet," says Dr. Rudd, so each hip will rotate in the same direction as you point each foot. Repeat this exercise ten times.

Then lie down on your side with your knees slightly bent, lift your upper leg off the bed as high as you comfortably can and slowly lower it. Lie on the hip that causes you the least pain, Dr. Rudd suggests, and repeat the exercise ten times. If you have pain in both hip joints, however, make sure you repeat the exercise on both sides.

If your knee is a problem, adds Dr. Rudd, sit on the edge of your bed with your knees bent and stretch out your leg until your knee is fully extended in front of you. Repeat the exercise ten times, suggests Dr. Rudd, and in succeeding weeks add weights to your ankle.

Start with a one-pound weight and increase your load by a pound every week until you can't possibly lift another ounce. The weights don't have to be autographed by famous athletes in order to work, either. A sock full of pennies or a sand-filled paint can weighed out on the bathroom scale will do the trick.

But exercise is the wrong thing to do if you should have a sudden pain flare-up, doctors say. Instead, rest the afflicted joint and take an anti-inflammatory drug such as aspirin. A nonsteroidal anti-inflammatory drug available at your local drugstore—ibuprofen, for example—is an alternative if aspirin is ineffective or causes side effects.

An ice pack applied to a painful knee for 15 minutes two or three times a day can also relieve the pain of walking up stairs or getting out of chairs. And if the pain is in your back, arms and legs, a hot bath—or a shower if you have trouble getting in and out of the bathtub—can help.

Superficial radiant heat—heating pads or hot packs, for example— can relieve a muscle spasm but has no lasting effect on the joint. And radiant heat that penetrates more deeply—infrared devices or ultrasound— doesn't really do any good, researchers feel.

If your pain continues despite these treatments and interferes with sleep, work and the movements of everyday life, you may want to consider replacing a troublesome joint. At one hospital, between 85 and 95 percent of arthritis sufferers who underwent surgical replacement of the hip, knee, shoulder or elbow said goodbye to their pain, doctors say.

ACCOMPANYING SYMPTOMS: A joint that suddenly becomes painful, hot and swollen may be under attack from bacteria. Check with your doctor. You may need bed rest, antibiotics, drainage of the joint and even hospitalization.

You should also check with your doctor if you have a pain deep inside your shoulder that gets worse at night, won't let you lie down and seems to limit the motion of your arm. You may have a "frozen shoulder" —which means that the muscles and tendons inside your shoulder can't do their job because there are bits of tissue stuck together inside the joint. Generally, doctors say, rest, heat and a gradually challenging schedule of exercises will bring your shoulder back into business. A shot of anesthetic into the joint may relieve your pain until those other methods work.

SYMPTOM: **Shoulders, Round.** *See* Symptom: Hunchback in chapter 2

SYMPTOM: **Stiffness**

COMMON CAUSES: Stiffness, particularly in the morning when you get out of bed, is usually a symptom of arthritis, tendinitis or bursitis (see Common Bone, Joint and Muscle Conditions).

BEST RESPONSE: Hot baths help to relieve stiffness caused by tendinitis and bursitis, says Lawrence Pottenger, M.D., whereas arthritis sufferers usually find taking a nonsteroidal anti-inflammatory medicine such as ibuprofen (Advil or Nuprin) more effective.

Usually, people with arthritis take two ibuprofen tablets four times a day, says Dr. Pottenger. But if you can take the last dose right before bedtime, it will help you wake up without stiffness. (Be sure to take the tablets with food or milk.) Moving and stretching your joints before you get out of bed also seems to help.

Another strategy to relieve morning stiffness due to rheumatoid arthritis, researchers report, may be to increase the amount of eicosapentaenoic acid (EPA), which is found in fish, in your diet. (Two rich sources of EPA, for example, are bluefish and Atlantic salmon.) A group of 23 arthritis sufferers in a 12-week study reported significantly less morning stiffness following a 12-week diet that, in addition to being high in polyunsaturated fat, was supplemented with fish oil capsules amounting to 1.8 grams of EPA every day.

A second study indicated that a seven- to ten-day partial fast reduced symptoms of rheumatoid arthritis in one-third of the patients. A third study suggested that avoiding foods to which you may be sensitive may reduce the duration of morning stiffness from 60 minutes to 10 minutes.

ACCOMPANYING SYMPTOMS: Check with your doctor if you have muscle stiffness combined with a low fever, throbbing headache and pulsating lumps along one side of your head. You could have an artery disease that requires medication. A hot compress along the side of your head or a gentle massage to the back of your neck may reduce your pain.

Common Bone, Joint and Muscle Conditions

Arthritis. There are two common forms of arthritis—osteoarthritis and rheumatoid arthritis.

Osteoarthritis, or degenerative joint disease, as it is sometimes called, is a product of wear and tear on the joints, says Lawrence Pottenger, M.D.

Normally, the end of each bone has a smooth layer of cartilage that acts like a shock absorber, he explains. "It has no blood supply and no nerves, so if you break it or if you put a crack in it, its ability to heal is extremely limited. Then, as you grow older, you just sort of wear out the pad. You can wear it down almost completely and it won't hurt because it has no nerves.

"But some of the tissue that's being worn off can cause an inflammation in the joint, so that the joint becomes hot and swollen."

Fortunately, the inflammation can be treated with anti-inflammatories like aspirin and ibuprofen (Advil or Nuprin), says Dr. Pottenger. Eventually, however, the cartilage pad wears away. "It's like having a bald tire," Dr. Pottenger says. When the cartilage is gone, he adds, bone starts rubbing on bone. And bones have nerves.

"Then it really starts to hurt. Under those circumstances, arthritis medicines can eliminate the swelling pretty much entirely but still leave you with about half of the pain."

So what can we do to retard the progress of this disease? "If you put a patient in a wheelchair, the arthritis would never get any worse," says Dr. Pottenger. "But no one wants to sit still all the time, so the wheelchair is not the solution."

In fact, some physicians now say that inactivity actually *causes* osteoarthritis. So instead of sitting around, doctors suggest, you should regularly exercise your joints by stretching them through their full range of motion. That's because the cartilage sitting on the ends of your bones is surrounded by a fluid that sends nutrients into the cartilage and removes waste. Without movement, the joint begins to starve and waste products are trapped. The arthritis gets worse, pain is increased and range of motion becomes even more limited. With movement, doctors say, oxygen and nutrients work their way in, waste is removed and swelling and pain are reduced.

Rheumatoid arthritis is more insidious than osteoarthritis because it can cause pain and inflammation of every joint in your body. And if it's not effectively treated, it can leave every joint permanently damaged.

Generally, rheumatoid arthritis attacks people between the ages of 20 and 50—mostly women. Nobody knows what causes it, although scientists suspect that it may begin as a viral or bacterial invasion. The problem is that it causes your body's defense system to release chemicals that attack the cartilage at the ends of your bones. The cartilage becomes deformed or locked into position.

Food intolerances may contribute to flare-ups, which explains why fasting or eliminating specified foods from your diet may relieve symptoms. Flare-ups can also be caused by stress and cold or damp weather.

Frequently, treatment includes 10 or 12 hours of rest a day, aspirin and other anti-inflammatory drugs, joint exercises, massage and heat. Some people also report less stiffness when they sleep in a sleeping bag or wear thermal underwear and stretch gloves to bed. And in at least one study, 70 percent of the study participants found that sexual arousal and activity relieved their pain—for hours.

Bursitis.   Think of hundreds of baby jellyfish scattered about under the surface of your skin, and you've got a general idea of what bursae are. Now think of them acting as cushions between skin and bone, skin and muscle, skin and tendons, and you've a general idea of what a tough life they lead.

They do a good job, too, until they get abused by infection, injury, arthritis, gout or even calcium crystals. Then they fight. They become inflamed, they frequently swell and they hurt like the dickens. That's when you've got bursitis, a common condition that can mimic the symptoms of arthritis if it's located anywhere near a joint.

Fortunately, most bursae calm down when you take a nonsteroidal anti-inflammatory drug such as ibuprofen (Advil or Nuprin) and give them a rest. Antibiotics are necessary, however, if your bursitis was caused by infection.

Carpal tunnel syndrome.   A nerve that runs from your hand to your brain passes through a narrow tunnel in your wrist formed by the wrist bones (carpals) and a tough membrane that binds everything together.

If the tissues within the tunnel swell—from repetitive wrist motions, arthritis, diabetes, injury or pregnancy, for example—the tissues will pinch the nerve and cause carpal tunnel syndrome. The result is a pins-and-needles sensation in your thumb and index and middle fingers, as well as numbness and pain, particularly at night.

Generally, doctors say, carpal tunnel syndrome is treated by wearing a wrist splint to bed, taking a nonsteroidal anti-inflammatory medication such as ibuprofen (Advil or Nuprin) or, under a doctor's supervision, therapeutic doses of vitamin B_6. If these treatments fail, surgery in which the carpal ligament is cut almost always relieves the syndrome. One aftereffect of surgery may be lingering fingertip numbness.

Gout.   Gout is a royal pain. That's because, traditionally, it's been experienced mostly by men, some of whom happen to have been kings.

Gout is actually a form of arthritis in which an inborn metabolic problem causes the production of more uric acid than your bloodstream can handle. The result is the formation of needlelike crystals that get dropped around the joints of your body (usually the big toe) like so much flotsam and jetsam. The crystals give your joints a lumpy appearance and, as they grow, become extremely painful.

Alcohol, low-carbohydrate diets and fasts are known to exacerbate or precipitate gout. To prevent an attack, doctors suggest, you should avoid all three of these, drink lots of water, exercise daily, maintain your appropriate weight and avoid purine-rich foods that produce uric acid, such as mussels, liver, asparagus, anchovies, sweetbreads, consommé, gravies, heart, kidney, meat extracts, herring and sardines.

Should you forget to maintain such a healthy life-style, a nonsteroidal anti-inflammatory medication such as ibuprofen (Advil or Nuprin) can reduce the pain of an all-out attack.

Myasthenia gravis.   Myasthenia gravis is a disease characterized by muscular fatigue and weakness. Probably caused by a malfunction in the immune system, which may be related to abnormalities in the thymus gland, it particularly affects muscles around your eyes, mouth and throat. It causes drooping eyelids and double vision, as well as difficulty in swallowing, speaking and breathing. Your arms and legs also may be weak.

There is no cure for myasthenia gravis, but remissions are common, and muscle weakness can usually be controlled by a class of drugs called anticholinesterases. Anyone with this disease should have an emergency supply in case they develop difficulty breathing or swallowing.

Osteomalacia. Osteomalacia is a bone disease doctors thought they had wiped out when vitamin D was added to milk. It's a disease in which bones soften and weaken because there's not enough vitamin D to help the body absorb calcium and phosphorus from food.

Unfortunately, a lot of older people do not drink milk. Nor do they go out into the sunshine or take vitamin D supplements—the other two methods of preventing osteomalacia. The result is fatigue, weakness and aching bones. And the symptoms get worse as the disease progresses.

Fortunately, osteomalacia responds well to daily doses of sunshine and doctor-supervised vitamin D therapy. After a bout with osteomalacia, however, doctors suggest you maintain bone health with a daily dose of 400 international units of vitamin D and 1,500 milligrams of calcium.

Osteoporosis. Bone is composed of a rich organic substance impregnated with minerals, largely calcium and phosphate. And far from being the brittle, chalky material you may remember from last year's Thanksgiving turkey, it's a living entity that constantly forms, disintegrates, re-forms and reshapes throughout life.

Yet it is this very process that makes it vulnerable. That's because there's a built-in balancing regulator that coordinates the breakdown of old bone and the manufacture of new. If you eat enough calcium, your skeleton is able to make more bone and make it denser (stronger). If you don't eat enough, however, the regulator that coordinates the bone loss/bone gain gets out of whack, and your skeleton begins to thin. Your body dissolves calcium from your bones into the bloodstream to prevent muscle cramps, maintain a normal heartbeat, facilitate nerve conduction and even aid in blood coagulation.

So what does that do to the bones? It hollows them out by reducing bone mass—what your doctor will label "osteoporosis." Unfortunately, the only way you know for sure you've got the disease is by going to a doctor for specific bone-density measurements or by breaking a bone. Loss of height and stooped shoulders are telltale signs of the disease.

The answer, some doctors say, is to bone up on calcium with supplementation. There's plenty of scientific proof to back up this advice. One such study was conducted on 80 women between the ages of 69 and 95—a kind of "worst-case" scenario for calcium-depleted bones. It indicated an increase in bone mineral content after supplementation. Moreover, it indicated that *exercise* also increases bone mineral content— even after the peak of bone growth at age 35.

These discoveries have stimulated a whole new effort to build bone mass in people of all ages. Experts are now recommending that the average person should get between 1,000 and 1,500 milligrams of calcium per day through diet and supplementation. There's not much point in going beyond that level, researchers say, because studies indicate that absorption plateaus at around 1,200 milligrams. Any excess is lost through urine, sweat and feces. And too much calcium in the urine can result in kidney stones in some people.

What kind of exercise is best? Walking, according to some doctors, wins hands down. But they probably mean a little more than an evening stroll. A study of 45 men and women aged 20 to 25 indicated, for example, that people who exercised six or more hours a week had denser bone than people who exercised less than three hours weekly.

Another strategy to fight osteoporosis for postmenopausal women is estrogen replacement therapy, both alone and in combination with calcium.

For the future, however, researchers are investigating the bone-loading effects of calcitriol, a hormone your body makes from vitamin D, and the chemical sodium fluoride. Sodium fluoride—in one study, at least—managed to increase bone density by 26 percent a year when it was added to a daily regimen of 1,500 milligrams of calcium and 400 international units of vitamin D.

Paget's disease.   Paget's disease is a bone disease that attacks people over 30. The lower spine, pelvis, legs and skull begin to manufacture new bone that is thick and deformed. It grows over old bone and produces pain, broken bones, an enlargement of the head, impaired hearing and loss of height.

Nobody knows what causes it, and there is no cure. Fortunately, however, the disease takes 20 to 30 years to develop, and even when it does, exercise can keep a wheelchair at bay, doctors say.

Tendinitis.   A tendon is actually not so much a separate thing as a geographic designation. It's the fibrous tissue at the end of a muscle that connects muscle to bone. For some reason—usually a minor injury—it can become torn, inflamed and painful. And that's when you've got tendinitis.

Unfortunately, it takes a few weeks or even months to heal, because the tendon is in constant use. That's why doctors suggest you rest the affected area and even use a sling if possible. Aspirin and firm bandages also help, and stretching a few days after the problem starts will keep your tendon from stiffening up.

Chapter 4
Breasts

SEE YOUR DOCTOR IMMEDIATELY IF:

- *You have unexplained discharge from the nipple*
- *You notice a red spot on your breast*
- *You find a lump in your breast*
- *You find a dimple on your breast*
- *You're beyond puberty and your nipple begins to retract*
- *The skin on your breast begins to thicken and the pores to enlarge, taking on the appearance of an orange skin*

When it comes to breast disease, what you don't know *can* hurt you. Lumpy breasts are common and, in most cases, are not a serious problem. But it's hard to know if you even have a lump—serious or otherwise—unless you regularly examine your breasts.

When we set out to do this chapter, time and again the experts we contacted emphasized the same thing—the importance of self-examination. Lumps frequently cause no symptoms. But self-examination can detect a lump, or at least raise some personal suspicions—if it's done *properly*. In fact, self-examination is so important to disease detection that we felt it worthy of a lesson right here:

Stand bare-breasted in front of a well-lit mirror and check for any visual abnormalities such as lumps, dimpling, change in skin texture or any changes in the appearance of your nipples. Lean forward slightly and, as you raise your arms slowly overhead, tighten your chest and arm muscles, again looking for any change in appearance.

Next, lie on your back with a pillow or folded towel under your right shoulder (this distributes the breast tissue more evenly). Put your right arm behind your head. Cup your left hand and use the flat of your fingers to feel for lumps, hard knots or thickening in the right breast. (A ridge of firm tissue in the lower curve of each breast is normal.) Begin examining at the outermost top and work in large circles around the nipple from the outside to the center. Always move in the same direction, and make sure you include the entire breast and nipple. Examine the armpit, too. Finally, squeeze your nipple to see if there's any discharge. Repeat the entire procedure on the left breast, using your right hand.

Repeat this practice once a month—preferably a week after your period. If you're no longer menstruating, do it at a regularly scheduled time, say the first of the month. Within a few months, you'll know how your breasts feel normally so you can detect changes more easily.

SYMPTOM: **Dimpling**

COMMON CAUSES: A dimple—one that looks much like a dimple on the cheek—can be a sign of breast cancer (see Common Breast Conditions). It can also be the result of an injury.

When the breast is bruised by a bump or blow, a fatty lump sometimes forms beneath the skin, explains Anne Rosenberg, M.D., a specialist in breast surgery at Thomas Jefferson Medical College in Philadelphia. The lump pulls the skin, causing it to dimple.

BEST RESPONSE: "A dimple in the breast as a result of an injury is not cancer and it will not cause cancer," says Dr. Rosenberg. In fact, it is not a serious symptom. The injury itself will heal and the dimple will go away, she says.

However, if you find a dimple on your breast, even if you can connect it to a recent injury or bruise, you should contact your gynecologist or family doctor, says Dr. Rosenberg. It could be an early sign of cancer.

ACCOMPANYING SYMPTOMS: If you're a nursing mother and have a dimple that is red and sore, and you also have a fever and chills, you could be suffering from mastitis (see Common Breast Conditions) or a breast abscess. You should see your doctor, who may put you on antibiotics to clear the infection or incise and drain the abscess.

SYMPTOM: **Lump(s)**

COMMON CAUSES: There are several causes for lumps in the breast, but only one of these is the one everyone fears—cancer. If you have just found a lump in your breast, the odds are that it is *not* cancer. Statistics show that about 80 percent of breast lumps turn out to be something other than cancer.

First of all, is your lump *in* your breast or *on* your breast? A lump that shows up *on* the breast—that is, you can feel a bump when running your finger over the skin—is usually a skin or sebaceous cyst or a boil (see Symptom: Lumps and Bumps in chapter 15). A sebaceous cyst is nothing more than a fluid-filled sac caused by a blockage in the sebaceous gland beneath. This type of cyst can become infected, causing a painful boil. They're often found on the areola, the pigmented area around the nipple.

The next question you should ask yourself is if you've detected *a* lump or a *lumpy breast*. If your breasts feel lumpy (you probably also feel pain), you could have fibrocystic disease (see Common Breast Conditions), a benign disease most common in women between the ages of 35 and 50. It tends to involve several lumps (actually fluid-filled cysts) of varying sizes that are usually located in the breast tissue nearest the armpit. The lumps tend to be movable. Sometimes the cysts can form deep in the tissue and can be confused with more serious lumps.

Now what if you've found *a* lump *in* your breast? The likely answer here is that it is a tumor, and the most likely kind of tumor is a benign (noncancerous) one. There is more than just one type of benign lump, each with its own characteristics.

A lipoma, for example, is slow-growing, soft, movable and painless. The tumor can vary from the size of a dime to the size of a quarter and most often develops in older women. A fibroadenoma is firm, movable, painless and usually oval shaped. It's most common in women between the ages of 15 and 30.

Another type of benign lump is termed traumatic fat necrosis and usually forms as a result of a blow or injury to the breast (see Symptom: Dimpling). This lump is firm, round and painless. Also, the skin around it may be red or bruised.

A lump can also be a malignant tumor (see breast cancer under Common Breast Conditions). It may or may not be painful, it is firm, stationary and feels as if it's attached to the surrounding breast tissue. It most often appears in the upper, outer part of the breast. It will gradually grow. Sometimes the skin over the breast will dimple, and you may see a change in the nipple.

Pregnant women may also feel lumpiness in the breast. This is due to the swelling of the milk-producing glands and is quite normal.

Lumps can always change in firmness, location and size. For example, the lump you felt before your menstrual period may feel completely different afterward. This is largely due to the hormonal changes taking place in the body at this time. Also, cystic lumps could disappear altogether.

BEST RESPONSE: "*Never* attempt to diagnose a lump in the breast by yourself," says Anne Rosenberg, M.D. "It is impossible to do."

Rather, the first thing you should do is make an appointment with your gynecologist or family doctor, who will see you as soon as possible. The first thing he or she will do is a breast exam to make certain that what you found is actually a lump. "The breast examination will tell the doctor if a lump exists, but it will not tell the doctor what kind of a lump it is," says Dr. Rosenberg.

If a lump is detected, your doctor may order you to have a painless, low-dose x-ray known as a mammogram. A mammogram will give the doctor a picture of the lump—its size, shape, etc.—but it cannot tell whether it is cancerous or noncancerous, says Dr. Rosenberg. Only a biopsy can show that.

If your doctor suspects a cyst, he or she may decide to aspirate it. In this procedure, which can be done in your doctor's office, a needle is inserted into the lump's cavity to withdraw any fluid that is present. If the fluid is clear and the lump disappears following aspiration, says Dr. Rosenberg, the lump is considered a cyst, and no further treatment is needed except for routine checkups. If the fluid is bloody, if there is no fluid, or if the mass doesn't disappear or disappears but returns, a biopsy will be necessary to further evaluate the lump.

In a biopsy, which can be done on an outpatient basis, all or part of the lump will be removed. If it proves to be benign, nothing further needs to be done. If the lump is cancerous, however, further surgery will probably be scheduled. The kind of surgery will depend a lot on the size of the lump, the location and the stage of the cancer. It may mean a mastectomy, in which the breast is removed, or a lumpectomy, in which the lump and a portion of the surrounding tissue are removed. A lumpectomy is almost always followed up with radiation therapy.

The best candidates for lumpectomy are those with cancer in the early stages, explains Dr. Rosenberg. The lump is small, less than three-fourths inch, and the disease has not spread. Lumps that have grown to about two inches can also be removed by this method, if the disease has not spread. "However, the method of treatment recommended is related to the individual case," says Dr. Rosenberg. "A mastectomy could be the safer method of treatment in some circumstances. For example, if the tumor is on the muscle. Or if the breast is small and a lumpectomy would remove most of the breast. Or if the breast is large and radiation treatment would not be as effective. Or if there's an underlying medical problem."

If the disease is more advanced—if the lump is larger than two inches and suspicious lymph nodes can be felt in the armpit—current treatment can vary, says Dr. Rosenberg.

"In our medical center, we first use chemotherapy and, if there's a favorable response, we operate," she says. "If there's no response to chemotherapy, then radiation is used. Other doctors may operate first."

In the most severe stage, where the cancer has spread to other parts of the body, surgery usually is not performed. Radiation is often the treatment of choice, says Dr. Rosenberg.

Dr. Rosenberg says you should discuss all your options thoroughly with your surgeon before deciding on a course of treatment. Also, as with any major surgery, don't hesitate to get a second opinion.

ACCOMPANYING SYMPTOMS: If you're a nursing mother and you find a painful, reddened lump in your breast, and you feel feverish and have chills, you could have mastitis (see Common Breast Conditions) or a breast abscess. You should see your doctor, who may put you on antibiotics to clear up the infection or drain the abscess.

SYMPTOM: **Nipples, Cracked**

COMMON CAUSES: If you're a nursing mother, you needn't be told that cracked nipples are painful. They're usually caused by an overzealous infant or one who is only sucking on the nipple rather than the areola, the pigmented area surrounding the nipple. Cracked nipples can make it easier for germs to enter the breast and cause mastitis (see Common Breast Conditions).

If you're not a nursing mother and have a cracked nipple, you could have Paget's disease of the breast, a rare type of cancer. It looks somewhat like a dermatitis of the breast, with flaking and dryness around the nipple.

BEST RESPONSE: If you're a nursing mother with cracked nipples, you should change your baby's position when he or she feeds, says Anne Rosenberg, M.D. Hold the baby's head an inch or so higher against your shoulder or nurse lying down instead of sitting up—or sitting up instead of lying down. And nurse more frequently. This will relieve fullness, which can aggravate the pain of cracked nipples.

Nipples can also be exposed to the air for 15 minutes after nursing. If these measures don't work, you should contact your doctor, who may recomend an ointment to promote healing.

"If you have an eczema-type condition of the nipples and it doesn't go away within several weeks, you should see your doctor," says Dr. Rosenberg. "I would be especially concerned if one nipple was more cracked than the other. Paget's disease of the breast is not a common problem, but if it's discovered early, treatment—which is the same as that for breast cancer—will be more effective."

SYMPTOM: **Nipples, Discharge from**

COMMON CAUSES: Medically it's termed galactorrhea, and it's very normal at certain times in a woman's life. A clear, milky discharge from the breasts is very normal during pregnancy, after pregnancy and at puberty. In fact, it can persist for up to two years after giving birth. It's also normal as a result of stimulation during sexual activity.

Certain medications, such as blood pressure pills, antidepressants and tranquilizers, can cause galactorrhea. And taking or stopping birth control pills can bring it on. Hypothyroidism (see thyroid disease under Common Whole Body Conditions in chapter 19), shingles (see Common Skin Conditions in chapter 15), a breast injury or breast surgery can also cause the breasts to secrete.

A discharge that is from only one breast and is bloody or brown, green or yellow in color is usually associated with some problem within the breast. Fibrocystic disease (see Common Breast Conditions) and, in rare cases, tumors are often the cause. A bloody discharge is often associated with cancer (see Common Breast Conditions).

BEST RESPONSE: Any discharge, bloody or watery, from your nipple should be reported to your doctor, says Anne Rosenberg, M.D.

Your doctor most likely will test the discharge to determine if it contains milk, a nonmilky substance such as pus from an infection or fluid from a cyst. He or she may also test you for a thyroid condition or, if you're experiencing headaches or vision problems, check for a possible pituitary gland tumor.

If the discharge is bloody, your doctor most likely will order a mammogram or biopsy.

SYMPTOM: **Nipples, Retracted**

COMMON CAUSES: Designed as nature intended, nipples will stand up, out and firm when stimulated. Nipples that are retracted or inverted won't. For some women, retracted nipples arrive with puberty. For these women, they are not a problem to health. They're only a problem if you want to breastfeed your baby.

However, an "outie" that suddenly becomes an "innie" can be a problem. It could be a symptom of breast cancer (see Common Breast Conditions).

BEST RESPONSE: If puberty presented you with retracted nipples, and you want to breastfeed your baby, you should speak to your obstetrician or your nearest chapter of La Leche League International, an organization that counsels breast-feeding mothers, about possible solutions to your problem. Sometimes gentle massage of the nipples during the last three months of pregnancy can help "train" the nipples to accept a baby's suckling. Also, the La Leche League markets a plastic breast shield that helps make nipples erect. Such a device can be purchased through the La Leche League catalog.

However, if one nipple has inexplicably retracted, you should see your physician, who will probably order a mammogram for detection of a possible tumor.

SYMPTOM: **Pain**

COMMON CAUSES: Breast pain is common before a menstrual period. It's also common in the early stages of pregnancy. In both cases, tenderness or soreness is the result of hormonal changes created by these conditions.

But painful breasts can also be a sign of fibrocystic disease (see Common Breast Conditions), says Anne Rosenberg, M.D. The pain is caused by fluid-filled cysts present in the breast.

Women runners and athletes, especially those with large breasts, can sometimes experience pain because of the jarring of the breast that occurs with an ill-fitting bra.

"Painful breasts are generally not a sign of cancer," says Dr. Rosenberg.

BEST RESPONSE: A well-fitted bra that provides plenty of support is helpful in alleviating breast pain, no matter what the cause, says Dr. Rosenberg.

If your pain is related to your menstrual cycle, a salt-free diet may help eliminate breast swelling associated with the pain. Some physicians prescribe diuretics ("water pills") to relieve excess fluid. Some doctors believe that reducing the amount of fat in your diet is also helpful.

One study showed that, for some women, the symptoms of fibrocystic disease can be reduced by avoiding the caffeine found in tea, coffee, cola and chocolate. Vitamin E has also been shown to relieve symptoms in some women.

A prescription hormone called danazol is being used to treat the disease. However, because of its side effects, including acne and menstrual irregularities, and because it is extremely expensive, it is only recommended for severe cases, says Dr. Rosenberg.

ACCOMPANYING SYMPTOMS: If you're a new mother and experience breast pain and swelling several days after delivery, the cause could be engorgement or local congestion of the breasts related to the production of milk. Heat and/or ice packs can help relieve the pain. Also, nursing your infant on demand will prevent the breasts from overfilling, which can alleviate the pain.

If you're breastfeeding and your breasts are painful, red and warm to the touch, and you feel feverish and have chills, you could have mastitis (see Common Breast Conditions) or a breast abscess. See your doctor, who may drain the abscess or prescribe antibiotics to treat the infection.

SYMPTOM: **Redness**

COMMON CAUSE: A red spot or a reddened area of any size on the breast that does not go away could be a sign of mastitis or cancer (see Common Breast Conditions).

BEST RESPONSE: Unexplained redness of the breast cannot be self-diagnosed, warns Anne Rosenberg, M.D. You should see your doctor as soon as possible.

SYMPTOM: **Swelling.** *See* Symptom: Pain

SYMPTOM: **Tenderness.** *See* Symptom: Pain

Common Breast Conditions

Breast cancer. Statistics show that a malignant, life-threatening breast tumor will develop in approximately 1 out of every 11 women. So it goes without saying that early detection—that means monthly self-examination of the breasts—is important for *all* women to practice (see the beginning of this chapter for instructions on how to do this).

Breast cancer starts with the development of a single lump, which is usually painless, hard and stationary, that appears to be attached to the surrounding breast tissue. It occurs most often in women past the age of 40.

No one knows why a cancerous lump develops, but there are certain risk factors that make some women more susceptible than others. These risk factors include a family history of the disease, childlessness or first pregnancy after age 30, a history of menstrual periods before age 12, menopause after age 50, obesity and a high-fat diet. Whether those with a history of fibrocystic disease are at risk is still a matter of controversy.

Currently, many doctors are recommending a screening mammogram for women after the age of 35 or 40 (depending on the doctor). A mammogram is believed capable of detecting breast lumps or other suspicious abnormalities up to two years before they can be felt by physical examination.

Treatment almost always includes surgery, either removal of the breast itself (mastectomy) or removal of the lump and surrounding tissue (lumpectomy). Radiation and chemotherapy are common follow-up treatments.

Men can also get breast cancer, although it's less common. Only 1 percent of breast cancer occurs in men. In 1985, according to one report, approximately 900 cases of male breast cancer were diagnosed in the United States.

Fibrocystic disease.   The most common affliction of the female breast, fibrocystic disease is a benign condition characterized by painful, lumpy breasts. The lumps are actually fluid-filled cysts that can vary in size and number. The condition usually occurs in women between the ages of 35 and 50, and the cysts often disappear after menopause, suggesting that hormones play a big role in the cause.

The cause of this condition, however, is uncertain and treatment is controversial. Some experts suggest that cutting down on caffeine found in coffee, tea, cola and chocolate will help alleviate the symptoms. Some recommend taking vitamin E, diuretics or hormones. These measures, however, do not help all women.

Some experts consider women with fibrocystic disease to be at higher risk for the development of cancer. However, the cancer committee of the College of American Pathologists disagrees, and feels that only a small percentage of those with fibrocystic disease run a risk of developing breast cancer. Nevertheless, those with this condition should have their breasts examined at least three times a year.

Mastitis.   Mastitis is a breast infection that most often occurs in nursing mothers. It usually results from an infection entering cracks in the nipples. It is characterized by painful, red and warm breasts. In mild cases, treatment includes bed rest, warm, wet compresses to the breast, frequent nursing and wearing a supportive bra. Aspirin is often prescribed to relieve pain. In more severe cases, antibiotics may be prescribed to clear up the infection.

Sometimes an infection can result in a breast abscess, although this is uncommon. An abscess is characterized by pus from the nipple. In such cases, draining the abscess is often required.

Chapter 5
Circulation, Heart and Lungs

SEE YOUR DOCTOR IMMEDIATELY IF:
- *You feel pain or pressure in your chest for more than five minutes*
- *You have recurrent chest pain*
- *Your regular heartbeat is replaced by rapid "twitching" or irregular skipping*
- *You cough up blood*
- *You're struggling to breathe, there's swelling around your neck and maybe some red, itchy lumps on your skin*

Heart disease and lung cancer. Together they form a malevolent image of death that rises, unbidden, every time you feel a twinge, a stitch or a heaviness anywhere between waist and throat. And it's no wonder—they were responsible for more than 900,000 American deaths in one recent year.

But the point of this chapter is that they needn't give you a feeling of doom. By practicing certain preventive measures, you can decrease your chances of getting either disease.

According to the National Heart, Lung and Blood Institute, there has been a 29 percent drop in death rates from coronary heart disease and stroke in the last ten years. The key to preventing heart disease, most doctors agree, is to stop smoking, control high blood pressure, cholesterol and diabetes, and maintain desirable weight. Exercising regularly, increasing your intake of fruits, vegetables, whole grains and fish and decreasing your intake of fat may also help.

The outlook for lung cancer, however, is not so favorable. It is treated much less successfully than other cancers. The best way to fight lung cancer is to prevent lung cancer. This means don't smoke. If you do—stop.

SYMPTOM: **Angina.** *See* Symptom: Pain

SYMPTOM: **Breathing, Difficult**

COMMON CAUSES: Trouble getting a deep breath, trouble getting enough air, rapid breathing, shallow breathing, shortness of breath and breathlessness are all different ways that people describe this symptom, says John Phillips, M.D., Lassen professor of cardiovascular medicine and chief of the Cardiology Section at Tulane University Medical Center in New Orleans.

"Trouble getting air out usually means asthma," adds the cardiologist. "Trouble getting air in and sighing frequently means anxiety."

But difficult breathing that is otherwise unexplained by such normal things as exertion, anxiety or excitement, he says, can be caused by pneumonia or heart failure (see Common Circulatory, Heart and Lung Conditions); asthma, bronchitis or emphysema (see chronic obstructive lung disease under Common Circulatory, Heart and Lung Conditions); an inability of the blood to carry enough oxygen, which could be caused by severe anemia (see Common Whole Body Conditions in chapter 19); a disease of the nervous system; a blood clot in your lungs or cancer.

But what does your heart have to do with breathing? If your heart isn't pumping efficiently, blood begins to back up in the lungs' millions of tiny capillaries, swelling them stiff with retained fluid. The fluid prevents close contact between air and blood, which means that the oxygen in the air you just inhaled is having a difficult time getting to your bloodstream. The result is a painful gasping for air.

And what's the connection between anemia and difficult breathing? Most anemia is caused by a lack of iron, and iron is an essential part of hemoglobin, the vehicle in which oxygen hitches a ride to the rest of your body. If there's not enough hemoglobin to provide transportation, the rest of your body does not get enough oxygen and you feel breathless.

What does *not* cause difficult breathing, however, is aging. The idea that your ability to take in oxygen is diminished as you get older is simply not true.

BEST RESPONSE: "If you're having a breathing problem you should see your doctor," says Robert G. Loudon, M.D., CHB., professor of medicine and director of the Pulmonary Disease Division of the University of Cincinnati College of Medicine. Shortness of breath can be triggered by so many diverse causes that only your doctor—aided by a stethoscope and possibly an electrocardiogram, an x-ray, the read-out from one or two pulmonary function tests and a blood test—can determine exactly what you should do.

For example, if you have heart failure—which, by the way, does *not* mean your heart has stopped beating—your doctor may recommend that you get plenty of rest. You can sometimes help your breathing by propping yourself up with pillows while you're in bed. Moving your legs around when you sit or lie down will help blood circulate.

Your doctor may also tell you to cut down on your daily intake of salt and may prescribe diuretics ("water pills"), drugs designed to take a load off your heart by reducing the amount of fluid your heart has to pump.

If you have a lung condition associated with irritable or hyperactive airways, such as asthma or bronchitis, avoid irritants such as tobacco smoke, perfume, air pollution and fumes from paint or household cleaners. Other common medical advice includes walking a mile every day to increase your body's ability to use oxygen, and maintaining good health with proper nutrition and sufficient rest. Your doctor may prescribe bronchodilators to keep your airways open or corticosteroids to reduce any inflammation or swelling.

Steam or mist from a vaporizer may also help make breathing easier. Only those people who are strong enough to cough, however, should do this.

If blood tests reveal you're anemic, you may need a dose of iron, vitamin B_{12} or folic acid, doctors say, depending on what caused your anemia in the first place.

ACCOMPANYING SYMPTOMS: If you're lightheaded and dizzy, have chest pain and feel like you're smothering, you may be one of the estimated 25 percent of the population who has episodes of hyperventilation, which means abnormally prolonged and deep breathing. These are also symptoms of a heart attack (see myocardial infarction under Common Circulatory, Heart and Lung Conditions), however, so if you're experiencing them for the first time, see your doctor immediately. If it turns out you're a victim of hyperventilation, trying not to worry about the episodes and learning to relax may be the best long-term solution. For temporary relief during the episodes, cover your mouth and nose with a paper (not plastic) bag and breathe normally.

SYMPTOM: **Pain**

COMMON CAUSES: Most people who get chest pain immediately wonder if they're having a heart attack—what doctors call a myocardial infarction (see Common Circulatory, Heart and Lung Conditions). And maybe they are. But it's just as likely that that chest pain is caused by the raspberry Slurpee you just drank. Or the follow-through on your golf stroke. Or even the chewing gum you were just popping.

The problem is that there are so many different kinds of chest pain and so many different causes that it takes a doctor to tell you what the pain means. And sometimes even your doctor's going to have trouble. Chest pain is that complex.

Pain that's related to the heart, for example, is frequently described as sustained, viselike and agonizing. It's usually—but by no means always—located in the upper third of your breastbone. It almost always gets worse when you exert yourself, doctors explain, and most often radiates out from the heart. It usually does *not* get worse when you move your shoulder, is usually not altered by breathing and is rarely relieved by vomiting, belching or passing gas.

Besides heart attack, heart problems that can cause chest pain include leaky or narrowed heart valves or valves that have slowly stiffened; weakened arteries that balloon out and slow or even stop the flow of blood; inflammation, infection or even swelling of the heart muscle or the membranous bag in which it sits; and angina, a common chest pain that is triggered by too little oxygen reaching the heart.

Typically, doctors say, angina pain is described as a pressing or squeezing sensation that begins in the center of your chest and spreads to your shoulders or arms—frequently along the left side—or even to your back, neck or jaw. Less commonly, the pain may occur only in your arms, wrists or neck.

It usually lasts only a few minutes and is most often triggered by exercise, emotional upset, exposure to the cold or any other situation that increases your heart's workload and subsequent demand for more oxygen. And, although angina is occasionally caused by a coronary artery spasm, it usually happens because the coronary artery is blocked with so much "sludge" that the flow of blood—and its precious oxygen cargo—is reduced to less than 40 percent of normal. In either case, however, blood flow and oxygen availability are usually restored within 5 to 15 minutes, and the pain disappears.

The pain of a heart attack is almost always more severe than that of angina, doctors say, and it usually lasts longer—sometimes for hours. The pain can vary in intensity from mild discomfort to excruciating pain, and it is frequently accompanied by sweating, nausea, vomiting, dizziness or fainting, even a feeling of impending doom. Keep in mind, however, that at least 10 percent of those who are having a heart attack never feel a thing. A heart attack doesn't have to hurt.

Chest pain that's not related to your heart, doctors say, may feel as though someone stabbed or poked you with a finger. It may be dull, and it's often at the lower end or below your breastbone, even under your nipple. It's unlikely to get worse with exertion—sometimes it can even be relieved by physical activity—although in many disorders the pain will get worse when you move your shoulder.

If you have pain in your chest and you can reproduce the pain or make it worse by touching the sore spot, chances are it is not due to your heart. Some kinds of chest pain that are not related to the heart may be made worse with breathing and better with belching, vomiting or passing gas.

Chest pain that's not caused by your heart, doctors say, can come from the lungs, esophagus or even your abdomen (see Symptom: Pain, Abdominal, Recurring in chapter 1). It can be caused by a virus, fungus disease or mold. It also can be caused by drinking cold liquids, indigestion (see Symptom: Indigestion in chapter 1) or swallowing air while eating, talking or chewing gum. It can be caused, especially in teenagers, by minor malfunctions—perhaps by inflammation from a stretched ligament—in the bones and cartilage of the chest wall, brought on simply by bending forward, stretching, reaching for an object, turning over in bed or playing tennis or golf. Sometimes it's even caused by the way you sit.

BEST RESPONSE: Because pain can mean so many things, diagnosis should be made *only by your doctor.* If you're bothered by any pain in your chest, says John Phillips, M.D., contact your doctor immediately.

ACCOMPANYING SYMPTOM: Chest pain accompanied by a cough that frequently produces blood-stained mucus can be a sign of pneumonia (see Common Circulatory, Heart and Lung Conditions), tuberculosis, a blood clot in your lung or lung cancer. Call your doctor.

SYMPTOM: **Palpitations**

COMMON CAUSES: Palpitations are nothing more than an awareness of your heartbeat, explains John Phillips, M.D. Generally, they're not a cause for concern.

What's causing your palpitations depends a lot on the way they *feel.* Is your heart beating hard? Or is it beating irregularly?

If it feels like your heart's beating hard, says Dr. Phillips, it could be due to stress or anxiety and not heart disease. "I can tell you that the most common manifestations of stress and anxiety are lightheadedness that feels like floating but not turning, the sensation of a lump in your throat that prevents swallowing saliva but not a beefsteak, little black and white spots in front of your eyes, numbness of the hands, feet, lips or one side of your left arm and hand, difficulty getting air in but not out, sighing, and sticking and stabbing chest pains."

But what if your palpitations feel as though your heart's beating irregularly? Everyone, doctors say, experiences a skipped beat or periods when the heart seems to race or flutter or flip. That's because momentary arrhythmias, as they're called, can be triggered by excessive caffeine, tobacco smoke, alcohol, worry, drugs or deficiencies in thiamine or potassium (particularly among alcoholics), as well as deficiencies in vitamin B_{12}, iron, magnesium and folic acid.

Less likely but more serious causes of palpitations are myocarditis (see Common Circulatory, Heart and Lung Conditions), an overactive thyroid (see thyroid disease under Common Whole Body Conditions in chapter 19), congenital heart defects, heart disease or lung disease. With true heart ailments, doctors explain, palpitations are usually a minor complaint. Pain and difficulty in breathing are likely to be more noticeable symptoms.

Some palpitations, however, can be life-threatening. That's because the heart is not unlike couples lined up for a square dance. They join hands and circle to the left, pause, circle to the right, pause, then hook elbows and swing one another around. But if just one of the four couples in a circle cannot keep to the rhythm of the dance's music, the whole circle disintegrates into chaos, with everyone running into everyone else.

The same thing happens when the four chambers of your heart don't keep in step. If your palpitations are caused by an arrhythmia called atrial fibrillation, for example, the muscles in your two atria—the upper chambers of your heart—do not contract effectively because of disorganized electrical signals. Unfortunately, this puts you at risk for a blood clot that can travel through your circulatory system until it blocks an artery or vein. It can even cause heart failure (see Common Circulatory, Heart and Lung Conditions) because of a decrease in blood flow through the heart.

If your palpitations are caused by an arrhythmia called ventricular fibrillation, the muscles of the lower chamber twitch instead of pump. The result is usually sudden death.

BEST RESPONSE: You need to see your doctor for any kind of palpitations, says Dr. Phillips. Don't just assume it's something minor—anxiety, for example—and not go. Your doctor will have a list of roughly 25 questions that will help him or her pinpoint your problem and make some suggestions. Probably, he or she also will give you a physical examination, chest x-ray, electrocardiograms and a couple of tests that may involve walking on a treadmill and wearing a portable heart monitor.

There are at least 100 different ways for your heart to beat, adds Dr. Phillips, and every one of them can have a different treatment. Sometimes all that's necessary is to cut out a precipitating agent such as tobacco or caffeine. Sometimes you need to correct an underlying condition, such as high blood pressure or atherosclerosis (see Common Circulatory, Heart and Lung Conditions). Sometimes you need to have an artificial pacemaker implanted just under the skin of your chest to jump-start your heart's electrical system. And sometimes, when you get that rapid pounding feeling in your chest that characterizes paroxysmal tachycardia (a type of arrhythmia), all you need to do is slow down a few nerve impulses by holding your breath, slowly drinking a liquid or even bathing your face in cold water.

If your palpitations are triggered by ventricular fibrillation, however, you and your doctor may have to do some heavy-duty thinking. More than 400,000 people die from ventricular fibrillation or ventricular tachycardia (rapid beat of the heart's lower chambers) every year, doctors say, yet the use of medication to control this condition is controversial.

The problem, they explain, is that between 5 and 15 percent of those who try to control their ventricular fibrillation or tachycardia with drugs will actually experience worse arrhythmias. Other side effects can also cause problems.

A study at the University of Virginia School of Medicine, for example, revealed that 29 percent of 123 study participants experienced major reactions to treatment by antiarrhythmic drugs. Significant side effects occurred in 20 to 50 percent of the drug trials in this study. As a result, researchers concluded that these drugs should not be given to people who do not have serious arrhythmia and who experience occasional palpitations. The drugs should be reserved for someone whose daily survival is at stake—someone who may drop dead without them.

Doctors also are trying to minimize adverse reactions by initiating drug treatment in the hospital, where you can be carefully monitored and where the effectiveness of any prescribed medication can at least be evaluated. Doctors at Thomas Jefferson University Hospital's electro-physiology laboratory in Philadelphia, for example, can insert a thin plastic tube into your veins and heart under local anesthesia, then give your heart one, two or three electrical twitches to see if they can trigger an arrhythmia. If they can't, says the lab's director, Arnold J. Greenspon, M.D., they know the drug has significantly increased your chance of survival over the next year. If they can, they know they need to find you another drug.

Fortunately, even if you have ventricular fibrillation or tachycardia that doesn't respond to medication, your heart doesn't have to quiver until it stops or gallop until you faint. Implanted defibrillators that kick your heart into action with a jolt of electricity if it stops beating and the surgical removal of a small piece of heart muscle from which a rapid ventricular heartbeat may originate have both given new hope to those who do not respond to medication.

ACCOMPANYING SYMPTOMS: If your palpitations are accompanied by difficulty in breathing, chest pain, abnormally frequent urination, fainting spells and even a false sense of impending death, you could have a particular arrhythmia known as paroxysmal tachycardia. But despite the frightening manifestations of paroxysmal tachycardia, it's not usually indicative of a serious problem.

SYMPTOM: **Sighing.** *See* Breathing, Difficult

SYMPTOM: **Wheezing**

COMMON CAUSES: Wheezing is a whistling sound that seems to come from your throat when, during exhalation, something constricts or obstructs your airways. It's usually caused by asthma (see chronic obstructive lung disease under Common Circulatory, Heart and Lung Conditions), doctors say, although it also can be caused by chronic bronchitis (see chronic obstructive lung disease under Common Circulatory, Heart and Lung Conditions), lung cancer, heart failure (see Common Circulatory, Heart and Lung Conditions) or even a foreign object lodged in your throat.

BEST RESPONSE: For most of those suffering from asthma or bronchitis, drinking a lot of fluids and using a vaporizer, steam kettle or hot or cold mists at the first sign of a wheeze will be helpful. This will prevent the secretions in your airways from drying out and blocking the passage of air. But those people who are too weak to cough up phlegm should not use vapor, steam or mists: Use of such methods can actually cause more problems. In any case, if you are too weak to cough up phlegm, you should be seeing your doctor.

When you see your doctor, says Robert G. Loudon, M.D., he or she will ask a number of questions, examine you and perhaps order a chest x-ray and run a pulmonary function test as well. During the test you will be asked to breathe in deeply from a machine, then to exhale as hard as you can back into it. The machine will calculate how much air your lungs can hold, how much of it you can exhale and how quickly you can exhale—a set of numbers that indicate just how well your lungs are working.

Your doctor may also ask you to inhale a substance that may help open up your airways to see how well it works in your case, or may ask you to inhale a substance that triggers wheezing if you're not actually doing so when he or she examines you.

If you have asthma, your physician is likely to suggest you use a metered-dose inhaler containing a medication that opens up your airways. Another frequently prescribed medication is theophylline, although its side effects—nausea and nervousness—have encouraged some doctors to suggest other medications as alternative treatments for mild to moderate asthma.

Because there is a lot of variation in the course of asthma itself and among the people who suffer from it, no one treatment regimen will work for all people. For some, a relaxation technique like yoga may help. In one study, 53 asthmatics who were trained in yoga practiced rhythmic deep breathing techniques, simple body movements, meditation and devotion. As a result, researchers concluded, the asthmatics had fewer attacks per week, used less medication and breathed easier than asthmatics in another group who were not practicing yoga.

For others, though, exercise may be helpful. Yes, you read it right—exercise. Despite the fact that in many asthmatics an attack of wheezing can be *triggered* by exercise, it can also sometimes relieve symptoms. Your asthma may actually trouble you less if you maintain good physical fitness and exercise to the level that your condition permits.

Common Circulatory, Heart and Lung Conditions

Arteriosclerosis.   Arteriosclerosis is hardening of the arteries. As you age and develop atherosclerosis, the disease causes your arteries to become increasingly narrow and brittle. They're less able to expand and contract and, as a result, the flow of blood through your body is impaired.

If your legs are not getting enough blood, for example, you may have pain in your calves when you walk or in your toes when you're taking a nap. If your brain isn't getting enough blood, you may get dizzy when you move your head, or you may periodically lose your vision.

Generally, doctors say, you can slow down arteriosclerosis the same way you delay the life-threatening effects of atherosclerosis: Reduce the amount of cholesterol and fat in your diet, avoid tobacco and take care of underlying problems such as diabetes or high blood pressure.

Asthma. *See* Chronic obstructive lung disease

Atherosclerosis. Atherosclerosis is a disease in which bunches of small blood cells clump together with cholesterol, a white, waxy substance in the walls of your arteries. There is some evidence that atherosclerosis forms in areas of arterial injury. No one knows where the injuries come from, scientists say, although it seems that they occur at arterial stress points—the branching of one artery from another, for example—and that some of the injuries may be caused by high blood pressure and the chemicals in tobacco smoke.

The problem is that the small blood cells don't know when to stop clumping. They continue to build the patch from blood cells, cholesterol and other odds and ends roaming your arterial highways until the patch—called an atheroma—bulges out from the arterial wall and reduces the flow of blood. If the artery is further narrowed by smoking and tension, both of which constrict blood vessels, or a buildup of cholesterol, or if it's damaged by diabetes or even a virus, there's a good chance that a vascular logjam will occur and the flow of blood—with its precious oxygen cargo—will be reduced or even stopped.

And then you're in trouble. If blood is cut off to your brain, for example, you'll have a stroke. If it's cut off to your arm or leg, you'll get gangrene. If it's cut off to your heart, you'll have angina or, if circulation is not quickly restored, a heart attack. Fortunately, blood flow is usually restored within a few seconds or minutes, and the part of your body that was affected resumes its normal function.

What are your chances of getting atherosclerosis? Researchers studying a group of New Orleans Caucasians found that 30 percent showed early manifestations of coronary atherosclerosis between the ages of 15 and 24. Between the ages of 35 and 44, the study showed more than 85 percent of the group had some manifestation of coronary atherosclerosis.

"The kinds of symptoms you might have that are short of catastrophic occurrences like a heart attack or stroke include dizzy spells that last for some time and weakness in an arm or leg," says Virgil Brown, M.D., chairman of the Atherosclerosis and Metabolic Disease Division at the Mount Sinai School of Medicine in New York.

Whether or not atherosclerosis that's progressed this far is reversible is debatable. Scientists suspect it is. "It's certainly reversible in animals," says Dr. Brown,"and some anecdotal data suggest that it's reversible in humans." But there is one thing that doctors know for sure: You can slow down the progress of the disease.

One effective way, says Dr. Brown, is to lower the amount of saturated fat and cholesterol in your diet. In large-scale studies where saturated fats were reduced to less than 10 percent of calories and cholesterol was reduced to less than 800 milligrams a day, blood cholesterol levels fell by approximately 15 percent. And another study indicated that for every 1 percent drop in blood cholesterol, there's a 2 percent drop in the incidence of heart disease.

Why all the fuss about cholesterol? Because every time you take a bite of some cholesterol-rich food such as egg yolk or hamburger, you give your body more cholesterol than it probably needs. Your liver already makes around a gram a day, and enough is enough.

Think of your bloodstream as a crowded highway. Every time cholesterol is needed somewhere—to produce hormones or insulate nerves, for example—it's wrapped in a protein packet and transported via your arterial highways to its destination. Then, when its work is over, it's wrapped in another protein packet and transported back to the liver for disposal. Anything that's left hanging around in your arteries is what can cause a problem.

Generally, researchers refer to the packet carrying cholesterol that's on its way to do a job as low-density lipoprotein (LDL) cholesterol. The packet carrying cholesterol that's on its way back to the liver is called high-density lipoprotein (HDL) cholesterol, and doctors like it because it's the trash truck for cholesterol. It escorts cholesterol to your liver, which, in this case, acts as the town dump.

Now it may seem as though researchers are splitting hairs—or fats, as the case may be—and they are. But they've got an excellent reason: 75 percent of the cholesterol roaming the arterial highways is LDL. And *not* coincidentally, LDL is the cholesterol that seems to keep building those logjams of atheromas. If you can reduce the amount of LDL in your blood, researchers claim, you can reduce the incidence of atherosclerosis and its killer offspring, heart attack and stroke.

That's why you need to know one kind of fat from another. It's not enough to reduce your total intake of cholesterol, cautions Dr. Brown. You also need to reduce the *saturated* fats that encourage LDL traffic.

But how can you tell saturated fat from unsaturated? Saturated fat is any fat that remains solid at room temperature. Dairy products, such as butter, and marbled meats are good examples. Think about the steak you broil in the oven. When you pull it out of the oven, the pan is full of hot, liquid oils. Leave the pan on the counter overnight, however, and the fatty oils congeal.

But some saturated fats are hidden. Bakery goods, for example, contain a lot of fat, most of it saturated. Bakers and other food manufacturers like saturated fats because they're easier to preserve than unsaturated fats, extending the food's shelf life. Saturated fats are also used to add crispness to foods ranging from pie crusts to crackers to "natural" cereals.

Prevention doesn't only mean cutting out the bad foods, says Dr. Brown. It means adding good foods to your diet as well. Fiber foods such as corn, beans, oats and fruit pectin have been shown to reduce cholesterol in your bloodstream by 5 to 10 percent. Fish, too, have a heart-protecting capacity. The reason is not fully understood. It may be because many fish contain large amounts of omega-3 fatty acids, fats that help thin your blood and slow down the tendency of your blood cells to clump together, says Dr. Brown. In larger amounts they can actually lower triglycerides—a form of fat—roaming your bloodstream.

One study revealed that even people on normal diets could reduce their triglycerides by 60 percent when they took 40 one-gram capsules of fish oil every day. That's a lot of pills, and when you think about the equivalent amount of fish—nine three-ounce servings of salmon—that's a lot of fish, too. But recent evidence from a long-term study in the Netherlands indicates that more moderate consumption of fish may also help reduce mortality from heart disease. Eating fish as infrequently as once or twice a week may help prevent coronary heart disease.

Diet, however, is only part of the prevention program. Prevention also includes exercise. The American Heart Association recommends that you do some sort of regular heart-pumping activity, such as walking, climbing stairs, running, bicycling or swimming for at least 15 to 30 minutes every other day.

If you already *have* the disease, your doctor may suggest heart by-pass surgery or a percutaneous transluminal coronary angioplasty (PTCA).

In bypass surgery, cardiac surgeons create a new pathway around the arteries that are partly blocked by atheromas. In PTCA, they maneu-ver a narrow tube with an uninflated balloon on the end into the blocked artery. When they subsequently inflate the balloon with fluid, the pressure opens the blocked vessel by splitting or cracking the atheroma.

At least one study indicates that bypass surgery may be overused, according to Constance M. Winslow, M.D., a researcher for the Rand Corporation, which conducted the study. Out of 386 patients in the study, 14 percent of the procedures were considered "inappropriate" and 36 percent were termed "equivocal," in other words, questionable.

Moreover, neither bypass surgery nor PTCA is without risk, doctors caution, and neither is a cure. Your blocked arteries can act up again within one to three years, and a second procedure may become necessary. In the future, doctors say, you may be able to have your arterial logjams zapped with a laser or ground up with the surgical equivalent of a vascular roto-rooter.

Bronchitis.   *See* Chronic obstructive lung disease

Chronic obstructive lung disease.   Chronic obstructive lung disease (COLD) is the umbrella term applied to asthma, chronic bronchitis and emphysema. They're usually lumped together because all three share a common characteristic: the airflow either into or out of the lungs is obstructed—sometimes even both ways.

The most common cause of chronic bronchitis, which is an inflam-mation of your larger airways, and emphysema, which is destruction of your smaller airways, is tobacco smoke, although both conditions are exacerbated by the nitrogen and sulfur dioxides characteristic of urban air pollution. Aerosol sprays we use in our homes may also contribute to COLD, as does occupational air pollution.

But nobody's quite sure what causes asthma. An attack of wheezing and coughing, doctors say, is usually triggered by exposure to an allergen, medicine (aspirin especially), infection, chemicals, tobacco smoke (whether you're doing the smoking or not), perfume, air pollution, fumes from paint or household cleaners, cold air, sudden changes in temperature or humidity, sinus inflammation and polyps. Exercise and laughing can also trigger an attack, as can strong emotions.

That does not mean that asthma is psychological, however. Asthma begins in your lungs, doctors emphasize, not in your head.

In the workplace, asthma can also be triggered by exposure to birds (feathers, excreta); insects (bees, insect dye, locusts, mites, weevils, silkworms); mammals (danders, urinary proteins, pancreatic enzyme supplements); seafood (crabs, oysters, prawns); vegetable matter (grains, tobacco, woods); microbes (enzyme detergents, baking products); pharmaceuticals (penicillins, tetracycline) and chemicals (platinum salts, formaldehyde, amines).

In fact, occupational asthma, as researchers usually refer to this problem, affects 3 to 15 percent of our industrial work force—50 percent in such high-risk industries as platinum refining and enzyme detergent manufacturing.

Fortunately, exercise and medicines that open up your airways can often help you stay ahead of the wheezes and gasps. Sometimes, however, only a change in occupation will solve the problem.

Coronary thrombosis.   *See* Myocardial infarction

Croup.   Croup is an upper respiratory illness in which children emit a shrill wheezing or grunting noise as they struggle to breathe. The noise usually occurs because a respiratory infection has narrowed the child's throat. It is accompanied by a harsh, barking cough and hoarseness. Croup symptoms can also develop in a child who has inhaled a foreign object.

For croup attacks, some doctors suggest you humidify the environment with a steaming kettle or vaporizer, or even the steam from a hot shower. But a child who is having trouble breathing may also need to be hospitalized and given oxygen. If the infection is caused by bacteria, the child may also need antibiotics.

Any child who has difficulty breathing and turns bluish—especially around the mouth—should be taken to a hospital immediately.

Emphysema.   *See* Chronic obstructive lung disease

Heart attack. *See* Myocardial infarction

Heart failure. Heart failure does *not* mean that your heart stops. It means that a problem such as atherosclerosis or a leaky valve has weakened your heart so that it can't pump effectively.

If you have left-sided heart failure, for example, blood accumulates in the veins that carry blood from the lungs, and your lungs fill with fluid. That's why its primary symptom is difficulty in breathing and sometimes a kind of bubbling sound when you inhale or exhale.

If you have right-sided heart failure, blood accumulates in veins that lead from other parts of your body to your heart. That causes lower parts of your body—your legs or ankles, for example—to swell. In long-standing left-sided heart failure, however, you can also develop leg swelling. With severe heart failure, you may also lose your appetite and become confused.

Fortunately, you can usually control heart failure with rest, a low-salt diet and drugs that force fluid out of your tissues, dilate your blood vessels and control your heart's contractions. A new drug—perhaps in the form of a nasal spray—that imitates a hormone naturally produced by your heart may perform all three of these tasks in the future.

High blood pressure. Hypertension is the $12 word for high blood pressure, which means that your heart is working overtime. It's usually defined as any blood pressure reading higher than 140/90. The 140 refers to how hard your heart is pumping out blood, and the 90 refers to how quickly it's filling back up.

Doctors can rarely tell you what causes high blood pressure unless it's related to an underlying disease. But they can tell you that those over the age of 45 with high blood pressure are three times as likely to have a heart attack, six times as likely to have heart failure and seven times as likely to experience a stroke as those with a lower pressure. It's a disease that shortens lives by an average of 10 to 20 years.

Yet half of those afflicted don't even know they have a problem, because this is one disease that has no symptoms during the early stages. That's why you should have your blood pressure checked once a year, and more often if you're taking oral contraceptives or estrogen, if you're pregnant or if hypertension runs in your family.

If your blood pressure is high, doctors say, you may want to cut your total salt intake down to one teaspoon a day, exercise 30 to 60 minutes three times a week, lose a few pounds and learn to relax.

Those with severe hypertension may need the help of medications. If the bottom number on your blood pressure reading is 100 or more—say 180/100—your doctor may want to reduce the load on your heart and blood vessels and bring it down quickly by giving you a diuretic ("water pill"), a drug that flushes excess fluid out of your body and into your bladder for excretion.

But although these diuretics and a group of drugs called beta-blockers have traditionally been the treatment of choice, their role has now become controversial. That's because doctors have been trying to figure out for years why these drugs will reduce your risk of heart failure, kidney failure and stroke but *not* your risk of atherosclerosis, heart attack or angina. It has come to the point, in fact, where some doctors are asking if diuretics and beta-blockers are not actually *increasing* the risk of heart problems among people with high blood pressure.

No one's really sure. More research is necessary before diuretics and beta-blockers are abandoned, researchers say. But in the meantime, they suggest that only low-dose diuretics be used and the "indiscriminate" use of beta-blockers be questioned. There are, they point out, other anti-hypertensive drugs (clonidine, guanabenz, prazosin, nifedipine, diltiazem, verapamil, captopril, enalapril) that can also lower blood pressure.

Myocardial infarction.   A myocardial infarction is a heart attack. It means that something—a blood clot, an arterial spasm, a logjam of cholesterol and other arterial debris—has blocked the flow of blood into your heart, and a part of your heart, maybe big, maybe small, has died.

Fortunately, it can take up to 24 hours for your heart to die when, as is frequent, a heart attack is triggered by a blood clot. It can vary from person to person, but usually "sudden death" due to a heart problem is from a type of arrhythmia called ventricular fibrillation, not from a heart attack.

That doesn't mean you can delay calling an ambulance or getting to your hospital emergency room when the symptoms—pain or a feeling of tightness in your chest, possibly dizziness, difficult breathing, sweating, chills, nausea or fainting—hit. Almost half of all people who have a heart attack die before treatment can be started.

That's why prevention is a must. Most heart attacks are caused by atherosclerosis, doctors say, so the only way to prevent one is to slow down or stop the buildup of fatty deposits inside your arteries that characterize this disease. And that means you should avoid tobacco smoke, eat a diet low in saturated fats and cholesterol and maintain proper weight.

You may also wish to talk to your doctor about taking a single coated or buffered aspirin a day. An aspirin a day may be able to keep heart attacks at bay. But don't take more than a single tablet. Taking more doesn't increase your protection, doctors have found out.

If you've already *had* a heart attack and you're alive one month later—even after a severe attack—you have an estimated 85 percent chance of surviving for at least a year and about a 70 percent chance of surviving for five years, statistics estimate. If you're one of the increasing number who make it past ten years, your life expectancy will be the same as if you'd never had an attack.

You can increase your chances of making it to that ten-year mark, doctors say, if you and your physician, after appropriate testing to determine your capabilities, develop an individually tailored exercise plan. At the University of Toronto, for example, researchers studied more than 600 post–heart attack people who exercised regularly. Compared to heart attack people who didn't exercise, the exercisers had nearly *five times* less chance of a second heart attack.

Myocarditis.   Myocarditis is an inflammation of the heart that strikes between 1 and 5 percent of those who get certain major viral infections, says Walter H. Abelmann, M.D., professor of medicine at Harvard Medical School in Boston. Sometimes the inflammation is just in a single spot, and sometimes it covers a wider area.

The problem, says Dr. Abelmann, is that when people refuse to slow down and rest during a viral attack with fever, that small area of inflammation can spread throughout the heart and lead to heart failure or irregular heart rhythms. Myocarditis, he adds, is responsible for at least 4,000 deaths every year.

If your recovery from a bout of flu is unusually slow, if you find it hard to breathe when you walk, or if you notice that your heart seems to pound for a long time after you've walked up a flight of stairs, you may have the problem. Fortunately, doctors can fight myocarditis with careful monitoring for life-threatening complications, and with fever-reducing medications, oxygen and rest.

Phlebitis.   Phlebitis is an inflammation or a blood clot in a vein. Major causes of phlebitis are injury, infection, cancer, prolonged incapacity, pregnancy and birth control pills. If it is in a superficial vein (one that is near the skin's surface), it is characterized by pain, redness, tenderness, itching and a hard, cordlike swelling along the vein. You may also have a fever.

Fortunately, you can ease the pain of phlebitis with aspirin and a hot water bottle. If you have an infection, your doctor will prescribe an antibiotic. You should also rest, elevate your feet and wrap the affected area of your leg with an elastic bandage. Eventually the clot will dissolve.

If the clot is in a deep vein, there is a possibility that this clot could break off and travel to the lungs. Your doctor will probably treat you with anticoagulants to prevent new clots from forming while your body dissolves the ones already present. Since the symptoms of phlebitis in a deep vein are similar to those of a clot in a superficial vein, you should see your doctor if you have any of the symptoms mentioned above.

Pneumoconiosis.   Pneumoconiosis means dust in the lungs, and it's not the kind of dust you find under your bed. It's the kind found in quarries and coal mines as well as workplaces where aluminum, asbestos, beryllium, iron, talc, cotton, sugar cane and synthetic fibers are handled.

Symptoms of difficult breathing and a cough with phlegm may take 10 to 25 years to develop. If you are exposed on an occupational basis to any of the dusts known to cause pneumoconiosis, doctors say, you should have a chest x-ray once a year. And you should seriously think about leaving your occupation if the test shows any abnormalities. Occupational lung disease, says the American Lung Association, is the number one cause of work-related disease and injury.

Pneumonia.   Pneumonia is not one disease but many—some caused by bacteria, some by viruses, some by fungi or other agents. Their common denominator is that they should all be taken seriously: Pneumonia is the leading cause of death from infectious diseases.

Legionnaire's disease, for example, is now known to be caused by bacteria that thrive in water. *Pneumocystis carinii* is a major killer of those with acquired immune deficiency syndrome, or AIDS.

Depending on the type of pneumonia you have, you may experience chills, pains in your chest, cough, fever, headache or just a general case of the blahs. In some cases your symptoms will come on suddenly; in others they take their time. If your symptoms are severe enough, or you're weak enough, you could easily end up in the hospital. Unfortunately, 20 percent of those admitted to a hospital with the most common bacterial types of pneumonia never make it back home. This is because they often have other underlying health problems such as heart disease, chronic obstructive lung disease, liver disease or a past history of stroke.

Ninety-five percent of those with other types of pneumonia *do* survive, however, in large part because of antibiotics.

Raynaud's disease.   Raynaud's disease is a circulatory problem that occurs when the small arteries that supply blood to your fingers, and occasionally your toes, become hypersensitive to cold. The arteries contract whenever you're exposed to low temperatures—whether caused by throwing snowballs or handing out ice pops—and reduce the flow of blood to the affected area, which becomes white, then blue, then red. As the disease progresses, small ulcers may form on the tips of the affected fingers, and disability may occur.

Raynaud's can also be caused by conditions other than cold, such as high pressure in the blood vessels of your lungs, an emotional disturbance, certain drugs, connective tissue disease, inflammation of the arteries themselves or injury to the blood vessels from vibrations of powerful equipment such as chain saws and pneumatic drills.

Fortunately, Raynaud's can be helped by drugs that dilate your blood vessels or by an operation in which your doctor snips the nerves that control the contraction of the arteries. More frequently, doctors suggest, Raynaud's can be controlled simply by avoiding cigarette smoke and keeping your hands and feet warm and dry.

It would also be nice if you could move to a warm climate, but if the Bahamas are not in your future, at least try to stay indoors during the coldest weather. An alcoholic drink once in a while also seems to help, doctors say.

Varicose veins.   Varicose veins are veins that have become twisted and swollen, either because of a weakness in the vein wall or a faulty valve somewhere in the vein itself. In either case, aching legs with unsightly bumps and discolored skin are usually the result.

Sometimes wearing support stockings, particularly if you put them on in the morning before you get out of bed, and keeping your feet raised above the level of your chest can make you feel better.

But a varicose vein will not go away until your doctor either removes the offending vein in a surgical procedure with multiple incisions, or injects it with a substance that plugs it up. Between 33 and 45 percent of those who have the injections will need them repeated, doctors say, while surgical complications such as scars and nerve injury occur in 5 to 20 percent. But no matter which procedure you choose, your body will rechannel blood through other vessels.

Chapter 6
Ears

SEE YOUR DOCTOR IMMEDIATELY IF:

- *You experience unexplained, sudden hearing loss*
- *Your ears become itchy and painful*
- *You get an object or insect lodged in your ear*
- *You're experiencing extreme discomfort or pain in your ear*

Remember the first time you heard your own voice coming out of a tape recorder? Sounded just awful, didn't you—sort of like a whiny eighth grader. Could that skin-crawling squeal you heard really be you?

You bet. You may *think* you have a voice as sexy as Lauren Bacall's or Richard Burton's, but the plain truth is that the tape recorder told it just like it is—and the way the rest of the world hears you.

There's no need to start blushing about it all over again. It's true for everyone: When you hear your own voice on tape, you hear quite a different tune than the one you hear coming out of your mouth. It's higher. And it sounds just awful to you because it's far from the sound you've been used to all your life.

The reason for this is that your ears pick up vibrations in two different ways, through airwaves (a method known as air conduction) and over the bones of the head (known as bone conduction). You hear through both methods all the time, but air conduction carries most of the load—except when you're speaking. When you talk, your voice hits your ears by both methods, and the resonance off the bones gives your voice a deeper pitch.

To better understand this, cup your hand over one ear and speak. You're cutting out even more air conduction and your voice will appear lower. Cover both ears and it's even lower yet.

So why are we telling you all this? Certainly not to make you feel uncomfortable about your voice. We're simply illustrating what an intricate organ the ear structure is. Your ears, which contain the smallest bones and muscles in the body, are responsible for two of your most important sensations—equilibrium and hearing. It's your ears that keep you on balance in a dark room when your eyes can't help. Or on rough terrain when sensations can't get through unsteady footing. The remarkable Helen Keller called her lack of hearing a far greater loss than her lack of sight because "it means the loss of the most vital stimulus—the sound of voice—that brings language, sets thoughts astir and keeps us in the intellectual company of man."

Ears are nothing to take for granted. They need to be treated with care. When we interviewed specialists to come up with the information for this chapter, they asked us to emphasize one thing: Protect your ears from loud noises—radios, headsets, jackhammers, jet engines, you name it. It will help preserve your hearing for a lifetime.

SYMPTOM: **Discharge**

COMMON CAUSES: Discharge from the ear can be thick or it can be brothy; it can be yellow or white, green or red-streaked, creamy or clumpy. It's sometimes profuse and it's sometimes only a small dribble. It is seldom a dire emergency, but it does require medical attention.

"If you wake up at 2:00 A.M. and find that your ear is draining, don't feel compelled to rush to the emergency room," says Jason B. Surow, M.D., an ear, nose and throat specialist at Cedar Lane Medical Group in Teaneck, New Jersey. "You should, however, call your doctor and let him or her know what happened so that appropriate therapy may be started."

If you notice discharge from your ear, it means you probably have an infection that involves the outer ear. Swimmer's ear (see Common Ear Conditions) can cause discharge, as can wounding the ear. In fact, ears are wounded easily. They're tender. So try not to scratch them too enthusiastically. You can't effectively relieve itching or remove earwax that way, Dr. Surow says. But you can give bacteria a nice, moist sore to infect and give yourself more discharge to contend with.

Sometimes, though, ear discharge is the result of a middle ear infection (see Common Ear Conditions). When a middle ear infection is acute, you're likely to feel strong, pounding pain; pressure is building inside the infected ear. Suddenly, almost with a pop, the pain is relieved. White or yellow discharge often follows. What's happened? Your eardrum has just ruptured. What should you do? Not panic. The term "ruptured eardrum" (see Common Ear Conditions) sounds somewhat horrifying. The problem itself may be minor.

Gray or yellowish pus occasionally seeping from the ear can signal a far more serious problem. In this case, you probably have a chronic middle ear infection. The condition may not sound as awful as "ruptured eardrum," but, untreated, it can cause permanent hearing loss.

Rarely, ear discharge is caused by something other than an infection. The outer ear, for example, can harbor a tumor, either benign or malignant (see Symptom: Growths) that will produce bloody discharge.

BEST RESPONSE: When your ear decides to drain, let it. "Don't try to wipe away the pus or, worse yet, plug the affected ear with anything," Dr. Surow stresses. "You should never put Q-tips, tissues, bobby pins, your finger or anything else into your ear any deeper than you can see. *Never* push anything, at any time, into your ear canal." Doing so could easily puncture your eardrum or cause other serious damage to the very delicate ear.

What you *should* do is consult a doctor, either a general practitioner or an otolaryngologist, a specialist in ear, nose and throat diseases. "Ear infections are relatively easy to clear up," Dr. Surow says. "But you can't do anything at home to cure one. Your doctor can treat the problem effectively." Remember, untreated ear infections can become chronic ear infections, and "chronic infections are no fun," as Dr. Surow says.

Listen to his advice and keep your hearing healthy: If pus or discharge is coming from your ear, see your doctor soon.

SYMPTOM: **Earache.** *See* Symptom: Pain

SYMPTOM: **Earlobe, Wrinkled**

COMMON CAUSE: Elephants aren't the only ones with wrinkled ears. In fact, a kind of wrinkle, crease or line running from where the earlobe attaches to the head and angling diagonally downward toward the back edge of the ear was, for several years, actually thought to be a predictor of heart disease.

Incredible as it may seem, a series of studies conducted over a number of years and involving thousands of people indicated that more than 60 percent of those with an earlobe wrinkle also had heart disease. More recently, however, a study from the University of Massachusetts Medical School has revealed that the correlation between wrinkled earlobes and heart disease is nothing more than a coincidence. Of 268 men checked for heart disease at the university, reports Joel M. Gore, M.D., director of the coronary care unit, 85 percent of those with *and* 85 percent of those without heart disease had wrinkled earlobes.

So what led earlier researchers to the conclusion that wrinkles indicated a heart problem? As people get older, explains Dr. Gore, they're more likely to get heart disease. And as they get older, they're more likely to get wrinkles. The ears are not exempt. Spotting both wrinkles and heart disease in so many of the same people, guesses Dr. Gore, led researchers to think they were just putting two and two together.

Unfortunately, they came up with five.

BEST RESPONSE: Since wrinkled ears aren't indicative of anything other than aging, there's nothing to worry about, says Dr. Gore. You don't need to do anything.

SYMPTOM: **Growths**

COMMON CAUSES: Boils, warts, benign tumors and, in certain cases, dangerous cancerous growths can all appear in or on the ear. A growth on the outside of the ear is most likely a wart or benign tumor. However, a tumor *can* be malignant, warns Jason B. Surow, M.D. In the early stages of growth they are almost indistinguishable.

Boils can appear outside or be snuggled just inside the ear canal. They typically produce pain about on a par with a toothache, pain that's more piercing when you move your jaw or the outside part of your ear.

Sores anywhere on or in the ear that bleed, ulcerate or simply won't heal are serious. They can mean a malignant growth. Malignant tumors are like skin cancer; the cells multiply uncontrollably. They may bleed and cause pain.

BEST RESPONSE: A persistent sore means you should see your doctor.

"You shouldn't diagnose yourself or play doctor when you have ear problems. Ears are just too complicated and delicate," explains Dr. Surow. "Only a doctor can accurately diagnose and thereby treat the cause of a sore ear or an ear with a growth on it." Even minor problems such as an ear boil may require medical treatment.

While you're waiting to get to a doctor, though, you can help relieve any soreness by putting hot water bottles against the affected ear. Don't wipe away pus or put anything into the ear. And, if the ear sore does turn out to be a boil, you might listen to what it's trying to tell you. Boils pop up when you're rundown, explains Joan Gomez, M.D., author of *A Dictionary of Symptoms.* The best ways to prevent them from occurring again are to rest, relax and eat a good diet. In other words, work at getting and keeping yourself happier and healthier.

ACCOMPANYING SYMPTOMS: If you have a growth on your ear that itches, aches intensely and has bloody drainage, you could have a malignant tumor and should see your doctor.

SYMPTOM: **Hearing Loss**

COMMON CAUSES: Helen Keller, who was both blind and deaf, once said that deafness was much the worse of her afflictions. Stanley N. Farb, M.D., author of *The Ear, Nose, and Throat Book,* would agree. "Toward one who loses sight, we extend every possible kindness," Dr. Farb points out. "With those who have lost a significant degree of hearing, we are often less than patient." We get tired of shouting or making an effort to communicate, and we simply stop talking to the person.

Luckily, if you're not hearing as well as you used to, you can probably be helped—depending on the kind of hearing loss you're experiencing. First, ask yourself, *in what way* am I hearing differently? Do you find your own voice unusually loud but everyone else's muffled? Can you understand other people's words without distortion when they speak loudly, but "loudly" is getting ever fainter? Is your hearing loss sudden but traceable to a recent trauma or accident? Has anyone in your family had surgery for otosclerosis, a disease causing progressive hearing loss? Any of these could be an indication of what is called "conductive" hearing loss.

Conductive hearing loss results from a mechanical breakdown somewhere in the middle ear. For various reasons, the eardrum or the bones of the middle ear that should telegraph the sound waves to the inner ear, don't. You never hear the sound because it's short-circuited. It never reaches the nerves that would have carried it to the brain.

This condition may sound dismal, but it shouldn't sound hopeless, because you can still hear some sounds. In other words, conductive hearing loss is rarely total. The bones of the skull can conduct a certain amount of sound. That's why you can often hear telephone conversations well and also why your own voice may seem louder than any other sound.

What causes conductive hearing loss? Any of a whole smorgasbord of ear disorders, says Steven Gray, M.D., an ear, nose and throat specialist at the University of Iowa Hospital and Clinics in Iowa City. Not surprisingly, most of these involve the middle ear. Chronic middle ear infections, a ruptured eardrum, cholesteatoma, barotrauma (see Common Ear Conditions) can all affect hearing, as can serous otitis media, another type of middle ear infection, Dr. Gray says. "Children are especially prone to these problems because of the narrowness of their eustachian tube." This tube, the small but busy conduit between the middle ear and the nasal passages, is easily blocked by nasal congestion. Ear infections result. Conductive hearing loss can follow.

But conductive hearing loss is an infrequent problem in adults. Far more common—affecting as many as 30 percent of all people who are over age 65 and a great many other people who are younger—is sensorineural hearing loss. Sensorineural hearing loss is caused by nerve failure or damage to the inner ear. Although the sound waves reach the inner ear, they never get "heard," because they are not transmitted to the brain.

"High-frequency sounds are affected first, causing difficulty in hearing consonants," according to Dr. Farb. In the early stages of sensorineural hearing loss, you may think that everyone around you is mumbling. They're not. They're enunciating; you're just no longer hearing the sounds *P, K, T, G* and *D*. Women's voices will be especially troublesome. They're naturally higher pitched than men's. So if a female friend says "Good day" to you, but what you hear resembles "Oo-ay," you may be developing sensorineural hearing loss.

The leading causes of this condition are aging and noise. As the hearing nerve gets older, it simply gets less efficient and less sharp. Of course, very little can be done to combat the problem of aging. It's an irreversible but gradual process, occurring over many years. Noise, however, is a different story. For example, doctors point out that if you listen to music through headphones or a headset, and the music is loud enough for someone else to hear it, you could be causing gradual hearing loss.

When the process is not gradual, hearing loss has some other cause. Infections, including measles and mumps, can result in sudden, permanent, profound nerve deafness. So, too, can certain drugs. Antibiotics such as gentamicin and streptomycin, some diuretics ("water pills") and even aspirin can affect hearing.

These drugs can produce unwanted, irritating sounds in the ears (see Symptom: Tinnitus), or they can cause deafness. Some diuretics needed to treat heart failure, for example, can cause sensorineural hearing loss. But if you have heart failure, don't decide on your own to quit taking diuretics. "Tell your doctor about any hearing losses you have before he or she prescribes drugs for you," advises Dr. Gray. "Don't make the decision to take or not take drugs solely on your own."

And don't self-diagnose your hearing problem, either. Conductive and sensorineural hearing losses may seem easy to differentiate in a book, but are difficult for people to differentiate by themselves. "Either one can be gradual or sudden, partial or profound," says Jason B. Surow, M.D. "Or they can be mixed; you may have conductive hearing loss together with nerve damage. Or the whole problem may be that your hearing is distorted, not lost."

Having distorted hearing, he adds, is like listening to an unreliable radio. You may at any time begin to pick up static instead of sound. Or you may notice sounds fading in and out, as happens on a car radio when you're traveling. Distorted hearing sometimes accompanies sensorineural hearing loss, or it may occur on its own. In this case, your "hearing trouble" may mean big trouble—trouble that has nothing to do with the ears. "Your brain may not be processing sounds correctly, even though the sounds have safely reached it," Dr. Surow says. "Your ears are functioning perfectly well, but what you perceive is scrambled. This can indicate, among other things, serious central nervous system disorders."

BEST RESPONSE: "When your hearing changes in any way, you should respond in only one way—by seeing your doctor," Dr. Surow stresses. Preferably, you should see an otolaryngologist. But if you can't arrange that, see your family doctor as soon as possible. Your doctor will probably send you to an audiologist, a person trained to give hearing tests.

Only a licensed audiologist or otolaryngologist can accurately determine what kind of hearing loss you have and how severe it is. He or she can also, if necessary, fit you with a hearing aid. "Not all people who dispense hearing aids are licensed audiologists or otolaryngologists," Dr. Gray warns. "Make sure you go to someone who is."

Before you get any hearing aid or try anything else on your own to help your hearing, visit an otolaryngologist. Armed with the results of your hearing test, he or she can help you decide how best to treat your problem. "Both conductive and sensorineural hearing loss are potentially treatable today," Dr. Surow explains. "But they're much more successfully treated in their early stages."

Drugs, surgery, hearing aids or implants that directly stimulate the hearing nerve—any of these may be able to help you hear better. "But not if you wait too long," Dr. Surow emphasizes. Hearing loss is your ear's way of shouting for help. It's a clear warning that something is wrong in there somewhere.

Listen to your ears. Doing so may help you keep your ability to listen. "When your hearing changes," Dr. Surow says in sum, "don't complain, don't worry, don't dream it'll get better and don't delay in seeking medical attention. Call your doctor at once."

SYMPTOM: **Itching**

COMMON CAUSES: Using headphones, piercing your ears, swimming in a pool or using a none-too-tender touch with a cotton swab can all cause ear itch. This itch is most probably the result of an allergy. But it can also be a sign of infection.

Allergies to poor-quality earrings or overused headphones are common. You could also be allergic to your shampoo, skin lotion, perfume, soap or anything else with which your ears come into contact.

Ear infections are equally common. Swimmer's ear (see Common Ear Conditions) will make your ear itch—and later hurt.

BEST RESPONSE: "If itchy ears are a problem, be careful to keep hair sprays, permanent wave lotions, hair dye, perfume, soap and water out of the ear canal and away from the ear opening," advises Stanley N. Farb, M.D. Don't scratch an ear that itches, and don't try to clean it by digging at it with a cotton swab.

The ear canal is self-cleaning, Dr. Farb explains. It doesn't need cleaning help from you, except for occasional removal of excessive wax (see Best Response under Symptom: Stuffiness, for tips on doing this safely). Poking at or scratching your ear when it itches just promotes the growth of infections, and infections just make your ear's itch worse.

SYMPTOM: **Lumps**

COMMON CAUSE: Pierced ears can be wonderful. There's the fun, for example, of wearing unabashedly bright globes on each earlobe when you're in an unabashedly bright mood. But sometimes pierced ears can be not-so-wonderful, like when they result in the development of lumps and scars.

"Certain people are just more susceptible to scarring than other people are," explains Steven Gray, M.D. "When scar-prone people get their ears pierced, they often form hypertrophic scars and/or keloids at the site of the pierce." These are large, ugly, sometimes lumpy scars that, in this case, form at the piercing site.

Earlobes don't damage easily. So if you don't have pierced ears and you have painful nodules in your earlobes, the problem could be a form of arthritis known as gout (see Common Bone, Joint and Muscle Conditions in chapter 3).

BEST RESPONSE: If you've recently had your ears pierced and are now developing a lump on the back of your earlobe, see a doctor. "A doctor can remove the scar," Dr. Gray says. "But the process is difficult and the results aren't always cosmetically perfect."

A better treatment, he says, is prevention. "People who're always scarred easily or excessively should think twice—and then three or four or five times—about getting their ears pierced."

SYMPTOM: **Noises.** *See* Symptom: Tinnitus

SYMPTOM: **Obstruction**

COMMON CAUSES: Children are curious by nature. They wonder, "What would it be like to have a pea in my ear?" They answer this theoretical question promptly: They put a pea in their ear. And they discover that it's unpleasant to have a pea in there.

Of course, once you're past the age of scientific experiments with peas and the like, you rarely get them in your ears. But you may get other unwelcome visitors. Small insects, for example, sometimes fly into ears. They can cause intense irritation as they move about. They can also produce a loud buzzing. This sound should be immediately identifiable as coming from an insect and not as just mysterious buzzing. The latter could indicate a serious ear problem (see Symptom: Tinnitus).

BEST RESPONSE: If your child (or, for some reason, you) gets an object stuck in the ear, tilt the head sideways so that the affected ear points down. If the object falls out, fine. But if not, do not try to remove the object, cautions Joan Gomez, M.D. Instead, she advises, go to the doctor.

If an insect is the problem, drop *warm* (not hot) olive oil into the ear, suggests Dr. Gomez. The oil will kill the bug. If the bug doesn't fall out after tilting the head, gently syringe the ear with water to flush it out. "Do *not* try to get the insect out by poking anything into the ear," Dr. Gomez emphasizes. You could, in poking, do more damage than a swarm of insects in your ear ever could.

SYMPTOM: **Pain**

COMMON CAUSES: Ear pain can be intense or it can be minor. It can feel worse when you tug on your outer ear or it can feel better. It can be throbbing or it can be piercing. And above all, it can have any number of different causes.

Infections of the outer ear canal, such as swimmer's ear (see Common Ear Conditions), can cause an earache. The pain is usually throbbing and is increased by pulling on the external part of the ear. Middle ear infections (see Common Ear Conditions) can also cause throbbing pain, says Steven Gray, M.D. "But when you have a middle ear infection, you don't make the pain any worse by tugging at the affected ear."

If, when you pull at your ear, it hurts severely but isn't throbbing, you probably have a boil nestled inside the ear canal. It may or may not be visible. The same boil or some other type of sore on the outside of the ear (see Symptom: Growths) can also cause the ear to ache.

And, just to keep your ear's life interesting and make any diagnosis of its problems difficult, an ear often hurts when there is nothing wrong with it. Many earaches are, in fact, sore throats or misaligned jaws in disguise. "The ear is subject to a lot of 'referred pain,' " Dr. Gray says. "Because of the complex way in which our nerves intersect on the way to the brain, a problem in one part of the body can appear as pain in a totally different part of the body."

The ear is commonly affected by referred pain from what Dr. Gray calls "the five Ts": the teeth, tonsils, throat, tongue or temporomandibular joint (the hinge that joins the upper and lower jaws in front of the earlobes). "Whenever you have a persistent earache and an ear exam shows that your ear is normal, your doctor should consider the possibility of referred pain," Dr. Gray advises. You may, in fact, need a dentist to cure your earache, since an ear's pain can easily be caused by jaw misalignments (see temporomandibular joint disorder under Common Facial, Jaw and Mouth Conditions in chapter 8) or by tooth decay.

BEST RESPONSE: Whatever you call it—earache, sore ear, tender ear, pain-wracked ear—it's not normal, and it shouldn't be ignored. When it comes to an earache, a good physical exam, including a medical history, is the best bet for finding the cause.

"Ear pain is a signal that something is wrong," Dr. Gray stresses. "Whenever your ear hurts, you should see a doctor as soon as you can." Only a complete ear examination can reveal what's causing the ache. "Most problems, such as ear infections, are fairly easy to treat while they're still minor infections."

Untreated, even minor infections can cause major complications. Middle ear infections, for example, can become chronic and eventually interfere with your hearing. When your ear first begins to bother you, let your ear doctor know. It may save you a lot of discomfort later.

ACCOMPANYING SYMPTOMS: Any earache is trouble. But an earache that's accompanied by fever, headache, vomiting, dizziness or hearing loss could indicate an especially serious ear infection, such as acute otitis media (see middle ear infections under Common Ear Conditions). This is common in children and requires prompt medical treatment, doctors warn.

In adults, an earache accompanied by weakness of the facial muscles, headache and dizziness can mean cholesteatoma (see Common Ear Conditions), a condition that often requires surgery. If uncorrected, cholesteatoma may result in the roof of the middle ear cavity being eaten away, sometimes leading to meningitis (see Common Neurological System Conditions in chapter 12).

Finally, an intense earache that's coupled with bloody drainage from your ear may mean that you've developed a malignant growth on your ear (see Symptom: Growths). If you have any of these symptoms, see your doctor at once.

SYMPTOM: **Redness**

COMMON CAUSES: Like a lump on the earlobe, a reddened earlobe is almost always a symptom of a poorly healed ear piercing. The redness means that the puncture has become infected. Most of the time, this infection is nothing to worry about. "As long as the puncture is in the lower, fatty part of the earlobe, an infection is a minor problem," says Steven Gray, M.D.

But with the increasing popularity of piercing ears in two or even three places, the dangers of infection have also increased, especially when the cartilage that forms the rigid part of the outer ear is pierced.

"The ear's cartilage has a poor blood supply," Dr. Gray explains, "so infections here are frequent and very tough to clear up." In fact, a doctor may have to cut the infected cartilage out of the ear. "And let me tell you, this is not an insignificant thing to have happen," Dr. Gray emphasizes. One of his teenage patients, in trying to be trendy, triple-pierced her ear and wound up losing most of the lower part of her ear to an infection of the cartilage.

If you've never had your ears pierced even once, let alone two or three times, and your ears turn red, it could be the result of a nervous habit of playing with your ears. Hard-core tweakers play with their ears constantly, the way other people twirl their hair or chew their pencils. If you, in secret or openly, are a tweaker, your red ear could be a sign of earlobe abuse.

Red ears can also be a symptom of dermatitis (see Common Skin Conditions).

BEST RESPONSE: Ask yourself whether you really need to have your ear look like a dart board. "I wish everyone were more aware of the danger involved in having an ear pierced over and over," Dr. Gray says. "But I also know that horror stories about the chances of losing an earlobe aren't going to stop anyone from having quadruple-piercing done if it's fashionable. So please, when you do have multiple piercing done, make *sure* that whoever does the piercing puts *each* hole through the fleshy part of your ear."

If you've already had the extra piercing (inexpertly) done, or if your one and only ear hole is now red and sore, see your doctor. "Washing the infected area regularly with hydrogen peroxide will probably clear up a simple infection of the lower lobe," Dr. Gray says. "You should have the ear checked by your family doctor, though, to avoid any complications. And if you know the infection involves your ear's cartilage, get to a physician as soon as you can."

If your lobstered earlobes are the result of earlobe abuse, you might want to try some relaxation techniques to get rid of your tension. Or you could always try pencil chewing for a few days.

ACCOMPANYING SYMPTOMS: Crustiness on your reddened earlobe, sometimes with and sometimes without pain, is another symptom of a poorly healed or infected ear piercing. Dr. Gray recommends that you see your physician if you develop either of these problems.

SYMPTOM: **Stuffiness**

COMMON CAUSES: Have you ever caught a cold, flown in an airplane, climbed a mountain or been hurtled up 15 stories in an elevator? Of course you have. And you've also experienced stuffed-up ears. "Most people get stuffy ears at some point in their lives," says Steven Gray, M.D. "In fact, it's uncommon not to have a feeling of fullness in your ears during a cold, allergy or other upper respiratory infection."

Your ears become blocked when you have a cold because the eustachian tubes (the short, narrow tubes that connect the middle ears to the nasal passages) swell shut. Children are especially susceptible to this; their eustachian tubes are smaller than those of adults.

When the eustachian tube swells, pressure in the middle ear cannot be equalized. The air in the middle ear gets absorbed, resulting in a vacuum. If the tube stays blocked, the vacuum will pull in fluid from the surrounding tissues, meaning fluids will not drain normally. Instead, they will accumulate within the ear, causing stuffiness. This condition is known medically as serous otitis media (see middle ear infections under Common Ear Conditions).

Rapid altitude changes also affect ears. To function normally, the ear requires air in the cavity *behind* the eardrum. This helps equalize pressure from the air on the other side of the drum. Airplane travel is a good example. Takeoff is much easier on the ears because they are under high pressure, allowing the eustachian tubes to equalize almost instantly. However, descent is a different matter. That's because the ears are now under low pressure, making it more difficult for the eustachian tubes to equalize, especially if they are blocked.

If you have a cold or sinus infection, for example, air won't get through, and the pressure on one side of the eardrum won't equal the pressure on the other. Your ear will feel badly "plugged."

Sometimes, of course, a feeling of fullness in your ears is more than a feeling. It's a fact. It's a symptom of waxy yellow buildup inside your ear canal. "Excess accretion of earwax may block your ear canal, making your ear feel uncomfortably full and possibly affecting your hearing," says Jason B. Surow, M.D.

BEST RESPONSE: Your response should depend on the reason for your problem. If you're on an airplane, you can be reasonably sure your full ears are a side effect of jet-setting. Your best response? Before and during descent of the airplane, swallow frequently, experts advise. If your ears still refuse to pop, try swallowing with your nostrils pinched shut. Chewing gum also helps.

Should all of these techniques fail, "a more forceful method is to pinch your nostrils shut, take a mouthful of air, close your lips tightly and try to blow out against your closed nose and mouth," suggests Stanley N. Farb, M.D. Your fellow passengers may stare. Smile back at them serenely, secure in the knowledge that *your* ears are clear.

Your best response when you have a cold is not so picturesque. In fact, your best response is to do almost nothing and wait for the cold to go away. "Once your cold has cleared up, your ears should also clear as the eustachian tube reopens," explains Dr. Surow.

But you can help ease your ears' symptoms while you wait, according to Donald Vickery, M.D., and James Fries, M.D., coauthors of *Take Care of Yourself.* "Moisture and humidity are important in keeping the mucus thin. Use a vaporizer if you have one," they advise. They also advocate "curious maneuvers," such as gently hopping up and down in a steamy shower while shaking your head and swallowing. (A shower mat and caution are a must for this technique.) This should clear out excess mucus. Over-the-counter antihistamines and decongestants can also decrease the amount of nasal secretion, allowing the eustachian tubes to expand.

If your symptoms persist for more than ten days or two weeks, see your doctor. Normally a trip to the doctor won't be necessary. Fluid in the ear can usually be treated at home, say doctors.

Home treatment alone will usually work against wax buildup as well. Proper home treatment begins with common sense. "Never put anything smaller than your elbow into your ear," Dr. Surow stresses. "You can't clean your ear with cotton swabs or bobby pins. You can only injure it."

You *can* clean your ear safely with a program of what Dr. Farb calls "preventive maintenance." First, put several drops of hydrogen peroxide or mineral oil into your ear canal twice a day for two or three days. "Then," he says, "using a soft ear syringe with lukewarm water, gently irrigate your ear canal to remove the softened wax." The wax should come out easily. If not, see your doctor. "You may also need a doctor's help if the wax is very hard and packed tightly in the ear canal," Dr. Farb admits.

ACCOMPANYING SYMPTOMS: The stagnant fluid that collects behind your eardrum when you have a cold provides a congenial home for bacteria. As a result, you can develop serious ear infections. Beware of these symptoms: pain, usually in one ear only, fever, a feeling of illness, or partial hearing loss. Any of these, together with a full feeling in your ear, can indicate an acute middle ear infection (see Common Ear Conditions). If you have any of these symptoms, see a doctor as soon as you can.

If atmospheric changes bother your ears and you can't make them "pop," you feel a little pain and dizziness and can't hear properly, you could have developed barotrauma (see Common Ear Conditions), a minor annoyance that should go away by itself in a few hours.

SYMPTOM: **Swelling**

COMMON CAUSES: A career in boxing is one sure-fisted way to contract swollen ears. But even those of us who could no more float like a butterfly than we could knock out Ali can find ourselves with swollen ears.

"Strong, glancing blows to the outer ear may cause swelling of the auricle (the external part of the ear)," explains Jason B. Surow, M.D. Sports injuries, falls or standing in the pathway of an opening door can all lead to swelling.

This swollen, injured ear needs to be tended, because if it's not—or if it is, but, by profession or inclination, you reinjure it over and over—the ear will become deformed. It will become a "cauliflower ear." Cauliflower ears sprout because of unchecked bleeding and clot formation under the skin, and they look like the vegetable they're named for: lumpy, plump and strange. The deformity is, unfortunately, often permanent.

BEST RESPONSE: "Anytime your ear swells, you should have it seen by a physician," advises Dr. Surow. If possible, you should go to an ear specialist, but if one isn't nearby or available, your family doctor should be able to assess the seriousness of the injury and begin to treat it.

"Early treatment will help ensure that the ear or your hearing won't be damaged," Dr. Surow says. It will also ensure that you don't produce a crop of unsightly cauliflower ears. Plastic surgery is the only treatment for these, and may only partially improve the damaged ear's appearance.

SYMPTOM: **Tinnitus**

COMMON CAUSES: Crackling, cracking, roaring, ringing, buzzing, hissing, pounding; say this string of words ten times very fast and they'll probably start to sound like annoying nonsense sounds. Now imagine hearing that kind of annoying nonsense no matter where you are or what you're doing—whether you're working, talking or trying to sleep.

Medically, this symptom is known as tinnitus, and it means hearing noises that aren't really there. No doorbell or telephone is making the ringing sound, and no one else can hear the ringing. In rare cases, another person (preferably your doctor) can actually hear a strange clicking or ringing inside your ears. This is called objective tinnitus, and it's caused by abnormalities in blood vessels around the outside of the ear, or by muscle spasms. These muscle spasms produce odd little clicking sounds inside the middle ear or in the eustachian tube, the thin tube that joins the nasal passages and the middle ear.

In the vast majority of cases, though, the sounds exist only for you. They can be exasperating. They can, if persistent, be maddening. They do *not* mean you need to worry about being crazy. "Tinnitus will not . . . result in losing your mind or your life," advises the American Academy of Otolaryngology—Head and Neck Surgery. Having tinnitus even puts you in good company. Nearly 36 million Americans live with it every day; over 7 million of them have the problem so severely they can't lead normal lives.

What causes tinnitus? Wax buildup in the ear canal can cause the problem. So, too, can excess environmental noise and a huge array of problems unrelated to the ear itself. High blood pressure (see Common Circulatory, Heart and Lung Conditions in chapter 5); diabetes and thyroid disease (see Common Whole Body Conditions in chapter 19); allergy (see Common Nasal Conditions in chapter 13); low blood pressure; a tumor; trauma to the head or neck; smoking; and certain drugs, such as gentamicin, streptomycin, diuretics ("water pills") and even aspirin, can all leave you suffering in sound, rather than in silence.

Or the trouble may originate within the structures of the ear. Certain diseases, including Meniere's disease and otosclerosis (see Common Ear Conditions) can cause a ringing sound in the affected ear. Both of these are potentially serious conditions. Otosclerosis, for example, can lead to deafness. Thus, tinnitus is sometimes the earliest symptom of approaching hearing loss.

"The onset of tinnitus may indicate the presence of an associated ear problem," explains Jason B. Surow, M.D. "Noises in your ear are like pain in your ear—your ears are telling you to see a doctor. Listen to them."

Yet often, Dr. Surow adds, even a complete ear exam may fail to find a cause for the sounds. "Most cases of tinnitus are simply not caused by any treatable problem," he says. Aging contributes to the problem, as does listening to loud music or living under stress. Any of these can undermine the health of your hearing nerve and, according to the academy, cause or worsen tinnitus.

"Unfortunately," Dr. Surow admits, "an awful lot of the time, people simply have to learn to live with the noises."

BEST RESPONSE: If you've been to a rock concert or have been exposed to a barrage of loud noises and develop tinnitus, there is nothing to worry about. The noises will go away in a day or two.

If you haven't been exposed to loud noises or your post–rock-concert internal siren doesn't disappear after 48 hours, you should see a doctor, says Dr. Surow. This is an indication something may be wrong. You need to have your tinnitus evaluated to find out whether it's treatable or not.

"If an otolaryngologist finds on examination that your tinnitus has a specific cause, he or she may be able to remove the cause and thus eliminate the noise," according to the American Academy of Otolaryology—Head and Neck Surgery. But all too often, "there is no specific treatment for noises in the ear or head."

In lieu of a cure, you *can* learn to cope. First of all, keep in mind that your ear and the auditory system to which it belongs are among the most delicate and sensitive mechanisms of your body. "Since it (the auditory system) is a part of the general nervous system, its responses are affected to some degree by the anxiety state of the person involved," according to the Academy. Therefore, if you have tinnitus but are longing for the sound of silence, here are some suggestions from the Academy:

Avoid loud sounds and noises; get your blood pressure checked; avoid salty foods; avoid nerve stimulants such as coffee, colas, tobacco and marijuana; exercise daily to improve your circulation; get adequate rest and avoid overfatigue. Also, reduce nervous anxiety, which can upset an already tense hearing system.

And stop worrying about the noise. "Recognize your head noises are an annoying but minor reality," the Academy advises, "and then learn how to ignore them as much as possible."

To help reduce head noises, the Academy suggests a technique called "masking." Tinnitus is usually more noticeable when you're in a quiet place, so you may be able to control or "mask" it by keeping your surroundings full of competing noise. Try listening to music at low volume. Or, if you're not in the mood for music, set your radio's dial between two stations, so you hear a constant low and humming static. This "white noise" should help subdue the unwanted sounds in your ear. Consider it radio-activity of the most beneficial sort.

Common Ear Conditions

Barotrauma.   This is a minor problem that results from not being able to equalize the pressure in your ears. It can happen when you have a cold or allergies and you go through rapid altitude changes, like airplane travel or diving. Normally, the air pressure in the middle ear is the same as the pressure in the outer ear. But when the airplane's cabin is depressurized before takeoff and then repressurized before landing, the balance of pressure within the ears is upset. The pressure on the outside of the eardrums becomes greater, and the eardrums are pushed inward, like a bongo drum being sat on. The ears feel full or stuffed up.

Suspect barotrauma if, in addition to a plugged-up feeling, you feel pain in the ear, have some hearing loss and are dizzy. Don't worry if you do have the problem. The symptoms usually clear up by themselves within a few hours. You may also be able to forestall them. If you have a cold and are going to be traveling by air, consider arming yourself with a decongestant. Sucking candy or chewing on gum can also help. But if you're habitually prone to the condition, see a physician, recommends the American Academy of Otolaryngology—Head and Neck Surgery. You may need to have fluid drained from your middle ear.

Cholesteatoma. Cholesteatoma sounds unpleasant and feels worse. It results from a malfunction of the eustachian tube, which connects the nasal cavity to the middle ear. The tube may never have opened in infancy. More often, it's become blocked because of repeated middle ear infections. Imagine it as a cave whose entrance was covered by a landslide. The air left behind, with no way to vent itself, soon becomes isolated and stagnant.

In the middle ear cavity, this sluggish air is gradually absorbed by the cells that line the cavity. Since the eustachian tube is blocked, no new air can arrive to replace it. So the air pressure inside the cavity drops. Higher pressure in the outer ear then punches the weakest part of the eardrum inward, forming a pocket in the membrane. Skin cells that are routinely shed by the eardrum begin to collect in this pocket, and soon they clump into a tight little cell ball—a cholesteatoma.

This cholesteatoma inevitably becomes infected. It begins oozing pus. The cholesteatoma erodes the lining of the middle ear cavity and damages the delicate bones housed there. The unpleasant upshot, should this condition remain untreated, is that the cholesteatoma will eat away the entire roof of the cavity, possibly leading to meningitis, an inflammation of the membranes covering the brain, or an epidural abscess, a collection of pus just outside of the spinal cord or brain.

If you had a history of ear trouble as a child, you should be especially wary of cholesteatoma. Watch for such symptoms as mild or moderately severe hearing loss and seepage of pus from your ear. Cholesteatoma can also cause headaches, earaches, weakness of the facial muscles and dizziness.

It can be treated effectively, though the treatment isn't always simple. If the cholesteatoma is small or in an early stage, it's possible to remove it through a minor operation. But if the cholesteatoma has been allowed to grow large, then the damage to your middle ear can be extensive. In this case, you'll require a more complicated operation; your middle ear and its tiny bones will have to be rebuilt. Surgery and skin grafting can sometimes help restore hearing.

Meniere's disease.   Because it is a disorder of the inner ear, Meniere's disease leaves you intensely dizzy. It does so by damaging the labyrinth, a delicate structure deep within the ear that controls your sense of balance. When you have Meniere's disease, fluid collects in the labyrinth. As the fluid increases, so does pressure within the ear. This pressure builds and builds until it finally swells, distorts or ruptures the membrane of the labyrinth wall.

If reading that unappealing description made your head spin, you now have some idea of how Meniere's disease makes you feel. It can also cause noises in your ear, muffled hearing and nausea. An attack of the symptoms will usually blaze up suddenly, incapacitate you totally and then go away, not reappearing for months or even years. The attacks themselves may last from several minutes to several hours. They usually become less frequent and less severe over time (in most cases), though you may find increasing deafness replacing them.

Meniere's disease is more common in men than in women and hardly ever appears before you're in your forties. It is recurrent and frustrating, but it is manageable. If you have Meniere's disease, your doctor will probably prescribe medications to help ease nausea and vomiting during an attack. You can do your part, too, by lying down and staying still when you first feel dizzy. Cutting down on your intake of fluids and salt will also help, since fluid retention seems to increase the severity and frequency of the attacks.

Middle ear infections.   Known to doctors by the generic term *otitis media,* middle ear infections are common, especially among children. The infections can be acute, chronic or serous.

Acute infections are one-shot flare-ups. They normally follow colds, sore throats or other upper respiratory problems. Adventuresome viruses or bacteria from these infections climb the eustachian tube (which connects the nasal cavity to the ear) and enter the middle ear. Once there, they inflame the cells that line the ear cavity, leading to stabbing pain and a feeling of fullness in the ear, as if cotton were stuffed deep inside it. You'll probably also have a fever and some hearing loss. Also, pus from the infection can cause the buildup of enough pressure within your ear to burst, or rupture, the eardrum.

Aside from this occasional threat to your eardrum, acute infections are a minor problem, annoying but not dangerous. But bacterial (as opposed to the more common viral) infections can be serious. If they remain untreated, they often become chronic, or they infect the mastoid process (a portion of the bone behind the ear). Should this happen, you may need an operation called a mastoidectomy, in which the infected bone is removed. Early treatment will help avoid this. Your doctor will probably prescribe antibiotics to clear up the infection. Aspirin and a little pampering will help relieve the pain of your infected ear. Try warming its cockles with a heating pad set at a low temperature. (Don't sleep with the heating pad under you, and clean away any pus that collects on it to avoid reinfecting your ear.)

Chronic infections require more work to cure. They can be stubborn and relentless. They develop slowly, even quietly. But the damage they do is permanent. If you have a chronic middle ear infection, you could, as a result, permanently lose part of your hearing. However, microsurgery can do much to cure the problem and restore normal hearing.

You can't correctly treat chronic infections yourself. See a doctor, who will probably clean the ear and prescribe antibiotic ear drops. In most cases, these will eliminate the infection, dry out the ear and prevent further recurrence. If you have an especially resistant case, you may need mastoid surgery. If your hearing has been impaired, you may *want* reconstructive surgery. Ear surgeons today can actually rebuild the tiny damaged bones in your middle ear.

"Serous" otitis media is one more variation on the ear infection theme. In this case, the ear's trouble is caused by an accumulation of fluid within the middle ear. The fluid buildup occurs because the eustachian tube has become blocked, usually because of a cold or allergy. Your ear becomes flooded, and it feels plugged, but you probably won't have a fever, as you would with an acute middle ear infection. You will hear less well, with one notable exception: Your own voice may become louder than you'd like. It may seem to echo over and over within your head.

Try speaking softly (or saying nothing you wouldn't want to hear repeated) while you're waiting to see your doctor. And do see your physician if your ear remains plugged for more than a week, recommends Jason B. Surow, M.D. Though serous otitis media can often be helped with decongestants, your doctor may want to prescribe antibiotics if there is an underlying infection, and/or drain the collected fluid from your ear.

Middle ear problems are notorious for returning. Discuss with your doctor how best to deal with yours. He or she may suggest that you see an allergist. Stubborn cases in children sometimes mean the child needs to have his or her tonsils or adenoids removed.

Otosclerosis.   This is a gradual, progressive, sometimes insidious disease that affects your ability to hear. Its first symptoms usually appear between the ages of 15 and 30. Left untreated over a number of years, it could result in deafness.

Otosclerosis is caused by an abnormal and unwanted growth of spongy bone at the entrance to the inner ear. As it grows, this bone impinges on the stirrup, the tiny bone through which sound waves pass into the inner ear. The stirrup, immobilized, can't transmit all of the sound waves that reach it. Conductive hearing loss results. About 80 percent of the time, otosclerosis will affect both of your ears, either at the same time or one after the other.

The disease was once synonymous with deafness. "This used to be a tragically incapacitating disease," admits Joan Gomez, M.D., "but now it is nearly always curable." An operation called a stapedectomy will improve hearing significantly about 90 percent of the time. In rare cases, though, the operation doesn't lessen deafness but causes it. In place of the partial hearing loss you had before the operation, you'll have profound deafness.

The first thing you should do if you notice a change in your hearing is consult a physician at once. "Medicine today can help an awful lot of people who couldn't have been helped even a few years ago. But, of course, we can't help anyone who doesn't come to us," says Steven Gray, M.D.

Ruptured eardrum.   A ruptured eardrum, as you'd probably guess, occurs when the eardrum bursts or is torn. Often the rupture follows unauthorized forays into the ear with cotton swabs, bobby pins or other objects. "*Never* push anything into your ear canal," emphasizes Jason B. Surow, M.D. You can't effectively remove wax or relieve itching with a swab. You can only hurt your ear.

An eardrum can also rupture because of a nearby explosion, a glancing blow to the ear or a severe middle ear infection. When the cause is an infection, you'll first feel intense ear pain as pus builds within the ear. Then the pain, suddenly and blessedly, will be relieved. Your ear will ooze a bit. Your eardrum has just burst.

The discomforts of a ruptured eardrum, whatever its cause, are usually slight. You should have only a nagging earache, some loss of hearing and discharge. The risks of the condition are a bit more serious. Bacteria, for example, can penetrate to the middle ear through the rupture. If you suspect that you have a ruptured eardrum, it's best to see your physician as soon as possible. The condition is usually more serious in an adult than in a child.

Until you get to your doctor, you can relieve any pain by covering the affected ear with an electric heating pad set at a low temperature. Nonaspirin painkillers such as acetaminophen (Tylenol) may also help. But *never* use ear drops. When you do see your doctor, he or she may prescribe antibiotics or patch your eardrum, and will suggest that you be gentle with the ear while it heals itself, a process that normally takes one to two weeks. Once the drum is ready, your ear's beat can again go on. You should have no lingering problems, and any hearing loss should be temporary.

Swimmer's ear.   The joys of summer: long swims, light clothing, lingering daylight . . . and acute infections of the outer ear canal.

Well, maybe acute infections aren't one of the joys, but they *are* one of the results of long swims and any activity that allows water to enter the ear canal. "Water remaining in the ear canal after swimming macerates the skin, permitting bacteria or fungi to infect it," explains Stanley N. Farb, M.D. These bacteria were either floating in the water or already living in your ear, waiting for the chance to get under your skin. The dampness, in softening your skin, gave them their chance and left you with the painful infection known as swimmer's ear.

When you have swimmer's ear, you'll probably notice some pus in your ear, and you'll have an earache. "If pushing on the piece of cartilage (tragus) in front of the ear opening causes pain, there is almost always an infection of the ear canal," Dr. Farb explains. Your best response at this point is to see your family doctor, who will probably prescribe antibiotics.

Once the infection is cleared up, you should start thinking prevention, unless you want to give up getting wet altogether. "A do-it-yourself earmold made from Silly-Putty will keep water out of ears," suggests Dr. Farb. "Be sure that your homemade mold fills the ear opening, but do not try to push the material down into the ear canal, as it may fragment." Since you personally tailor the molds, they fit better and are more watertight than plastic earplugs. Wearing a bathing cap helps hold them in place.

But if you refuse to wear a bathing cap or feel inadequate as a sculptor, Dr. Farb points out that you can instead try putting four or five drops of isopropyl alcohol (70 percent) in each ear canal after swimming. This dries out any water remaining in the canal and also creates an inhospitable environment for bacteria. Taking these few precautions should get you and your ears through the summer swimmingly.

Chapter 7
Eyes

SEE YOUR DOCTOR IMMEDIATELY IF:

- *You see halos around lights or flashes of light*
- *You have severe eye pain*
- *You lose part or all of your vision*
- *You have double vision*
- *Your eyes begin to bulge or protrude*
- *You suspect a foreign body is embedded in your eye*

Y ou can throw smoldering glances over your shoulder as much as you like. But if your baby blues are rimmed in red, weeping or twitching with fatigue, they're not going to communicate the message you expect. Not even if they're smudged with shadow, fringed with mascara or framed by Cartier.

Fortunately, most eye problems are easy to solve—as long as you quickly get working on the solution. So whenever your eyes seem to lose that healthy sparkle, take a close look in the mirror. Then check any problems by checking them out in the following pages.

SYMPTOM: **Black Eye**

COMMON CAUSE: "Black" eyes are a misnomer. They're more likely to be red, purple or—after a week or so—a striking green and yellow. You may worry because they look awful, but a black eye is rarely a symptom of eye damage. It's a symptom of tissue damage—usually from a blow.

BEST RESPONSE: Any blow to the eye strong enough to cause bruising may also cause internal bleeding, doctors say. So you may want to apply cold compresses to the injured eye—cold will constrict blood vessels and help prevent further bleeding—then get yourself to an ophthalmologist as soon as possible.

Expect the bruise to last about two weeks, kaleidoscopically changing colors. Nothing you can do will speed the healing process, but if you're bothered by the eye's appearance, cover it with flesh-colored makeup.

SYMPTOM: **Blood Spot(s)**

COMMON CAUSES: When a spot of bright red blood suddenly appears on the white of the eye—and doesn't interfere with vision or cause any pain—it is almost always a symptom of a "subconjunctival hemorrhage." This is a frightening name for a harmless condition. The bleeding is usually reabsorbed within seven to ten days, explains Ira A. Abrahamson, Jr., M.D., associate clinical professor of ophthalmology at the University of Cincinnati College of Medicine.

The hemorrhage can be caused by injuring or rubbing the eye, or even bursting one of its innumerable small blood vessels by violently coughing, sneezing or vomiting. Bleeding can also indicate a serious disease such as arteriosclerosis or high blood pressure (see Common Circulatory, Heart and Lung Conditions in chapter 5) or leukemia (see Common Whole Body Conditions in chapter 19) elsewhere in the body. Excessive use of some medications, most frequently aspirin, can also cause these spots.

BEST RESPONSE: If you're not sure what caused the hemorrhage, see your ophthalmologist, says Dr. Abrahamson. Then, once you're certain it indicates no real problem, sit back, relax and wait for your body to reabsorb the blood.

SYMPTOM: **Blurred Vision**

COMMON CAUSES: Blurred vision can indicate a problem within the eye itself or it can indicate a mix-up elsewhere in the body. Cataracts and glaucoma (see Common Eye Conditions), for example, can cause vision to blur. But so can anemia or diabetes mellitus (see Common Whole Body Conditions in chapter 19), kidney trouble, nerve diseases and even tobacco and certain drugs—especially those containing cortisone.

A foreign object in the eye can also cause sudden blurring or misting of vision (see Symptom: Foreign Body in Eye), as can an inflammation (see Symptom: Redness).

Fuzzy, blurry vision may also be the result of an uncorrected vision problem, especially nearsightedness. About one person in five needs glasses to correct it. If you're nearsighted, you have to squint to see objects that aren't close to you. You'll be handicapped if you want to play golf (not the kind of handicap golfers want), do any bird watching or see a school blackboard.

Farsightedness causes the opposite problem: You literally can't see what's right in front of your nose. In this case, you can see the school blackboard, but you can't read your textbook. Farsightedness is usually present from birth. If the condition is severe and remains undiagnosed, it can lead to crossed eyes as a child tries to compensate (see Symptom: Crossed Eyes).

BEST RESPONSE: "Any change in vision should be evaluated—even if this change is temporary," emphasizes Richard S. Koplin, M.D., ophthalmic microsurgeon and director of the Bio-Engineering and Computer Science Department at the New York Eye and Ear Infirmary in New York City. This is especially true if you are beyond age 50.

Some diagnoses can even be reassuring. "If your vision is being affected by cataracts, don't worry unduly," suggests Merrill Knopf, M.D., an ophthalmologist in Long Beach, California. "Cataracts can be successfully removed surgically. But you needn't be in a big hurry to have the operation. You don't need surgery until your changed vision keeps you from doing things you'd like to do."

Considering all the serious possibilities, a diagnosis of nearsightedness or farsightedness is also cheering. Both of these conditions can be corrected with eyeglasses or contact lenses, Dr. Knopf says. Your doctor will help you decide which corrective measure is best for your eyes.

SYMPTOM: **Bulging**

COMMON CAUSES: Staring—at beautiful people or peculiar modern art—is normal. Involuntary, permanent staring is not, especially if your staring eyes seem to be protruding from their sockets. This condition is called exophthalmos, and it's caused by a swelling of the soft tissue that lines the eyeball's "bony nest"—its socket. The eyeball is pressed forward, exposing an abnormally large amount of the front of the eye.

Exophthalmos can occur in one or both eyes and almost always indicates a serious problem elsewhere in the body. Most commonly it indicates an overactive thyroid (see thyroid disease under Common Whole Body Conditions in chapter 19), although sometimes it's caused by a bacterial infection behind the eyeball. It can also indicate an aneurysm, blood clot or hemorrhage in the veins or arteries behind the eye.

BEST RESPONSE: Get to a doctor as soon as you notice any abnormal bulging. Early diagnosis and treatment of whatever is causing your sudden staring can help protect your vision.

If your problem is a thyroid imbalance, though, correcting the imbalance may not correct your eye bulge, doctors say. Surgery or medication may be needed.

ACCOMPANYING SYMPTOMS: Check with your doctor as soon as possible if you also have pain and vision changes—especially if your vision is steadily blurring. You may have a tumor.

SYMPTOM: **Crossed Eyes**

COMMON CAUSES: If you've ever worried that crossed eyes could be caused by looking at your nose and having your eyes "stick" that way, stop worrying. Eye muscles can't stick, and making funny faces can't cause crossed eyes. But several serious eye conditions can.

In children, crossed eyes are almost always what is medically called strabismus. A child with strabismus sees two separate images of everything. Such double vision is, of course, distracting. So the child's mind adjusts by choosing to believe only one of the images. And the child begins to see with only one eye. The other eye, ignored and left to its own devices, frequently begins to lose vision, a condition called amblyopia (see Common Eye Conditions), better known as "lazy eye."

If this condition is not treated before the child is six years old, "the child will never be able to learn to use both eyes together," warns John Eden, M.D., an associate clinical ophthalmologist at Columbia University College of Physicians and Surgeons. So crossed eyes in children should never be considered just a cosmetic problem. Nor can it be assumed that a child will outgrow them. That won't happen—and don't be fooled into thinking it has just because your child may eventually learn to position his or her eyes so that they appear to be straight.

The only exception occurs in infants. Babies sometimes appear to be cross-eyed. But as the bridge of a baby's nose expands, this illusion disappears. Any child whose eyes still appear crossed after age 1½, however, has strabismus.

If you're an adult and your previously aligned eyes suddenly appear crossed, you may also have strabismus. Or there may be a disorder elsewhere in your body that affects either the nerves between the brain and the eye or, less commonly, the muscles themselves. These disorders include diabetes mellitus (see Common Whole Body Conditions in chapter 19); high blood pressure and arteriosclerosis (see Common Circulatory, Heart and Lung Conditions in chapter 5); muscular dystrophy, a genetic, degenerative crippling disease; inflammation of the arteries at the temple; or a brain injury.

BEST RESPONSE: Should you (or your child) start to have double vision and suddenly notice that your eyes are crossed, an immediate trip to the doctor is in order. And on the way, you may want to patch one eye to eliminate the double vision.

After your doctor has checked for any underlying problem and, if necessary, treated it, your vision will probably correct itself within a few months, although in some cases eyeglasses or eye surgery may be necessary.

To protect against crossed eyes, all children should have an eye examination before the age of three, says Dr. Eden. Strabismus is not always pronounced enough for parents to spot, but it is usually easy to diagnose and correct if an eye doctor is consulted. "The examination at age three is, therefore, perhaps the most important visit to an eye doctor anyone can make," Dr. Eden concludes.

SYMPTOM: **Dark Circles**

COMMON CAUSES: Your eyes may be your windows to the world, but the delicate skin beneath them can be a window to your general health. The dark circles you see there are really small veins returning blue blood to your heart. These veins usually become visible only when you're tired, ill or pale or have lost a lot of weight.

In children, dark circles under the eyes are often caused by an allergy (see Common Nasal Conditions in chapter 13). Doctors call them "allergic shiners." Some people, though, are genetically prone to them, says Merrill Knopf, M.D. As you age, the shadows appear, and they won't fade.

BEST RESPONSE: If the problem is an allergy, keep your child away from the allergen, advises Keith W. Sehnert, M.D., a consulting physician at Trinity Health Care in Minneapolis. Common allergens include house dust, cat or dog dander and foods such as wheat, cow's milk, chocolate and peanuts. If you're not sure what your child is allergic to, adds Dr. Sehnert, take him or her to a doctor.

For yourself, a healthy life-style, with adequate sleep and a balanced diet, may help wipe away any circles. If you're genetically prone to dark shadows and are bothered by their appearance, you might try a specially modified makeup base or even glasses with tinted lenses to help hide them.

SYMPTOM: **Discharge.** *See* Symptom: Pus

SYMPTOM: **Double Vision**

COMMON CAUSES: If children complain of double vision, they very probably have crossed eyes (see Symptom: Crossed Eyes), whether their eyes actually appear crossed or not.

Double vision in adults is double trouble. It, too, probably signals the onset of crossed eyes. But in adults, crossed eyes are themselves often the symptoms of a more serious problem, such as diabetes mellitus (see Common Whole Body Conditions in chapter 19), high blood pressure (see Common Circulatory, Heart and Lung Conditions in chapter 5) or a brain injury.

BEST RESPONSE: Patch one eye so that you won't continue to see two images, doctors suggest. Then, without thinking twice about it, see your eye doctor.

SYMPTOM: **Dryness**

COMMON CAUSES: When your eyes are dry, they'll burn—feeling sandy, hot and grit-filled, as if your eyeball had become a desert. This dry-eyed feeling is a symptom, not surprisingly, of dry eye syndrome. More formally, the condition is called keratitis sicca, and it occurs when there are changes in the quantity or the quality of tears produced by the tear glands. Then, without its usual lubrication, the white of the eye becomes irritated, bloodshot and swollen, and scrapes against the eyelid with every blink.

The unpleasantness of dry eye syndrome can be caused by any number of things. Aging is the most common. "As we get older, tear production naturally diminishes," explains Merrill Knopf, M.D. And for people of any age, severe dermatitis (see Common Skin Conditions in chapter 15), rheumatoid arthritis (see arthritis under Common Bone, Joint and Muscle Conditions in chapter 3), allergies to eyedrops or other medications, vitamin deficiencies (especially a vitamin A deficiency) or a hot, arid climate can all cause dry eyes.

Dry eyes can also be a symptom of a serious eye problem such as an inflammation of the tear gland, a tumor in the gland or paralysis of the nerve that leads to the gland. They can also indicate some sort of hormonal disturbance elsewhere in the body.

BEST RESPONSE: If you've begun feeling an unusual grittiness in your eyes, see your ophthalmologist, suggests Ira A. Abrahamson, Jr., M.D. If the problem is in the eye itself or in your environment (if, for example, you're allergic to something), your doctor should be able to help you find and eliminate the irritant.

Yet frequently, dry eyes are forever. In this case, the solution *is* a solution: artificial tears. They're specially formulated to replace deficient or incomplete normal tears, says Dr. Knopf. They're safe and can be used indefinitely. Each patient can experiment and find the frequency or the number of drops needed to make his or her eyes feel comfortable.

You might also reduce the discomfort of dry eyes by using only white tissues when you wipe your eyes, using a humidifier where you live and work, wearing sunglasses and avoiding harsh chemicals, such as oven cleaners, whose fumes could get into your tearless—and therefore vulnerable—eyes. You might also want to let your family doctor know you've got dry eyes. Then he or she will be sure not to prescribe any medication that could exacerbate the problem.

But a new and promising treatment for dry eyes may someday help you kick the artificial tears habit. This treatment involves the use of vitamin A ointment. Since vitamin A is important in eyesight, Scheffer Chuei-Goong Tseng, M.D., of the Massachusetts Eye and Ear Infirmary in Boston, theorized that applying the vitamin directly to the eye might stimulate mucus-producing cells. He was right. He applied vitamin A ointment to 23 of his patients with chronic dry eyes.

"After treatment, clinical symptoms of dryness, irritation and light sensitivity were invariably relieved in all cases," Dr. Tseng reported. The best news about this treatment is that it is the first that can actually *treat* dry eye syndrome and not merely relieve its symptoms.

SYMPTOM: **Eyelashes, Turning in**

COMMON CAUSES: When the margins of the eyelids begin to turn inward, the eyelashes, along for the ride, also turn inward, featherdusting the eyeball with every blink. Such constant irritation can, in turn, lead to a host of new eye problems such as conjunctivitis (see Common Eye Conditions) and/or corneal ulcers. Although it most often affects the lower lid, it can happen to either the upper or lower lid.

This condition, known as entropion, most commonly affects older people. As you grow older, the fibrous tissue on the lower lids can become lax. This allows the muscles in the eyelid to contract excessively, pulling the margin of the lid in toward the eye.

Occasionally, the turning in of the eyelids occurs for reasons other than simple aging. Excessive scarring of the eyelid could be the cause; this scarring often follows chronic and untreated infections like conjunctivitis, as well as cuts or burns of the eyelids and face that have healed poorly.

BEST RESPONSE: If your eye is already irritated when your eyelashes begin to rub, see your doctor so he or she can treat both problems. Otherwise, according to the American Medical Association, your best response is a logical one: If your lower eyelid won't stay in place on its own, tape it. Attach one end of a piece of adhesive tape to the skin underneath your lower lashes. Tape the other end to your cheek. Leave the tape in place for a few days. Remove the tape and see whether the condition has cleared up of its own accord. If it hasn't, see your doctor. You may require minor surgery.

SYMPTOM: **Eyelid, Lower, Sagging**

COMMON CAUSES: If your lower eyelid hangs down, exposing your eyeball and its lining, you have a condition called ectropion. And it can be very irritating.

Like entropion—the turning in of the eyelashes—a sagging lower lid is usually the result either of aging or of scarring. The problem is that, in sagging away from the eye, the lower lid leaves the eyeball exposed. The eyeball, in response, often becomes dry and sore. Or it waters excessively. This happens when tears that normally lubricate the lining of the eyelids and the front of the eye aren't able to enter the tear duct in the lower lid. With no other outlet, the tears will run down your cheek.

BEST RESPONSE: See your physician. The condition rarely clears up on its own, according to the American Medical Association. A minor operation on the tissues beneath your eye will usually put a lid on this eye problem.

SYMPTOM: **Eyelid, Lump on**

COMMON CAUSES: If the lump is painful, swollen and itchy, it's probably a sty. If, on the other hand, the lump is painless, the problem is likely to be a cyst.

Harmless growths also manifest themselves as lumps on the eyelid. And some of these can be quite colorful. A papilloma, for example, which is an outgrowth of skin on the edge of the eyelid, can range in color from pink to black. Small yellow-colored lumps, though, are probably accumulations of fat. For some reason, these small globules of fat often gather beneath the outer skin of the eyelids, especially near the nose. The condition can be indicative of diabetes mellitus (see Common Whole Body Conditions in chapter 19) or high blood cholesterol.

Growths—or sores with scales that often crust and bleed—can indicate certain kinds of cancer. But rarely are lumps on the eyelid malignant.

BEST RESPONSE: Only a doctor can accurately diagnose an eyelid lump's cause. So if you develop a lump, see your doctor. Should he or she tell you you have a sty, relax. Sties go away. They're also less likely to recur if you *do* relax, since you usually develop them only when you're overstressed and underrefreshed.

But if you don't want to wait for the sty to go away by itself, medical experts say, you can make the sty burst early. Apply hot compresses to it frequently—as soon as the lump appears. The warmth will help "ripen" the sty, drawing the pus to a head. Do not squeeze the sty, though. Wash your eyelid carefully to remove any pus that drains.

Hot compresses are useful, too, in combating the irritation of a cyst, says John Eden, M.D. But though the compresses can make the initial infection subside, the cyst itself may remain. Usually, a doctor will have to remove it.

Any other growths should be checked by an ophthalmologist. Harmless lumps need to be removed only if you find them unattractive. Consult with your doctor before deciding.

SYMPTOM: **Eyelid, Red**

COMMON CAUSES: A red or inflamed eyelid is usually the result of what is medically called blepharitis. This is an infection of the eyelid's edges, which become sore, red and encrusted with scaly skin (see also Symptom: Scaling).

Blepharitis occurs often in children and recurs often in anyone who's had it once. A few of the problems that may have triggered the original infection include measles, scarlet fever, dandruff or rubbing your eyes.

Allergies—often to drugs, soaps or cosmetics—can also cause the eyelids to become inflamed.

BEST RESPONSE: See your doctor at the first signs of redness, suggests Merrill Knopf, M.D. Because blepharitis can be a stubborn problem, be sure you follow your doctor's instructions and use any prescribed medications as directed.

Women should also try to limit the use of eye cosmetics. Eyebrow pencils and mascara—even face powder—can interfere with healing, says Dr. Knopf. Mascara can, in fact, transmit infections. So it's important not to use other people's makeup and to discard mascara after six months.

Also keep your hands, face and hair clean, says Dr. Knopf, and if you have dandruff, use a shampoo especially made to combat it. If you have any other infection—a cold or acne, for example—get it treated and under control.

SYMPTOM: **Eyelid, Upper, Drooping**

COMMON CAUSES: A droopy upper eyelid, or ptosis, as doctors have named it, is a condition with many variations. It can occur in children or adults. It can involve one eye or both. It's usually unattractive, sometimes disrupts vision, and can indicate a serious problem elsewhere in the body.

In young children, ptosis is almost always the result of a congenital weakness of the muscles that raise the eyelid. In this case, it usually affects only one eye and grows no worse with age.

With adults, however, it can indicate a muscular disorder such as myasthenia gravis (see Common Bone, Joint and Muscle Conditions in chapter 3), or it can be due to facial paralysis or to the severe pain that accompanies a migraine headache. And when ptosis occurs suddenly in one eye, doctors say, disease of the brain must be considered.

BEST RESPONSE: If one or both of your previously normal upper eyelids begins to droop, see your ophthalmologist at once, urges Ira A. Abrahamson, Jr., M.D. Only a doctor can diagnose and treat the problem that led to the drooping.

To correct the droop itself, your doctor may prescribe eyeglasses with special supports built into them. Or, in some cases, surgery to strengthen the eyelid muscle is needed.

SYMPTOM: **Foreign Body in Eye**

COMMON CAUSES: The feeling that you have "something in your eye" sometimes means that you *do* have something in your eye. And sometimes it doesn't. Sometimes it means that you're seeing—or rather, feeling—"ghosts."

"Our bodies are clever," explains Merrill Knopf, M.D. "We've got wonderfully specialized ways of knowing what is going on in various parts of our bodies. We have highly sensitive nerve endings in our fingertips, for example, because we need to feel sensitively there."

But in the cornea, we have very few nerves designed to feel pain, so the sensations we do have are primitive. As a result, "Anytime *anything* irritates or affects your eye, you're likely to feel as if 'something' is in there," Dr. Knopf concludes.

Conjunctivitis or iritis (see Common Eye Conditions), dry eye syndrome (see Symptom: Dryness), corneal abrasion, or any number of other eye problems can leave you with these eye-ghosts.

Of course, sometimes when you feel as if you have something in your eye, you do. And foreign objects in your eye can cause serious damage. "The cornea of the eye is a glasslike, arched dome, similar to the crystal on a watch," according to Howard W. Lee, O.D., author of *Eye Care: What You Need to Know before You See the Eye Doctor.* Scratch it and you can't see clearly.

If, however, you're certain you have no foreign body in your eye, yet the "something is in there" feeling persists, you may have a condition in which the eyelashes turn in toward the eyeball and scratch the cornea (see Symptom: Eyelashes, Turning in).

BEST RESPONSE: When you think you have something in your eye, your first response should be to find out whether you're right, doctors say.

But first you should ascertain if the something is *in* the eye or floating *on* the eye. If the object is in the eye, do not attempt to remove it, say doctors. Gently cover *both* eyes and have someone take you to the doctor immediately. Both eyes need to be covered because your eyes work in tandem; looking around with the uninjured eye will cause the injured eye, even if patched, to follow. Such movement could cause additional injury or scarring.

If the object is floating on the eye, wash your hands thoroughly with soap and water and examine the eye in good light. But do not rub your eye! Pull the upper eyelid down over the lower lid, then let it slide back. This will produce tears and may flush out any particle. If there is an eyedropper handy, fill it with warm water and squeeze it over the eyeball to flush out any particles.

If nothing flushes out, look up while you pull the lower lid down and have someone else examine the eye and try to locate any objects. If the other person can see an object—and it's *not* embedded in your eyeball—have him or her pick it off with the corner of a clean, moistened cloth, handkerchief or paper tissue. Don't use cotton swabs to pick particles off the eyeball; their loose fibers will come off and stick to the moist eye.

If you still can't find the irritant, however, it might be underneath the upper lid. Look down while you place a cotton swab or a wooden matchstick across the upper lid and gently fold the lid up over it. If you or your friend can see the particle, pick it off with a clean, moistened cloth, handkerchief or paper tissue.

If the object can't be seen, doctors say to patch the eye with soft pads and get medical help.

SYMPTOM: **Itching**

COMMON CAUSES: An eye that itches is an eye that may be infected or have an allergy. Conjunctivitis (see Common Eye Conditions) or a sty can also cause distracting, even intense, itching, but less intense itching may be the result of anxiety, eyestrain or an uncorrected vision problem.

BEST RESPONSE: Since most itching is caused by allergies, you can use over-the-counter eyedrops containing naphazoline, such as Clear Eyes, to relieve the itching. However, warns Merrill Knopf, M.D., use them prudently to avoid a rebound effect, or you could make the problem worse.

Warm or cold compresses applied to the closed eye may help relieve the itch, says Ira A. Abrahamson, Jr., M.D. But don't rub your eyes and don't share your towels, tissues or handkerchief with anyone, since you could easily spread an infection. Do, however, share your complaint with an ophthalmologist.

Until you can get to a doctor, do *not* try to self-medicate with eyedrops that were previously prescribed for another infection or for other family members, adds Dr. Abrahamson. Also, don't patch the itching eye, since the warm, enclosed eye would become a perfect incubator for bacteria.

SYMPTOM: **Jaundice**

COMMON CAUSES: Jaundice—a yellowing of the whites of the eyes— almost always means liver disease. The yellow tinting of the skin is caused by an excess of a reddish-yellow pigment called bilirubin in the bloodstream. This substance is a by-product of the breakdown of aged red blood cells by the liver. Normally, most of the bilirubin the body produces is safely excreted. But when the liver is damaged, bilirubin builds up, and jaundice—with its characteristic yellowing—occurs.

Hepatitis (see Common Abdominal and Digestive System Conditions in chapter 1), in all its various forms, is one of the most frequent and serious of the liver diseases that can result in jaundice. Cirrhosis (see Common Abdominal and Digestive System Conditions in chapter 1) will also cause the eyes to become yellow, as will certain medications.

The source of jaundice may also be bile duct blockage. If your bile ducts are obstructed by gallstones or a tumor, for example, bilirubin can't be excreted as it should be, and jaundice follows.

Finally, hemolytic anemia (see anemia under Common Whole Body Conditions in chapter 19) allows an abundance of bilirubin to be released into the bloodstream. The result? Jaundice.

BEST RESPONSE: If the whites of your eyes are yellow, call your doctor immediately, say medical experts. Jaundice doesn't usually occur unless you have a serious health problem.

SYMPTOM: **Light Sensitivity**

COMMON CAUSES: When light makes your eyes ache, something is amiss. Light sensitivity, like pain or discomfort, is one of the eye's earliest—and sometimes most urgent—warning signals.

"Because an eye is designed for seeing and not for feeling," explains Merrill Knopf, M.D., "it has few ways of letting you know when it's not well." Light sensitivity is one of them. Never shut your eyes to what they're telling you.

Acute glaucoma (see Common Eye Conditions), a disease that can leave you permanently blind within 48 hours, may first have you wincing at the sight of light. Inflammations of the cornea can do the same. Often this inflammation is itself a symptom of a serious infection. Eyestrain can also make your eyes uncomfortable. So, too, can a cold, severe allergies, migraine headaches or stuffed sinuses. Certain drugs can also make the eyes sensitive to light as a side effect.

BEST RESPONSE: Don't take this problem lightly—see a doctor as soon as possible, urges Dr. Knopf. Many of the eye disorders associated with light sensitivity can be treated only if they're caught early.

"Always be wary when you develop any of the eye's most basic symptoms—discomfort, sudden vision changes, haloes around lights and/or a sensitivity to light. They're there for a reason; they're there to help save your sight," he says.

ACCOMPANYING SYMPTOMS: If your sensitivity to light is accompanied by severe headache, stiff neck, nausea, vomiting, drowsiness or confusion, call a physician at once. This condition represents a medical emergency. You may have meningitis (see Common Neurological System Conditions in chapter 12) or a hemorrhage of the brain.

SYMPTOM: **Pain**

COMMON CAUSES: Pain is an early symptom of a number of eye problems. You shouldn't ignore eye pain, but neither should you panic. First, decide what kind of pain it is you're feeling. Is it a dull, constant ache in both eyes? If so, you may have dry eyes (see Symptom: Dryness), eyestrain or even a bad cold.

A more piercing pain could indicate a foreign object in the eye (see Symptom: Foreign Body in Eye), while a vague feeling of pain in one eye only—especially if the eye is also red—may signal an infection such as conjunctivitis or iritis (see Common Eye Conditions), or an inflammation of the white part of the eye, such as scleritis.

Severe eye pain is a medical emergency. It can mean acute glaucoma (see Common Eye Conditions). "Acute glaucoma hurts," says Howard W. Lee, O.D. "It hurts a lot. It can come on rapidly and it can reduce vision rapidly." In fact, if the condition is not treated within 48 hours, you run the risk of losing vision in the affected eye.

BEST RESPONSE: "Pain is a message from your body to your brain that something is wrong," says Merrill Knopf, M.D. "And that message is given to you for a reason. If you have a broken arm, for example, it's in pain because your body doesn't want you to use the broken arm and make things worse."

The same thing is true with a pain in your eye. You can try taking a dose of aspirin or acetaminophen (Tylenol), says Dr. Knopf. But if the pain persists beyond that single dose—or if it's severe—you need to see your doctor to translate what the pain is trying to tell you.

SYMPTOM: **Puffiness**

COMMON CAUSES: Puffy eyes are the result of a collection of fluid around and under the eyes. Puffiness occurs for a variety of reasons. Keeping the head level with or below the heart can cause the area around the eyes to swell, says Thomas O. Burkholder, M.D., an ophthalmologist in Allentown, Pennsylvania. Anytime blood has to move "uphill" to get back to the heart, he explains, there is an increased tendency to swell. Sleeping, scrubbing floors or playing an intense game of marbles all put the eyes below or level with the heart. Puffiness can result, particularly as you get older.

"Skin tends to lose its elasticity as we age," Dr. Burkholder says, and so the tissues around the eyes become all the more susceptible to "tugs" from swelling or insistent gravity. Fatigue and hard drinking can make the problem even worse.

Severe swelling around the eyes, though, may be due to allergy, Dr. Burkholder says, particularly in young people.

BEST RESPONSE: An hour or so in an upright position, sitting or standing, normally will help unpuff your eyes, says Dr. Burkholder. Cold compresses—ice cubes wrapped in a towel, for example—can also speed recovery. Sleeping on your back and not on your stomach may prevent puffy eyes in the morning. And to combat hard drinking and fatigue, a couple of early nights back-to-back (and back-to-mattress) may put a speedy end to the puffiness.

SYMPTOM: **Pus**

COMMON CAUSES: Pus is never pleasant. But it can be beneficial. Usually composed of white blood cells—mixed with bacteria—it often acts as the body's police force, says Merrill Knopf, M.D.

"Pus appears at the site of insurrections or riots in the body," says Dr. Knopf. The pus indicates that the body is working to quell an infection. "It helps keep your eyes clean," adds Dr. Knopf, "and it lets you know when you do have an infection."

Conjunctivitis and iritis (see Common Eye Conditions) can also cause pus.

BEST RESPONSE: You'll need to see an ophthalmologist to find out what's actually causing the pus, says Dr. Knopf. The discharge itself often provides clues. By examining its composition, a doctor can determine what kind of infection you have and what kind of treatment is called for.

Let your eyes water freely until you can get to a doctor, suggests Dr. Knopf. Try not to rub them—and don't patch them either. "If you have bacteria or other unfriendly bodies in your eye," says Dr. Knopf, "covering the eye just gives them a homier environment. They like warmth, and patching an eye raises its temperature."

SYMPTOM: **Redness**

COMMON CAUSES: Eyes don't become red or inflamed without good cause, or, more accurately, bad cause. These bad causes include fatigue, infections, bacterial invasions, injuries and serious diseases. Where and how severely the eye is inflamed is usually an indication of the cause.

Inflammation of the inner eyelid, for example, is symptomatic of conjunctivitis (see Common Eye Conditions), whereas inflammation of the white of the eye probably indicates scleritis. And scleritis itself sometimes indicates a problem elsewhere in the body: rheumatoid arthritis (see arthritis under Common Bone, Joint and Muscle Conditions in chapter 3) and various kinds of infections can cause the white part of the eye to become inflamed.

Iritis, keratitis and acute glaucoma (see Common Eye Conditions) can also cause the eye to turn red.

BEST RESPONSE: Because red eyes are frequently caused by fatigue, a nap or a good night's sleep may be the best medicine you can take. But commercial eyedrops such as Visine, Murine Plus or Visine A.C. and the like can also help relieve the redness, says Ira A. Abrahamson, Jr., M.D.

These eyedrops contain a decongestant that constricts the swollen blood vessels, whitening your eyes. For cosmetic purposes, they're effective. But they shouldn't be used often, since the decongestant can cause a rebound effect. Your blood vessels then reenlarge in less and less time, and you may eventually find yourself with redder eyes than you had before you used the drops.

You should also be aware that these eyedrops cannot cure an eye infection or disease. If your eyes are still bloodshot five minutes after you use the drops, consider the red lines as red lights: Stop using the eyedrops and see your doctor. And keep your mitts off your eyes in the meantime. Rubbing them will only make the problem worse.

ACCOMPANYING SYMPTOMS: If you experience severe eye pain, headache, rapid change in vision, sudden appearance of floating spots, acute redness of the eyes, pain on exposure to light or double vision, get to a doctor—preferably an ophthalmologist—at once. You could have a serious eye condition such as acute glaucoma (see Common Eye Conditions).

SYMPTOM: **Scaling**

COMMON CAUSES: Scaling skin on the eyelids—skin that flakes, sticking to the eyelashes like dandruff—is very often a symptom of blepharitis, an infection of the eyelid (see Symptom: Eyelid, Red). Children and people with dry skin or dandruff on the scalp are especially susceptible to this condition.

If you've never had blepharitis before and have no skin problems elsewhere on your head or face, your dry, flaky skin could be due to an allergic reaction.

BEST RESPONSE: Visit an ophthalmologist as soon as possible. Left untreated, doctors say, blepharitis can spread, causing ulcers to form on your eyelid, and eventually causing your eyelashes to fall out. Or the flaking skin can get into your eye, leading to conjunctivitis (see Common Eye Conditions). .

In addition, says Merrill Knopf, M.D., keep the eyelid area clean. "When you apply medicine, any crusts or scales on the lid should be removed so that the medication can reach the infected places." The crusty material should first be softened with a clean, warm, moist washcloth or cotton swab and then *gently* scrubbed away from the edge of your eyelids with tearless baby shampoo.

"Removing the crusts this way may feel uncomfortable at first," Dr. Knopf acknowledges. "But keeping your eyelids clean may be enough to get rid of the infection."

SYMPTOM: **Spots before Eyes**

COMMON CAUSES: Are you seeing vague spots floating before your eyes? Are they maddeningly difficult to bring into focus? Then you probably have nothing to worry about. Minute particles—such as dust or bubbles in your tears—float constantly in the clear fluid of your eye.

From time to time, these particles float into such a position that they block some of the light entering the pupil. "This throws a shadow onto the layer of the eyeball known as the retina, just as a moth flying through the light beam of a movie projector throws a shadow onto the movie screen," explains Howard W. Lee, O.D.

You're most likely to see these "floaters" when you're tired, worried, run-down or anemic. "And the older we get, the more material there may be floating around in our eyes," adds Dr. Lee.

Sometimes, though, seeing spots means you'd also better see a doctor. The first symptom of a detached retina (see Common Eye Conditions), for example, is often floaters. Inflammation within the eye, internal hemorrhages, blows to the eye or a tumor could also be the cause. And black specks that remain fixed and unfloating could signify a scar on the retina.

BEST RESPONSE:　See your doctor if floaters appear regularly. If your doctor finds no problem, says Merrill Knopf, M.D., go back to leading a normal life, and, with time, the number of floaters will usually decrease.

If your floaters increase, however, or if you notice a sudden shower of small dots, flashing lights or a curtain moving across your field of vision, you should have your eyes reexamined. Sometimes there are microscopic changes that occur in the eye that may not be visible on the first exam.

ACCOMPANYING SYMPTOMS:　Flashes of light followed by floating black shapes, progressive loss of part of your peripheral vision and progressively blurred vision may indicate an eye emergency such as a detached retina. See an ophthalmologist at once.

SYMPTOM:　**Twitching**

COMMON CAUSES:　An out-of-kilter muscle in your eyelid usually corresponds to an out-of-kilter condition elsewhere in your life. Fatigue, stress, too much coffee or a drug you are taking can all cause muscular twitching, especially in the muscles of the eyelid.

BEST RESPONSE: Close your eyes and apply hot or cold compresses, says Ira A. Abrahamson, Jr., M.D. And get more rest. A shut eye usually cures a twitching one. If the twitching is persistent or bothersome, see your ophthalmologist for a complete exam.

SYMPTOM: **Watering**

COMMON CAUSES: "The external part of the eyeball is provided with a remarkable system of irrigation and drainage—the lacrimal system or tear glands," says Ira A. Abrahamson, Jr., M.D. Occasionally, this drainage system backs up, tears overflow and the eyes water.

In both infants and adults, for example, excessive tearing can be caused by mucus plugging the tear duct. Or it may be the result of irritation. A speck of dust (see Symptom: Foreign Body in Eye), an inflammation of the eyelid or eye (see Symptom: Eyelid, Red and Symptom: Redness), an infection of the cornea (see keratitis under Common Eye Conditions) or an allergic reaction (See allergy under Common Nasal Conditions in chapter 13) such as hay fever can make the eyes water.

Blocked sinuses or inward-growing eyelashes (See Symptom: Eyelashes, Turning in) could also be the villains. Finally, an obstruction of the tear ducts can result in lots of tearing.

BEST RESPONSE: You should first try removing any mucus plug in the tear duct, suggests Dr. Abrahamson. After washing your hands, place one finger (with a short fingernail) on the middle portion of the lower lid and gently move the finger—pressing in slightly—toward the tear sac, located at the inner corner of the eye, next to your nose.

Next, press firmly over the tear sac and—with a downward motion—bring the finger along the bone at the side of your nose. Hopefully, this procedure will empty the tear duct and force any mucus plug into your nose or eye (where it will be harmless). Try it, five or six strokes at a time, three or four times a day for a week.

Should your eye still be watering, Dr. Abrahamson says, consult an ophthalmologist.

ACCOMPANYING SYMPTOMS: If your eyes are swollen, red and tender over the tear sacs, and if you can produce pus when you apply pressure there, see your ophthalmologist as soon as possible. You may have developed acute dacryocystitis, an infection of the tear sac. Surgery is often required to permanently relieve this condition. In the meantime, Dr. Abrahamson suggests, apply warm compresses to the area for five minutes every two hours. This should temporarily relieve any discomfort.

SYMPTOM: **Yellowing.** *See* Symptom: Jaundice

Common Eye Conditions

Amblyopia. Amblyopia is commonly known as lazy eye, although the eyes are not really lazy at all. They're just underemployed. A lazy eye is anatomically capable of sight, but, for various reasons, the brain chooses not to notice the images this eye sends it. Being unused, the eye becomes useless.

Often, in children, amblyopia is the result of uncorrected crossed eyes. It can also develop if one of your eyes is significantly more nearsighted or farsighted than the other. Plus, certain diseases or injuries that affect the retina (the light-sensitive layer at the back of the eye) or the nerves connecting the eyes to the brain can destroy vision in the affected eye.

Lazy eyes don't always wander about aimlessly in their socket. Oscillating movements are only the most obvious symptom of amblyopia. Others to watch for, especially in children (who rarely complain about vision defects because they don't realize they have them), include a tendency to rub one eye frequently or to repeatedly bump into objects on one particular side.

As soon as any of the symptoms of a lazy eye appear, see your eye doctor. Amblyopia is serious, because if it develops in a young child and is not treated before the age of six or seven, the damage is usually irreversible; the child will never be able to see properly with that eye.

Luckily, early detection usually means early recovery. Patching the energetic eye, for example, forces the "lazy" one to accept its responsibility for seeing. Eyedrops, special glasses, special exercises and even injections of tiny amounts of botulism toxin (which paralyzes certain muscles, so the eye can't wander) have also been successfully used to treat amblyopia. Surgery is a last, but sometimes necessary, resort.

Cataracts. A cataract is a cloudy area that appears in the normally clear lens of the eye. Gradually, over a period of years, the cataract blocks or distorts light entering the eye. As a result, vision becomes progressively dimmer.

The most common cause of cataracts is aging. The lens in the eye simply begins to deteriorate. But young people can also develop cataracts, usually as a result of a complication from something else, such as iritis, an eye injury or diabetes mellitus. Cataracts occur most of the time in both eyes, but only one eye may be affected.

The cataract need not be treated if the vision loss it causes is slight. "When the loss of vision interferes with your life—and not before—you should consider cataract surgery," says Merrill Knopf, M.D. Early surgery offers no benefits.

If your vision has decreased to the point where you need surgery, however, today's technology has made cataract surgery an outpatient procedure with a 90 to 95 percent rate of success.

Conjunctivitis. Conjunctivitis is any redness, itching and swelling of the conjunctiva, a transparent membrane that lines the eyelids and outer eye. It can be caused by an infection or allergy, or by chemical irritation from something like chlorinated water in a swimming pool.

The treatment for this very common condition depends on its origin. Some forms of conjunctivitis are caused by infection and treated with antibiotic eyedrops. Other forms won't respond—you just have to wait for your body's own defense system to shoot them down.

But be wary of using cortisone drops to treat the infection. If you should have an undetected herpes infection in your eye, the cortisone will make the condition much worse.

Should allergies be causing your eye irritation, remove the cause of the allergy. If this is impossible—if you don't know what the allergen is or you know it's your cat but can't bear to be parted from her—your eye doctor can prescribe eyedrops that should help relieve your symptoms.

Detached retina.   The retina is a delicate layer of light-sensitive cells at the back of your eyeball. Beneath these cells is a second layer composed of blood vessels that provide the retina with nutrients and oxygen. A detached retina occurs when the retina pulls away from these blood vessels.

A hole in the retina is what leads to the detachment. This is as unpleasant as it sounds. The hole allows some of the jellylike mass of the eyeball, called the vitreous humor, to seep through, pulling the retina away from its normal resting place. As more and more vitreous humor seeps in, more and more of the retina will be lifted away. Eventually the retina becomes almost completely detached from the eyeball and, if left untreated, it can cause permanent blindness.

Luckily, retinal detachment is rare. It seldom occurs before middle age. It does occur more often in people who are nearsighted and in anyone who has had an eye lens removed because of a cataract. Surgery is needed to correct it.

Diabetic retinopathy.   This disease is a frightening complication of diabetes. It occurs in some diabetics when small blood vessels in the retina become narrowed and then die. The remaining vessels may begin to leak blood into the retina—causing a permanent blurring of vision— and fragile new blood vessels often grow on the retina. Unfortunately, these new vessels leak blood into the jellylike part of the eyeball, the vitreous humor, which will temporarily dim vision. The leaked blood is usually reabsorbed, but not before it has caused scar tissue to form on the retina. The scarring permanently blocks eyesight.

Treatment for this condition involves plugging the leaky vessels by using laser surgery. In severe cases, the vitreous humor must be drained from the eye and replaced with an artificial substitute.

Studies have shown that early treatment can prevent diabetic retinopathy. That's why diabetics should have their eyes examined yearly.

Glaucoma.   Glaucoma is a disease caused by increased pressure within the eyeball. To understand how it works, think of the eye as being like a bathtub. If you turn on a bathtub's faucets and leave the drain open, the water will empty from the tub. If you turn on the faucets and close the drain, the tub will soon overflow with water. But cover the tub with a tarpaulin, and the tarpaulin will bulge. This is exactly what happens in your eye when you develop glaucoma.

In a healthy eye, the fluid that the eye constantly produces drains out through a network of tissue, called the drainage angle, between the iris and the cornea. In some eyes, this drainage angle doesn't work well. The fluid either drains more slowly than it is produced or it simply backs up, not draining at all. Pressure then builds up in the eye, eventually reducing the flow of blood to the retina and the optic nerve. Vision may be permanently dimmed as a result. If left untreated, glaucoma can lead to blindness.

Glaucoma can be either acute or chronic. Acute glaucoma—sometimes called angle-closure glaucoma—is rare. It occurs mainly in farsighted elderly people. It is also an eye emergency. During an attack of acute glaucoma, the drainage angle becomes blocked suddenly and completely. Pressure builds quickly and destroys the fibers of the optic nerve. If the condition isn't treated within 48 hours, you run the risk of losing vision in the affected eye.

Treatment itself is fairly simple: The doctor uses a laser to make a small opening in the iris to relieve the pressure. If acute glaucoma is treated in time, vision should return almost to normal.

Chronic glaucoma is a quieter but no less devastating disease. In chronic glaucoma, fluid builds up in the eye over a period of years. The pressure within the eye also gradually builds up. Though the optic nerve is in effect being slowly strangled, there may be no symptoms at all. That's why doctors recommend an eye exam every year or two for everyone over the age of 40.

Fortunately, chronic glaucoma is treatable. Any vision that's been lost is gone forever, but your remaining sight can be saved if you use eyedrops or tablets that lower eye pressure. You may have to take these for the rest of your life. And if medication doesn't work, you can be treated with the laser or undergo an eye operation in which a surgeon creates an artificial drainage channel.

But remember, if you have chronic glaucoma, only early diagnosis can save your eyesight.

Iritis.   Iritis is any inflammation of the iris—the colored part of the eye—and other internal structures of the eye. Microscopic white cells, together with excess protein from leaky blood vessels in the eye, begin to float around aimlessly in the jellylike mass of the eyeball.

These wandering cells may attach themselves to the back of a transparent membrane at the front of the eye— the cornea—or they may settle to the bottom of the eyeball. If enough of them gather, however, they can block the opening through which liquid drains out of the eye. This can cause glaucoma. And long-standing, untreated iritis can lead to cataracts.

Keratitis. Keratitis is any inflammation of the cornea— the curved, transparent membrane at the front of the eye. Because light enters through the cornea, it's often called the "window" of the eye.

In most cases, keratitis is the result of an infection caused by a type of bacterium, virus, fungus or amoeba. It can also be caused by allergies to chemicals.

Infections of the cornea are serious. When an infection does occur, it can be a virus that's responsible—usually herpes simplex, the same virus that causes cold sores around your mouth. That's why you should never put your fingers to your eyes after touching your mouth when you have cold sores.

Another cause of corneal infections is contaminated contact lenses. If you wear contact lenses and develop a red eye, stop wearing the lenses immediately.

To treat the infection and resulting inflammation, you may be hospitalized. If you are treated at home, you will probably be given medicated eyedrops to use frequently.

Macular degeneration. The macula is the part of the eye that distinguishes fine detail in the center of your field of vision. It's what allows you to read newsprint or see fine embroidery.

With age, the small blood vessels in the eyes sometimes become constricted and hardened. The macula doesn't get enough blood and degenerates, which results in blurring of central vision. As the disease progresses, you will lose more and more of your central vision, until only your peripheral vision remains—like a picture with a hole in its center. But people do not go totally blind from macular degeneration.

There are two types of macular degeneration—wet and dry. The wet type is treatable; the dry type is not. An ophthalmological examination is needed to determine which kind you have. If you have the treatable kind, a laser is used to destroy the blood vessels growing in places where they shouldn't. Lasers are helpful in preventing the disease from getting worse.

Macular degeneration develops slowly. It's painless and it usually affects both eyes. Vision can sometimes be improved by eyeglasses with powerful magnifying lenses. Multivitamins may be helpful. If you experience a sudden change in vision, you should see your ophthalmologist. Such a change could signal the onset of macular degeneration.

Chapter 8
Face, Jaw and Mouth

SEE YOUR DOCTOR IMMEDIATELY IF:

- *You have a sore that lasts more than 10 to 14 days*
- *You have swelling accompanied by a fever*
- *You have difficulty moving the muscles of your face*
- *You have numbness or soreness on one side of your face*
- *Your face swells and you know you've already had the mumps*
- *Swelling sets in, pain gets worse or your upper and lower teeth just don't seem to meet after an injury*
- *Your mouth has been burned by chemicals*
- *You have extremely bad breath that does not go away*

Most of us only think about our jaw (as opposed to the teeth embedded in it) when it meets with an outside force—like when we accidentally get kicked in the chops by an eight-year-old who's practicing karate. Otherwise we ignore it.

But think what it would be like if you had to speak, kiss, eat or swallow *without* a jaw. Speech would be little more than a monotone. Kisses would be limited to the one-dimensional pucker-toward-the-cheek social ritual. And eating and swallowing would be so drastically affected that few people would be able to handle anything more sophisticated than soup broth.

Next time you tear into a steak with your teeth, give some thought to the supporting cast of muscles, joints and nerves that make up the jaw. And watch out for small boys practicing karate.

SYMPTOM: **Bad Breath**

COMMON CAUSES: Back in the tenth century, a Welsh woman who left her home within the first seven years of marriage couldn't make claims on her husband's property unless at least one of her reasons for leaving was a "good" one. Impotence was a good reason. So was halitosis, better known as bad breath.

Many medieval women must have gotten themselves back into circulation as a result. Oral hygiene wasn't too well advanced in the tenth century—you couldn't find tooth floss or fluoride toothpaste anywhere—and poor oral hygiene was and is the leading cause of bad breath.

"A huge percentage of all cases of halitosis are caused by fermenting plaque or by gum disease," says Cherilyn G. Sheets, D.D.S., spokesperson for the Academy of General Dentistry, practicing in Inglewood and Newport, California. Because as many as 90 percent of us have some degree of gum inflammation or periodontitis (see Common Tooth and Gum Conditions in chapter 16), most of us will also, at some time, have bad breath.

How can you tell whether your bad breath is caused by mouth trouble? For one thing, you may not have known at first that you had bad breath at all. Diplomatic (perhaps long-suffering) friends may have had to tell you. You rarely "taste" or are aware of this type of bad breath. But you can check whether you have the condition by performing a simple home "mouth odor test," according to Robert J. Mallin, D.D.S., a dentist in Metuchen, New Jersey. "Take dental floss and pull it gently between your teeth, then smell any debris on it," he says. "If it stinks, you have a problem."

What if, to your great relief, it doesn't stink? Well then, you may still have a problem, but a problem caused by something other than gum disease. A filmy tongue can lead directly to bad breath.

"If you look at the tongue under a microscope, it resembles a shag rug. It's covered with thin, hairlike papillae," explains Dr. Mallin. "Food debris gets trapped in these filaments and putrefies. The odor, of course, is unpleasant." An unclean tongue is, in fact, one of the most potent of all causes of halitosis.

If you practice good oral hygiene and still have bad breath, it may, instead, have a lot to do with your habits. Smoking, giving long speeches, sleeping (maybe sleeping *through* long speeches)—all of these can lead to drying of the mouth (see Symptom: Dry Mouth). This, in turn, causes bad breath. Also, a cold or a sore throat can give you bad breath.

Certain serious conditions elsewhere in your body could also be blowing an ill wind through your mouth. If your nose, for example, is blocked by a chronic sinus infection or a simple cold, you'll probably have to contend with bad breath as well. Also, lung problems, ranging from mild bronchitis to cancer (all compounded by smoking) can cause halitosis, as can indigestion or vomiting.

BEST RESPONSE: If you've just eaten a slice of garlic-and-anchovy pizza and now have bad breath, you've nothing to worry about—unless, of course, you've got a job interview or a date in the next few hours.

"If your bad breath doesn't last for more than a day, it's not a medical problem," Dr. Sheets says. "It may, though, be a social problem. You might try mouthwash or brushing with baking soda. They can cover the odor for a few hours." Don't use mouthwash to mask recurrent bad breath, however. Mouthwash lowers bacteria for an hour or two, but more grow back than before.

You also might try brushing your tongue. In one study, Joseph Tonzetich, Ph.D., a professor of oral biology in the faculty of dentistry at the University of British Columbia, found that when he asked people with "morning mouth" to brush their teeth regularly, their mouth odor was reduced by 25 percent. When they brushed their tongue, the odor was reduced by *75 percent.* And when he asked them to brush both their teeth and their tongue, their bad breath was reduced by 85 percent. Dr. Tonzetich's conclusion: "Tongue brushing is one of the most effective methods of decreasing breath odor."

But sometimes all the good oral hygiene habits in the world—admirable as they are—won't get rid of your bad breath.

"A healthy mouth won't produce odors," Dr. Sheets emphasizes. "Infections of the gum will." A good plaque control program should therefore help lessen the problem.

But, as Dr. Mallin says, "Brushing and flossing by themselves won't stop periodontal disease once it's begun. If you have persistent bad breath, see your dentist."

SYMPTOM: **Burning**

COMMON CAUSES: It may be a hot thrill for chili lovers or an occupational hazard for fire-eaters. But for most people, a burning mouth is an unpleasant symptom of health problems, some of which can be serious.

A burning sensation can have several causes, and more than one could be responsible for the condition.

A burned mouth is, not surprisingly, one cause of a burning mouth. Either hot food or caustic chemicals can cause mouth burns. More often, burns are simply a nuisance caused by overheated foods; your tongue and palate are especially susceptible. These burns are usually minor. In fact, you probably won't realize at first that you *have* been burned—that the swigs of boiling coffee you'd hoped would clear your head instead charred your tongue.

"Most people aren't always aware of the cause, since the pain may not develop until the burned skin sloughs off," explains Thomas McGuire, D.D.S., who practices preventive dentistry in Carmel Valley, California.

Even if you eat only ice cream and other nonflammable foods, though, you can still wind up with a mouth on fire. In this case, the fire is probably a feeling and not a fact. Many diseases and mouth problems can make you feel as if your gums are aglow. Diabetes or vitamin deficiencies, for example, could be at fault. Cold sores (see Symptom: Sores) can also cause a burning, smarting sensation in your mouth, even before the characteristic herpes blisters appear. You're at special risk for cold sores when your resistance is low, says Howard B. Marshall, D.D.S., a periodontist in New York City and author of *How to Save Your Teeth.* "The outbreak has been associated with trauma, allergy, menstruation, sunburn, emotional upset and fever."

Interestingly, several factors—in particular, menstruation, hormonal changes, trauma and depression—have been shown to cause a burning feeling in the mouth, without help from the herpes virus. And wearing dentures, which puts the mouth itself under special stress, can quickly set the mouth fires burning. In fact, wearing dentures is one of the most frequent causes of a burning mouth.

BEST RESPONSE: Decide if your burning mouth was actually burned. If hot foods *have* burned your mouth, you can cool the fire fairly easily, says Dr. Marshall.

"To get temporary relief while the tissues are healing, try rinsing with bicarbonate rinses made by mixing one teaspoon of sodium carbonate to one glass of warm water. Rinse with it several times a day, particularly before eating." But don't try to relieve this hurt by chewing (as opposed to swallowing) aspirin. "Aspirin is a strong acid and it *burns* the skin," stresses Dr. McGuire.

Eating foods that are not too hot or too acidic should also help healing. And avoid cigarettes; they reduce healing ability, and smoke by-products are direct irritants.

If, after doing all of this, the burn does not seem to be getting better, see your doctor.

Relax, though, if your mouth is burning only because a cold sore is erupting. In fact, relaxing may be your best possible response. "Because cold sores are caused by a virus, trauma, excitement and worry don't help them any," explains Dr. McGuire. "Try not to irritate them, and alter your diet to eliminate foods that bother them" (see Best Response under Symptom: Sores, for more tips on how to cool cold sores).

If your burns were caused by chemicals, call your poison control center or your physician immediately. Children especially are at risk from accidentally swallowing caustic household chemicals. This is an emergency and requires immediate action.

Your poison control center can give you specific instructions based on the chemicals that caused the burns, says Rutherford Rose, Pharm.D., of the Maryland Poison Center. You'll also be given some general instructions as well: Do first aid and get the child (or yourself) to a hospital or emergency room.

Immediate first aid is important, she says. Rinse the mouth, spit or wipe the chemical out of the mouth. Then dilute the chemical by drinking a couple of glasses of water. Do not induce vomiting. Get to the nearest medical facility as quickly as possible.

ACCOMPANYING SYMPTOMS: If a burning sensation in your mouth is coupled with numbness, swelling, bleeding or pain, also in your mouth, with no apparent cause, you should see your dentist at once. These symptoms could indicate oral cancer.

SYMPTOM: **Chapped Lips**

COMMON CAUSES: Do your lips resemble a lunar landscape, fissured with deep cracks? Are they sore and peeling, flaking like parchment?

"If you have dry, chapped lips, you've almost certainly not been drinking enough water," says Cherilyn G. Sheets, D.D.S. Your lips may become dry on the outside because you're dehydrated on the inside.

External factors also play an important role, of course. Sun, wind, dry air, caffeine and habitually biting or licking your lips can all do their part to parch them. So can allergy. Allergies are good suspects if your lips stay stubbornly chapped, refusing to heal, says Thomas Goodman, M.D., author of *The Skin Doctor's Skin Doctoring Book*. The possible allergens are many: chemicals found in lipstick; the flavoring used in your favorite toothpaste, mouthwash or chewing gum; or "anything else that you have a habit of chewing or sucking on, such as a pencil, pen, telephone cord or eyeglasses."

BEST RESPONSE: Dr. Goodman's farewell-to-chapping prescription is succinct and exact. Begin, he says, by applying nonprescription ½ percent hydrocortisone cream 20 times daily. Be careful not to lick the chapped area. And, according to Dr. Sheets, be sure to drink plenty of water and to avoid or cut back on caffeine.

Next, after your dry, cracked lips have begun to improve, switch from the hydrocortisone cream to plain old petroleum jelly (Vaseline) or to a lip balm (such as Chap Stick). Use this 20 times daily, and, again, avoid all temptation to lick your lips. After a few days, you should be able to reduce your applications of petroleum jelly or lip balm to 10 times a day, and, after a few more days, to 5 per day. You'll probably need or want to maintain this regimen indefinitely, Dr. Goodman says, adding, "and no licking."

If you suspect, though, that the original chapping was caused by an allergy, you should now experiment a little, trying to find the actual allergen. Eliminate all suspected allergens, such as lipstick, or a new brand of toothpaste or mouthwash. After your lips have been pink and healthy for a week or so, "go back (one at a time) to lipstick, toothpaste, mouthwash, etc., giving each a few days to react," Dr. Goodman suggests. You will probably find the culprit if you're careful. "Once you have found the problem-causing agent, you should never go back to using it again," he says. And hopefully, you shouldn't develop chapping again.

SYMPTOM: **Cheek Biting**

COMMON CAUSES: Putting tongue in cheek is fine. Putting teeth in cheek is not. "If you are tense or have generalized anxiety or hostility, this may manifest itself when you are sleeping, or even when you are awake." How? By biting your cheek, says Howard B. Marshall, D.D.S.

Tension is, in fact, the leading cause of cheek biting. But there are others, explains Thomas McGuire, D.D.S. Trauma from an accident, new fillings rubbing on the cheek or tongue, a bad bite (which will have you chewing your cheek when you mean to chew your food), fat cheeks that get in the way or wisdom teeth that have become "sensitive"—any of these factors can leave your cheeks in peril from your teeth.

Children and young adults are especially susceptible to cheek biting. The problem usually becomes apparent when, if pain hasn't already made the child complain, the wounded cheek begins to bleed.

BEST RESPONSE: "The treatment is partly your responsibility and partly the dentist's," Dr. McGuire stresses. You can ease any immediate discomfort by rinsing your mouth with a mixture of one part 3 percent solution of hydrogen peroxide and one part warm water. But after that, you're going to have to make sure you eliminate the real cause of the problem, he says.

Dr. Marshall agrees. "You should ask your dentist to help you in several ways. He can check the relationship of the upper to the lower teeth and see if there are any irregularities on the tooth surfaces that are contributing to your habit. If so, he can eliminate these. He also may find that you have a sharp cusp, or an incorrect relationship of teeth in the cheek area you keep chewing. Again, he can correct this."

But if the cause is more mental than dental, *you'll* need to take responsibility for your cheek's protection. "You can help yourself by examining your life-style and relationships to see what is tension producing," Dr. Marshall says. "Try to eliminate those areas or find other ways to release the tension so as to increase your general relaxation." In other words, relax and laugh. You'll be less tempted to bite your cheek, if you can look at life tongue-in-cheek.

SYMPTOM: **Cracked Mouth Corners**

COMMON CAUSES: Cracked corners are also painful corners—the simple exercise of opening your mouth is enough to make you wince.

The most common cause of the condition is a poor bite from tooth loss or poorly fitting dentures. Another common cause is excessive moisture at the corners of the mouth as a result of drooling. The saliva needs a place to go and often seeps to the corners of the mouth to dribble out. Sagging cheeks—the "hound dog look"—is another common cause. But cracked corners can also be caused by candidiasis, which is a yeast infection, or ariboflavinosis, which is a riboflavin deficiency.

BEST RESPONSE: To help relieve the pain and discomfort associated with cracked mouth corners, doctors recommend topical medications, such as antifungal, antibacterial or steroid creams and ointments. If the problem is associated with drooling, preparations containing silicone are recommended.

To get rid of the problem completely, however, you'll have to see a doctor to get the cause of the problem diagnosed. For example, if a bad bite is the cause, dentures may be required or refitted to correct the problem, or, if it's a vitamin deficiency, vitamin therapy will be necessary.

SYMPTOM: **Difficulty Opening Mouth**

COMMON CAUSES: Few people have difficulty opening their mouths, particularly at the wrong time. But when there is a problem, the cause is usually pretty serious. Tetanus (see Common Facial, Jaw and Mouth Conditions), quinsy (see Common Throat Conditions in chapter 17), tumors, infected wisdom teeth, or a dislocated jaw is frequently the problem.

So, too, is a bunch of muscle/nerve/joint symptoms that are frequently grouped by dentists and doctors under the term temporomandibular joint disorder—commonly referred to as TMJ (see Common Facial, Jaw and Mouth Conditions). TMJ often has other symptoms, however, including headaches, earaches, roaring noises and clicking sounds, neck and chest pains, backaches, dizziness and even mental lapses. TMJ has so many seemingly unrelated symptoms that doctors find it difficult to diagnose.

BEST RESPONSE: If you suspect you have tetanus, quinsy or one of the other serious problems that can make opening your mouth difficult, see your doctor immediately.

TMJ also needs to be professionally diagnosed. But once you know your problem is TMJ, there are a number of things you can do yourself to help relieve the symptoms until the problem is solved.

Take two buffered aspirin four times a day and put a heating pad over the joints located directly in front of your ears twice a day for half an hour each time, suggests David Fairbanks, M.D., spokesperson for the American Academy of Otolaryngology—Head and Neck Surgery.

"I also tell patients to quit grinding and gritting their teeth and to quit chewing gum or other hard, chewy foods," says Dr. Fairbanks. "And we make sure that they chew evenly—not just on one side."

People with TMJ should also exercise the joint by bringing their lower jaw forward and up in front of their upper jaw ten times before each meal and another ten times before bed, adds Dr. Fairbanks. And if that doesn't work, go see your doctor. He or she will get you into all sorts of other gadgets, such as occlusal retainers—plastic and wire devices that are also called occlusal splints, bite plates, night guards, bite guards or simply "appliances." Essentially, these devices are designed on the theory that you can't easily open your mouth because your jaw is not in the proper position. The occlusal devices are supposed to straighten the jaw, but whether or not they really work is still a matter of professional controversy.

Studies by dentists and doctors from around the world, however, are generally positive. A study at the University of Kentucky, for example, revealed that 12 people who were fitted with occlusal retainers experienced less pain and better mobility in their mouth within four to six weeks of treatment. A second study, this one at Georgetown University School of Dentistry, revealed that 84 percent of 17 men and women who wore retainers between three weeks and one year showed improvement. The problem with most of these studies, however, is that they are generally too small or not well done. In addition, sometimes just learning to relax can be almost as effective a remedy as anything else.

"TMJ is one of the most controversial issues I've ever come across," says Dr. Fairbanks. "We cannot get any semblance of accord within our own specialty or the orthodontic specialty on treatment."

SYMPTOM: **Discolored Tongue**

COMMON CAUSES: In some objects, in some instances, color changes are great. Leaves change colors and keep artists employed. Traffic lights change colors and keep autos intact. Chameleons change colors and keep themselves amused. But a tongue that changes colors won't interest artists or amuse animals. It will, like a traffic light, alert you to oncoming trouble.

This "trouble" sometimes turns your tongue black. A black tongue isn't attractive. It also isn't healthy. Bacterial overgrowths blacken the tongue. The bacteria fill the fissures on the surface of the tongue, making it appear black or deep brown. Smoking or taking antibiotics can also make the tongue look black or brown.

But black isn't the only color the tongue can turn. In its more patriotic moods, the tongue can become red, white or even blue. A red tongue is a warning sign. Stop, it says, and take stock of your health. You may have tongue trouble, including inflammations such as glossitis or geographical tongue (see Common Facial, Jaw and Mouth Conditions) or a viral infection. Or you may have a serious problem unrelated to your mouth. Pernicious anemia (see anemia under Common Whole Body Conditions in chapter 19) or a niacin deficiency can tomato-color your tongue, as can a reaction to certain medications. Or your red tongue can have no apparent cause. Worse, it can signal a precancerous condition.

A white, splotchy tongue may be a sign of a precancerous condition. White, usually wet, crusty patches, known medically as leukoplakia (see Common Facial, Jaw and Mouth Conditions) are caused by chronic irritation from such sources as smoking or syphilis. Though they will not always evolve into cancer, they do need to be seen and attended to by a physician.

A white tongue in children, especially a white tongue sprinkled with red spots, could mean scarlet fever. This early stage of the disease is known, appropriately, as the white strawberry tongue stage. Next, the white color will slough off, exposing the red, raw tongue beneath it. This is called the red strawberry tongue stage and, despite the whimsy of its name, it indicates a serious illness.

You probably needn't worry, though, if your tongue is blue. Tongues get blue. They snap out of it. In fact, a brightly colored tongue probably has a bad case of the sugar blues—or sugar greens or sugar oranges or whatever other color of sugar candy you've been sucking on. Dyes in foods are the number one cause of discoloration in tongues. Such discoloration will soon fade. And, if your tongue's blue color has been there since birth, it's probably a type of birthmark. Often slightly raised and hairy, a birthmark can be a nuisance, but it's not dangerous. Still, it would be prudent to have it checked by a physician.

There is at least one instance when a blue tongue might be a sign of trouble. It can be a sign of anemia (see Common Whole Body Conditions in chapter 19).

BEST RESPONSE: Most tongue disorders are minor and will clear up on their own. You probably have nothing to worry about if your tongue simply changes color and then fades back to its normal pink. If it doesn't, it could be a sign of disease and you should see your doctor, especially if any tongue problem persists for more than ten days.

Geographical tongue, however, will generally go away by itself. There really is no treatment or cure. Glossitis will clear up once your doctor finds the specific cause for the inflammation. In the meantime, however, doctors suggest that you avoid spicy foods and other things that can irritate the tongue, such as smoking and alcohol.

Leukoplakia is a more serious matter, however, since it can lead to cancer. Getting rid of the original irritant is essential. Surgical removal of the patchy lesions is simple and will usually arrest the disease.

ACCOMPANYING SYMPTOMS: If your tongue looks bright red and it is also swollen and painful, you may have a serious problem. The redness you're seeing is the real color of your tongue; normally this bright red color is masked by your papillae (tiny projections of tissue), so that it appears to be pink. When the papillae for some reason disappear, the redness shines through. If this redness or any pain persists, you should seek medical advice.

If the color change is accompanied by swelling and sores, you should see your physician or dentist as soon as possible. Rarely, such changes could indicate oral cancer.

SYMPTOM: **Droopy Mouth**

COMMON CAUSES: A droopy mouth is usually triggered by a disease that has weakened the facial muscles. The most common cause is Bell's palsy (see Common Facial, Jaw and Mouth Conditions), a disease that occurs in roughly 1 out of 5,000 people per year and recurs in about 1 in 10.

Although it was first described in 1821, scientists are just now beginning to figure out what causes it: a virus that inflames the nerves in the face—maybe even the same virus that causes fever blisters.

BEST RESPONSE: If you suspect you have Bell's palsy, check with your doctor. He or she will probably want to run a test that monitors how well your facial nerves are working.

"About 70 percent of those who get Bell's recover spontaneously," says David Fairbanks, M.D. "But a number of them don't have full resolution and they end up with an asymmetrical smile."

Currently, some doctors suggest that corticosteroid drugs will help minimize the virus's effects, while others suggest they are worthless. Surgery is also a controversial treatment for Bell's, performed on less than 10 percent of all people who experience facial paralysis, and there are some doctors who suggest that there are absolutely no indications for doing it—ever. The antiviral drug acyclovir is now being tested as a treatment.

As the nerves affected by Bell's palsy heal themselves, they may send inappropriate signals to other parts of the face, and drooling, tearing and a runny nose may accompany the initial weakness in the face. Sometimes the eye on the affected side of the face won't close properly. Moisturizing eyedrops from your local pharmacy will protect the eye from irritation, as will a temporary eye patch or a pair of sunglasses. At night, an ophthalmic ointment may soothe the eye, or your doctor may recommend a preformed piece of tape on just the upper lid that will allow you to stiffen the lid and close it.

SYMPTOM: **Dry Mouth**

COMMON CAUSES: In the next few hours, do you plan to give a major presentation to your firm's major stockholders? Say "I do" to the person you most want to do things with? Run the Boston Marathon or participate in anything that makes you nervous?

If so, then having a dry mouth is perfectly normal. "What doctors call 'situational dry mouth' can occur anytime you're under stress," explains Philip C. Fox, D.D.S., a senior investigator at the National Institute of Dental Research of the National Institutes of Health in Bethesda, Maryland.

If your dry mouth is something you wake up with in the morning, or if it wakes you up in the middle of the night, it almost always means you're sleeping with your mouth open. "Sleeping with your mouth hanging open will naturally dry out your mouth," Dr. Fox says. "You may sleep this way habitually. Or you may have some kind of nasal obstruction."

A dry, unlubricated mouth that lingers, though, bothering you throughout the day *and* night, is more than merely a nasal problem or a minor one. In fact, it's dangerous. "Dry mouth, or xerostomia, is more than just an unpleasant side effect," emphasizes Ira Shannon, M.D., professor of biochemistry at the University of Texas Dental Branch in Houston. "It's an extremely painful, potentially damaging condition that can produce serious problems for its victims."

Why? Because saliva is your teeth's salvation. "A variety of proteins in saliva can discourage bacterial growth or actively kill bacteria," according to the National Institute of Dental Research. When your mouth doesn't produce enough saliva to dampen their enthusiasm, these same bacteria will adhere to the teeth, multiplying merrily and causing severe tooth decay.

Saliva is also important because it bathes the teeth with calcium and phosphate minerals, replacing these minerals as they're lost and strengthening the teeth. Too little saliva means undernourished teeth. It can also mean an undernourished *you.* Saliva contains enzymes that start digestion of starches in food. It also moistens food, making it easier to swallow. A dry mouth therefore affects the ability to chew, to taste and even to speak.

What produces this very uninviting symptom? "There are four major causes of clinical dry mouth," Dr. Fox says. "The single most common is a side effect to medication." Over 300 frequently used drugs may produce xerostomia. These range from drugs used to treat high blood pressure and cancer to over-the-counter antihistamines and decongestants. Not all dry mouth is drug-induced, of course. Radiation treatment of the head and neck, such as would be necessary to combat oral cancer, is the second most common cause of malfunctioning salivary glands.

Also, many serious diseases or health problems, including glandular disorders and Sjögren's syndrome, a disorder that causes dry mouth and dry eyes and may also be associated with rheumatoid arthritis, can turn your mouth to dust. And finally, the fourth major cause of dry mouth is what doctors call idiopathic and what the rest of us call mysterious.

"Often," Dr. Fox admits, "doctors can find no clear cause for the problem. But that doesn't mean it isn't making life miserable for whoever has it."

BEST RESPONSE: Situational dry mouth is nothing to worry about, says Dr. Fox. It will disappear as soon as the stress is diminished. "Try drinking a glass of water or taking a few deep breaths," he says. "Your mouth should soon be well lubricated again."

You also needn't worry if your dry mouth strikes in the night. To find out whether it's habit or a nasal obstruction that's causing you to sleep with your mouth open, try this simple test: Close your mouth and breathe exclusively through your nose. If you feel you're about to strangle, you have an obstruction of the nasal passages. "The problem in this case is not with your salivary glands but with your nose, and it needs to be treated by an otolaryngologist [ear, nose and throat specialist]," Dr. Fox concludes.

If your dry mouth is an all-day problem, the first thing you should do is make a complete list of the medications you're currently taking, Dr. Fox says. "Next, call your dentist, complain loudly that your mouth is dry and tell your dentist what drugs you're using." If any of your medications is causing the dry mouth, you and your dentist, together with your physician, should confer about whether you can stop taking the drug or switch to a different one. Usually, once use of the offending drug is discontinued, your dry mouth will begin to irrigate itself again. In rare cases, after prolonged drug use, the condition is permanent.

Dry mouth is a symptom that deserves to be taken seriously. If you are not taking drugs and you have a dry mouth, you should have a complete workup to determine the cause.

Unfortunately, permanent dry mouth is a reality that many will have to face. "Unless your doctor finds some underlying systemic cause for your xerostomia and can treat that cause, your dry mouth is probably an affliction you'll have to learn to live with," Dr. Fox says. Luckily, not all of his outlook is so gloomy. "There *are* methods to combat the symptoms of dry mouth," he explains. "It's up to each person to try them and see what works for him or her."

The first and most important element in any anti-dry mouth program is scrupulous attention to dental hygiene. "I can't emphasize this enough," Dr. Fox says. "Anyone with dry mouth caused by changes in salivary function will probably require topical fluoride treatment in addition to very conscientious brushing and flossing." Your dentist can help you devise the best tooth-care regimen for you. "You may need to see your dentist fairly often," Dr. Fox adds. "But believe me, it's worth it."

Protecting your teeth is not the only aim of anti-dry mouth measures, though. You should also try to stimulate as much saliva output as you can. "Often, people with dry mouth still have some salivary gland function. It's just dropped way below normal," Dr. Fox says. Sucking on something, such as (sugar-free) candy or even ice can help. The best thing of all to put in your mouth may be sugarless gum. According to Dr. Fox, "It's flavored, which stimulates saliva secretion. Plus, the direct stimulation of your mouth that accompanies chewing can sometimes be helpful."

Potentially more long-lasting solace from dry mouth may come from a (still experimental) drug, pilocarpine. Dr. Fox, who is heading the research team studying the drug, says results thus far have been encouraging. "We've given the drug to people whose salivary glands were damaged by Sjögren's syndrome," he says. "And we found that it did stimulate increased saliva output for several hours."

But, cautions Dr. Fox, this is not a cure for dry mouth. "It's only an advance in the symptom's treatment, and it can only help people whose glands are still capable of being stimulated. It won't be of any use if you've lost all salivary gland function." If you think, though, that the drug might help save you from trauma associated with too little saliva, have your dentist refer you to Dr. Philip C. Fox, c/o the National Institute of Dental Research, 9000 Rockville Pike, Bethesda, MD 20892.

Of course, if your saliva stoppage is total, then swallowing drugs or chewing on gum can do nothing more than make your jaw sore. You might instead try artificial saliva, available over the counter in different forms. "It doesn't sound pleasant and it's really not," Dr. Fox admits. The saliva substitute usually has to be sprayed into your mouth often, sometimes every few minutes. It can be costly, and it isn't significantly better than squirting your mouth with water, according to Dr. Fox. "It mimics the wetness of saliva, but it doesn't contain saliva's protective proteins. Still, I wouldn't discourage anyone from using it. Try it. If it works for you and you're comfortable with it, great. By all means keep squirting," he says.

You might, as an alternative, try rinsing your mouth frequently with warm water or salt water. This is sort of the do-it-yourselfer's artificial saliva. And it's also a wise practice for anyone with a dry mouth. "Rinsing often is soothing to your mouth, good for your teeth and essential when you eat," Dr. Fox says. "You need liquid to wet your food and make it easier to swallow. Make sure you drink plenty of water at every meal."

Finally, remember that your fight against dry mouth should be a collaborative effort, involving you, your dentist and your physician. Don't undertake these measures without first seeing your physician or dentist. After that, though, the biggest share of the fight is yours.

"There's still not a lot that medical science can do to relieve dry mouth," Dr. Fox says, in sum. "Your health care practitioner can give you a list of options. But then you have to keep trying them until one works. This smorgasbord approach is state-of-the-art in dry mouth care. In other words, self-care for dry mouth is still the best care."

SYMPTOM: **Flushing**

COMMON CAUSES: Flushing can be caused by a number of fever-related illnesses such as the flu, scarlet fever, yellow fever, typhus or empyema, which is an accumulation of pus in a body cavity. It can also be a complication of diabetes mellitus (see Common Whole Body Conditions in chapter 19) or high blood pressure (see Common Circulatory, Heart and Lung Conditions in chapter 5). But it's also a condition that 80 percent of all women experience when they go through menopause.

Infamously known as a "hot flash," menopausal flushing is triggered by the body's response to the sudden decrease in estrogen production by the ovaries. The face and upper body—sometimes the entire body—become very warm and flushed as skin temperature suddenly rises 7° or 8°F.

Hot flashes usually last from two to three minutes, although some women have reported flashes that lasted up to an hour. They stop in the two to nine years it takes the body to get used to a lack of estrogen.

BEST RESPONSE: "The popular image of the middle-aged woman as an emotional wreck, drenched in sweat and unable to cope, has been played up by pharmaceutical companies to persuade doctors and their patients to use drugs for this condition," writes Sadja Greenwood, M.D., M.P.H., in her book *Menopause, Naturally.*

Instead, try to avoid anything that raises body temperature, such as alcohol, caffeine, hot drinks, hot meals, warm rooms and emotional upsets. Avoid smoking, since smoke reduces the amount of estrogen your body manufactures.

The point, says Dr. Greenwood, is to keep cool. Open a bedroom window at night when hot flashes and related sweats keep you from getting the rest you need. One reason that menopausal women seem to be tired or to have difficulty concentrating, states Dr. Greenwood, is that hot flashes keep them from getting enough sleep. Wear layers of clothes that you can easily peel off when a hot flash begins, eat frequent small meals, maintain your normal weight and drink iced water or juice after exercise.

Some doctors do suggest that there's a place for drug therapy with the roughly 25 percent of menopausal women who experience unbearably severe hot flashes. One of the most popular, called estrogen replacement therapy (ERT), does stop hot flashes while you're taking it. But ERT is a controversial treatment because of reports linking it to an increased risk of uterine cancer, gallbladder disease and high blood pressure. And hot flashes do return if you abruptly stop taking it. Getting several medical opinions and doing a lot of reading on your own can help you decide whether or not ERT is right for you.

SYMPTOM: **Hairy or Furred Tongue**

COMMON CAUSES: It may look like hair; it may feel like hair. But it's not hair. That hairy tongue you're sprouting is just a result of overgrown papillae, or tiny projections of tissue. These papillae normally cover the tongue, and everyone has them. But sometimes, for different reasons, the papillae begin to lengthen. They become lush and full; you begin to feel a need to mow your mouth.

What produces this "hair"? Fungal infections such as candidiasis (see Common Facial, Jaw and Mouth Conditions) can, as can taking antibiotics. Smoking, too, can act as a hair tonic for the tongue. Luckily, although a hairy tongue may not be especially attractive, it's also not serious. Nor is a related problem, a "furred" tongue.

As its name implies, this condition leaves you feeling as if your tongue has grown a pelt. And in fact, it has; you've probably got a whitish or yellowish coating on the surface of the tongue. The problem often accompanies illness and fever. When you're sick, you're eating less and talking less, meaning the tongue is less active. As a result, a film accumulates. Just as a snoozing animal in hibernation grows furry, so does your tongue. But your tongue's fur coat would not be pleasant to snuggle into. It's a mix of bacteria, food particles and excess cells. Your mouth tends to be dry during an illness, so it doesn't produce enough saliva to wash away this coating.

BEST RESPONSE: Having either a furred or hairy tongue is nothing to make the rest of your hair stand on end. Neither condition is serious. If your tongue's fur coat is the result of an illness, it should disappear when the illness clears up.

If your tongue is hairy, the best way to restore it to normal is gentle brushing. First soak your toothbrush in warm water to soften it, dip it in a diluted antiseptic such as mouthwash or hydrogen peroxide, then brush your tongue gently twice a day, if it isn't painful to do so. If you're a smoker, you might want to consider kicking the habit.

If this hairy situation persists for more than ten days, or if it bothers you significantly, talk to your physician or dentist.

ACCOMPANYING SYMPTOM: If you have a coated tongue and have been having bouts of indigestion, your problem may be reflux esophagitis, an inflammation of the esophagus resulting from the backup of acid and pepsin from the stomach. You should see your doctor.

SYMPTOM: **Lumps, in Mouth**

COMMON CAUSES: You've just found a lump in your mouth? Did you develop a matching lump in your throat as you stared at the thing, contemplating its causes?

Well, you can let the lump in your throat, at any rate, dissolve. Yes, a lump in your mouth may be a symptom of cancer. But probably it's not; mouth cancer is uncommon, especially in people under 40.

An unmistakable, lonely lump *might* be a tumor, benign or malignant. Benign tumors usually occur singly. This type of tumor makes its appearance as a small, pale lump. It may have been growing slowly, over the course of several years. If you have such a lump, it probably hasn't bothered you much; benign tumors are hardly ever painful.

Malignant tumors, though, are attention-grabbers. Like benign tumors, they may start as painless, small lumps. But they don't remain painless or small. A cancerous lump will metamorphose into an ugly ulcer with a hard, raised rim and a fragile center that bleeds easily. The ulcer will grow and erode the surrounding tissue in your mouth. The more advanced this cancer becomes, the more pain it'll cause. And the more danger it'll pose, explains the National Institute of Dental Research.

Oral cancers can spread to other parts of your body. They *can* be life-threatening. But they *are* uncommon. If you've never smoked or been a heavy drinker, the likelihood of any lump in your mouth being cancerous is remote, according to the institute.

Of course, what you call a lump may be what another person calls a sore (see Symptom: Sores), such as a canker or cold sore.

BEST RESPONSE: "Anytime you have a lump or sore in your mouth that doesn't go away within ten days to two weeks, go see either your dentist or your family doctor at once," advises Cherilyn G. Sheets, D.D.S. "Seeing your doctor should reassure you," Dr. Sheets adds. "You probably don't have a serious problem."

Cancer of the mouth would need to be treated with surgery and radiation. But if (as is more likely) your "lump" is a cold sore or a canker sore, no intrusive or drastic measures are necessary.

Whatever you do, don't ignore the lump, says Dr. Sheets. Lumps in your mouth, if not life-threatening, are also not normal and should be taken care of.

SYMPTOM: **Noises, Jaw**

COMMON CAUSES: Noises when you open or close your mouth, which usually sound like a kind of clicking or popping, do not mean anything unless they are accompanied by pain, says David Fairbanks, M.D. But clicking or popping *and* pain does mean something. It may mean that cartilage in the jaw's hinge is wearing down. Or, it could be a sign of temporomandibular joint disorder, or TMJ (see Common Facial, Jaw and Mouth Conditions).

BEST RESPONSE: Try to reposition the pressure point in your jaw by exercising your mouth with more than words, suggests Dr. Fairbanks. Bring your lower teeth out in front of your upper teeth ten times before each meal and before bed. Make sure you chew evenly on both sides of your mouth while eating, he adds, and stop clenching, gritting and grinding your teeth or otherwise abusing your jaw.

And if you're worried about TMJ, relax. A study at the University of Illinois's TMJ and Facial Pain Research Center revealed that clicking rarely progresses to the difficulty in opening the mouth that most people with TMJ experience. TMJ needs to be professionally diagnosed. If you have the condition, there are a number of self-help measures you can follow, including taking aspirin and wearing an occlusal retainer. (For more on how TMJ is treated, see Best Response under Symptom: Difficulty Opening Mouth.)

SYMPTOM: **Pain, Jaw or Face**

COMMON CAUSES: Facial pain is probably the most common medical complaint today. Possible causes include Bell's palsy, tic douloureux, and tetanus and temporomandibular joint disorder, or TMJ (see Common Facial, Jaw and Mouth Conditions); as well as quinsy (see Common Throat Conditions in chapter 17); arthritis (see Common Bone, Joint and Muscle Conditions in chapter 3); cancer; mumps; sinus or tooth infections; injuries and poorly fitting dentures.

BEST RESPONSE: Acetaminophen (Tylenol) and heat may temporarily relieve facial and jaw pain, says David Fairbanks, M.D. But you should still see your doctor, since the causes can be both serious and diverse.

SYMPTOM: **Pain, Tongue**

COMMON CAUSES: A sore tongue is often caused by an inflammation called geographical tongue (see Common Facial, Jaw and Mouth Conditions). A geographical tongue is usually dark red and smooth in patches. It's usually sorest when you eat spicy foods, but its cause is unknown.

Glossitis (see Common Facial, Jaw and Mouth Conditions) is a similar tongue disorder that also makes the tongue sore. But, unlike geographical tongue, it can have direct causes. Infection, injury or allergies can all lead to it. So, too, can anemia (see Common Whole Body Conditions in chapter 19). And, also unlike geographical tongue, glossitis will inflame the entire tongue.

But a sore tongue could simply be caused by tongue sores, such as canker sores (see Symptom: Sores). Or it may be that you're unintentionally chewing at your tongue all the time because of jagged teeth or poorly fitted dentures. This constant irritation would make the most cheerful of tongues pretty sore.

BEST RESPONSE: Clearing up a tongue-ache is usually a matter of patience. Most tongue disorders go away without any treatment except solicitude. Avoid very hot or spicy foods, alcohol and tobacco for a few days.

If, however, you have a tongue problem that lasts for more than ten days, you should see your physician. If your doctor finds that your sore tongue is being caused by an underlying disorder, such as an infection or a nutritional deficiency, this will need to be corrected. Your tongue should then heal quickly and completely.

ACCOMPANYING SYMPTOM: Very rarely, a persistently sore tongue, especially if it is accompanied by a lump that doesn't heal, can indicate oral cancer.

SYMPTOM: **Sores**

COMMON CAUSES: Most people misname mouth sores. They call their cold sores "canker sores," their canker sores "fever blisters" and their fever blisters "a pain in the neck" (when that's hardly the place that's sore).

Mouth sores come in a wide range of styles, sizes and colors. Is yours a small, blisterlike sore, yellowish-white in color, with a reddish border? Then it's almost certainly either a canker sore or a cold sore. The majority of mouth sores are one or the other. And the majority of people get them.

How can you tell which kind of sore you have? "Canker sores and cold sores typically crop up in different places in your mouth," explains Cherilyn G. Sheets, D.D.S. "You get canker sores *inside* your mouth—on your tongue, your cheek and the other wet tissue inside your mouth. In contrast to this, you get cold sores on the outer, dry parts of your mouth, particularly on your lips."

These two kinds of sores not only have different campgrounds, they also have different causes. Cold sores, which are sometimes also called fever blisters (because they often swell after illness), are caused by the herpes virus. "About 70 percent of us are exposed to the herpes simplex I virus in infancy," says Steven D. Vincent, D.D.S., M.S., an assistant professor in the Department of Oral Pathology and Diagnosis at the University of Iowa College of Dentistry in Iowa City. "Then we carry this virus the rest of our lives. It lives in the nervous system. It can't be cured and it can't be killed."

There's no need to panic, though. This isn't quite as horrific as it sounds. The immune system eventually establishes a balance of power with the virus, keeping it inactive most of the time. But when resistance is lowered for some reason, the virus rushes back into action, and you develop a cold sore.

Stress, frustration, exhaustion, menstruation, poor nutrition, food sensitivity (especially to arginine-rich foods, such as chocolate), emotional upset, fever and even sunburn—all of these have been known to precipitate a cold sore eruption.

Of course, some of the same problems can contribute to a canker sore's growth. A canker sore is medically called an aphthous ulcer, and "at this time, the exact cause is still unknown," says Howard B. Marshall, D.D.S. Genetic predisposition, hypersensitivity to certain mouth bacteria or stress and anxiety can lead to mouth ulcers. Food allergies, too, may be responsible for canker sores.

Citrus fruits lead the list of suspected allergens. But one study showed that, whereas food allergies played a part in canker sore formation, everyone's allergy was different. One person studied was allergic to figs, another to tomatoes, a third to milk, cheese and wheat flour. So if an allergy is promoting your canker sore outburst, you may have difficulty identifying the food.

Remember, not all sores are canker sores *or* cold sores. A small ulcerating sore, for instance, could be the result of poorly fitting dentures rubbing against the gums. Over a period of years, these same uncomfortable, uncorrected dentures lead to the formation of leukoplakia (see Common Facial, Jaw and Mouth Conditions), a potentially precancerous disease. Any constant irritation, including wearing dentures, smoking or heavy drinking will promote the development of leukoplakia.

If you have a series of tiny, whitish, lacy sores, you could have oral lichen planus (see Common Facial, Jaw and Mouth Conditions), while creamy white or yellowish patches that can be rubbed off easily can be a sign of candidiasis, or oral thrush (see Common Facial, Jaw and Mouth Conditions). Trench mouth, known in medical terminology as necrotizing ulcerative gingivitis (see Common Facial, Jaw and Mouth Conditions), also causes mouth sores. These mouth sores are especially unpleasant—painful ulcers that spread across the gums and often bleed.

BEST RESPONSE: If you're uncertain what kind of sore you have, if your sore doesn't heal or if it keeps recurring, you should see your dentist, Dr. Vincent says. "Oral cancer and other mouth disorders, including oral thrush and trench mouth, require medical treatment, and the sooner it's begun the better."

Medicine, however, can't do much to decrease the healing time of a cold sore or canker sore once it has actually developed, says Dr. Vincent. You simply have to wait for it to heal on its own.

This healing typically requires one to two weeks, Dr. Vincent adds. Over-the-counter anesthetics designed to combat mouth pain can sometimes help to reduce the irritation while the sore heals. But use these preparations cautiously and sparingly. "Many nonprescription cold sore medications serve as cauterizing agents. They may dry out the sore temporarily. They may make it feel less symptomatic for a few hours. But they're also likely to increase the healing time," Dr. Vincent warns.

What *can* you safely do, then, to soothe your mouth sores? "The best treatment I have found for canker sores is to rinse the mouth with a good mouthwash, then dry the sore with a cotton swab and then place denture adhesive paste over the sore," explains Dr. Marshall. This will ease the discomfort, although it is not a cure.

Cold sores are easier to control than canker sores. "In our clinical practice, the control of recurrent cold sores has proven possible," Dr. Vincent says, though he cautions that in order for the treatment to work, cooperation and commitment are required.

The treatment doesn't require much of your time. You simply must, at the onset of a cold sore's prodrome (its early warning signals, including tingling, itching and burning), apply topical acyclovir, a drug available by prescription from your dentist or doctor. "Acyclovir, applied early enough, can significantly decrease the size and severity of cold sores," according to Dr. Vincent. "It is by far the best treatment we've found."

Another potentially useful (perhaps supplemental) treatment may exist, though. It involves manipulating your diet. Several studies have found an apparent link between a diet high in the amino acid arginine and recurrent cold sore outbreaks. In these studies, arginine helped the herpes virus grow and reproduce. You, of course, don't want your herpes virus to do this.

Luckily, lysine, another amino acid, inhibited the activity of the herpes virus. Therefore, according to Craig S. Miller, D.M.D., and Clark N. Foulke, D.D.S., who published a paper on the lysine connection, you should be able to reduce the frequency of cold sore outbreaks by eating foods high in lysine and avoiding those high in arginine. Lysine-rich foods include milk, fish, chicken, brewer's yeast and soybeans. Foods that those prone to cold sores should avoid, say Dr. Miller and Dr. Foulke, are nuts, chocolate, popcorn, gelatin desserts, brown rice, raisins and seeds.

But whether changing your diet can really prevent cold sores is a topic of hot debate. The majority opinion in the medical world seems to be that it cannot. After all, many doctors note, the studies of arginine and lysine were conducted on cell cultures. Cell cultures do not necessarily behave like people. Yet, according to other doctors and many cold sore sufferers, the treatment helps.

If you'd like to try your luck with lysine, Dr. Miller and Dr. Foulke recommend that you not only follow the low-arginine/high-lysine food guidelines but also supplement your diet with L-lysine tablets, available in most health food stores. A dosage of between 312 and 1,000 milligrams daily, they say, just may help to cool the fire of your cold sore. Of course, this or any other supplement program should have the approval and supervision of your doctor.

Another tip to help make you a good sore loser is to always use a lip balm with a sunblock factor of 15; ultraviolet rays activate the herpes virus in certain people. Perhaps most important of all, "adequate oral health together with good overall health can do a lot to reduce your chances of developing cold sores or canker sores at all," says Dr. Sheets. Dr. Marshall offers his prescription for soreless living: "Rest, good nutrition and elimination of stress, to give the body a chance to recover and repair."

If none of these measures helps—if, in other words, your sore seems stubbornly determined to stick around—see your dentist or physician. Some sores can be quite serious, and any sore that persists for more than two weeks needs to be treated.

ACCOMPANYING SYMPTOMS: Mouth sores that are accompanied by fatigue, paleness and frequent infections could indicate a blood disorder or leukemia (see Common Whole Body Conditions in chapter 19). In children, these same symptoms may be accompanied by swollen neck glands, a purplish-red rash, pains in the limbs and severe headache. These are some of the main symptoms of acute lymphocytic leukemia (the type that appears most often in children).

If you or your child has these symptoms, it is necessary to see a physician. Proper examination and blood tests may well show that your fears were groundless.

Mouth sores that haven't healed within two weeks, sores that bleed easily or sores that seem to be growing can indicate oral cancer and should be seen by a dentist or physician. Malignant tumors in the mouth often don't cause pain until they're quite advanced, so don't ignore any lingering sore, even if it seems minor.

SYMPTOM: **Swollen Salivary Glands**

COMMON CAUSES: Salivary glands are usually complacent and co-operative. They gear up at the sight of appetizing food; they dry up at the sight of unleashed Dobermans; they quietly keep your mouth lubricated the rest of the time. In fact, you probably never think about your salivary glands at all, until they go into revolt.

The mouth is filled with salivary glands—any place where saliva appears, it has been pumped by a salivary gland. The biggest glands, called the parotids, are located below and in front of each ear.

Swollen salivary glands usually indicate one of several conditions. The swollen gland is probably either infected or blocked by a salivary duct stone. The two problems can be interrelated. Stones sometimes lead to infections. The so-called stone itself is a hard, pebble-sized bit of matter that's been encrusted by the chemicals in the saliva. You'll be most aware of it at mealtimes. This is because the stone partially blocks the duct and, when you eat, a great deal of the saliva produced cannot pass the stone. As a result, the gland swells. The glands that line the floor of your mouth may be especially susceptible to this problem, but the disorder is uncommon.

If one of your salivary glands is not only swollen but sore, if the lymph glands in your neck are also swollen or if you have a bitter taste in your mouth (from pus trickling down), then you probably have an infection.

A salivary gland most commonly becomes infected as a result of mumps. Bacteria can also invade the gland when you're run-down, or if the gland itself has been damaged by stones. Though the condition isn't serious, if left untreated it can cause scarring and, eventually, loss of function in the gland.

More serious is a salivary gland tumor. Luckily, such tumors are almost always benign. They grow slowly, often unnoticed, for years. The only symptom of the tumor is a lingering swollen gland. Very rarely, the swelling can be caused by a tumor that is, or may become, malignant and possibly life-threatening.

BEST RESPONSE: If you have any swelling in your mouth, under your chin or behind the angle of your jaw, see your doctor. If, for example, you have a salivary gland infection, you'll probably need treatment with antibiotics.

Salivary duct stones may need to be surgically removed, as do growths of any kind. And sometimes the whole gland will have to be taken out. But don't worry; your other salivary glands can usually compensate, keeping your mouth moist and healthy.

SYMPTOM: **Taste Abnormalities**

COMMON CAUSES: Having no taste is not just an affliction art critics need to dread. In fact, losing the ability to taste can be a symptom of a number of different problems, many of them serious.

Some of them involve the mouth, others the brain and others originate from farther afield. Some of them cause complete loss of taste, whereas others cause only partial loss. With some, you become unable to taste certain foods; with others, you're constantly saddled with a mysterious, phantom taste. This might not be unsettling if the taste were one you liked—if, say, you were haunted by the taste of peanut butter fudge. But more often, the ghostly taste is bitter, acidic, metallic or just plain ghastly. And it or any other taste abnormality is very disruptive. It affects your appetite. It affects your social life. So changes in your sense of taste are never unimportant.

Luckily, the most common cause of a loss of taste is also one of the most benign. The flu, when it's finally fleeing, will often temporarily rob you of the ability to taste. Over 25 percent of patients with taste abnormalities suffer from postinfluenzal hypogeusia—decreased ability to taste—and associated dysgeusia—distortion of the ability to taste, explains Robert I. Henkin, M.D., Ph.D., director of the Center for Molecular

Nutrition and Sensory Disorders at the Georgetown University Medical Center in Washington, D.C.

What does the flu do to take taste away? The usual agents that produce the symptoms of nasal stuffiness, fatigue and muscle aches, which are so common in the flu, also injure the taste buds. These same viruses may also injure smell receptors, causing a loss of smell. Hay fever and associated allergies, which produce stuffed noses, are also frequent culprits in taste robberies, mainly because they interfere with smell function, thereby reducing the flavor obtained from food.

The taste-robbers, though, needn't be strangers to your mouth. They can also be your mouth's sometime friends. Salivary glands, for example, may play a vital role in the process of taste. Any slowdown in the output of saliva may disrupt taste (see Symptom: Dry Mouth and Symptom: Swollen Salivary Glands).

And a rogue's gallery worth of unpleasant mouth disorders, though they don't steal your taste, can change it unpleasantly. Gum disease such as gingivitis and periodontitis (see Common Tooth and Gum Conditions in chapter 16) and tooth decay can leave a taste in your mouth that your mouth would rather not taste. So can necrotizing ulcerative gingivitis, or trench mouth (see Common Facial, Jaw and Mouth Conditions).

An even more irritating mouth problem is posed by dentures— irritating, that is, if you want to taste properly. New or tightly fitted dentures sometimes cause changes in taste. For one thing, they cover taste buds located on the roof of the mouth. This causes you to add more flavorings to food to obtain the expected taste.

You never "taste" things until your brain tells you that you taste them. Therefore, serious (though uncommon) neurological disorders, including brain tumors, cranial nerve abnormalities, strokes and head injuries can cause the sense of taste to diminish, disappear or become distorted.

A large range of other problems can do the same. Everything from ear surgery to vitamin and mineral deficiencies can affect taste, Dr. Henkin says. The hormonal disruptions that accompany pregnancy or menstruation can also make food taste peculiar. Or the side effects of certain drugs and the direct effects of last night's "excess" can cause the mouth to taste of mush.

Finally, nutritional deficiencies may announce themselves in the mouth. A lack of vitamin B_{12} or vitamin A sometimes causes loss of part or all of your taste. And a zinc deficiency almost always affects your sense of taste. "Clearly, zinc deficiency alters taste perception," concluded the authors of one comprehensive study.

BEST RESPONSE: "More often than not, the loss of taste is a medical and not a dental problem," says Robert J. Mallin, D.D.S. "It needs to be checked by a physician." *Any* sudden changes in your ability to taste or in how foods taste need to be evaluated, he emphasizes.

ACCOMPANYING SYMPTOMS: If you've lost your taste and also notice pain and redness around a wisdom tooth, it's a sign that the tooth might be infected.

You should be wise to the fact, though, that these same symptoms could indicate other problems. If you have the symptoms of an infected wisdom tooth, but with the telling addition of a small, flabby lump in your gum, a fever and possibly some swelling of your face and jaw, you may have an abscessed tooth.

In either case, you'll have to see your dentist as soon as possible.

Common Facial, Jaw and Mouth Conditions

Bell's palsy. Bell's palsy is simply a disturbance of one of the facial nerves. Each facial nerve starts out in the brain, then branches out from the main pathway toward the eyes, ears, tongue and chin. The palsy is believed to be caused by a virus, and it often follows a cold. Other causes are thought to be a tumor, injury, hereditary predisposition or the constriction or spasm of a blood vessel.

Bell's is slightly more common in women and is most likely to disappear without any residual effects if the nerve's paralysis—that's what causes the muscular weakness—occurs as a single episode, is painless, does not affect the whole face or begins gradually. Complete recovery is likely in 75 percent of those who have it, and satisfactory recovery occurs in another 15 percent. The nerve will not fully recover its ability to function in roughly 10 percent of those who get the palsy, but plastic surgery can frequently reduce any cosmetic problems.

Candidiasis. Also known as oral thrush, this condition is brought about by an invasion of fast-growing, yeasty fungus in the mouth. The fungus involved is one of the many microbes normally present in the mouth.

Normally, these microbes are kept in check by the body's immune system. But if natural resistance to infection is lowered, or if you're taking antibiotics that upset the balance of power among the mouth's microbes, the fungus will begin to multiply, and you'll develop oral thrush.

Candidiasis appears as creamy yellow, slightly raised, usually sore patches in the mouth. The patches can also sprout in the throat. If these patches are rubbed off while you're eating or brushing your teeth, they'll leave a painful, raw area.

The disease is especially troublesome for denture wearers, since the sores make dentures difficult to wear. But many people get it at some point in their lives. It's most prevalent among very young children and the elderly, and it sometimes indicates an underlying problem such as iron deficiency anemia or disorders of the immune system. Oral thrush has a disconcerting tendency to recur. But it's easily treatable. See your doctor, who will probably check for any underlying cause and then prescribe an antifungal agent in the form of lozenges.

Geographical tongue. This is a minor problem with a misleading name. It doesn't mean that your tongue has taken up globe-trotting. It does mean that part of your tongue is inflamed.

When you have geographical tongue, the papillae that normally cover the tongue no longer form properly. They no longer cover the whole tongue, leaving parts of it raw, red and often sore, especially when you eat spicy foods.

Geographical tongue occurs in patches that come and go, apparently at random. It has no known cause or cure. But it also has no known bad effects and will normally disappear in time.

Glossitis. This is a condition similar to geographical tongue, but with a less memorable name. Ironically, glossitis covers more territory than does geographical tongue; if you have glossitis, the entire tongue is inflamed, not just patches of it.

Like geographical tongue, glossitis is an inflammation of the tongue in which the papillae no longer cover its surface. Unlike geographical tongue, it has direct causes and can often be treated. Infection, allergies or poor nutrition can all produce glossitis, as can iron deficiency or pernicious anemia.

Once your doctor has identified the underlying condition responsible for the glossitis and has treated this problem, the glossitis should clear up without further ado. There are things, though, that you can do. Avoid hot or spicy foods and avoid anything else that would irritate your sore tongue—such as indulging in alcohol or tobacco.

Leukoplakia. This is a disease in which white, thickened patches develop inside the cheeks, on the lips or tongue or anywhere along the gums.

Leukoplakia most commonly occurs in middle-aged or elderly men. The white splotches it produces are often a reaction to a long-time irritant, such as tobacco, poorly fitted dentures or sometimes alcohol. The patches tend to become fissured and have an even stronger tendency to become malignant. If left untreated, they may grow or ulcerate, becoming acutely painful. Leukoplakia in the mouth will eventually interfere with the ability to swallow or speak.

Luckily, although leukoplakia is an unpleasant and unsightly disease, it's also a treatable one. Getting rid of the original irritant is essential. So, quit smoking (and, if necessary, drinking), have your dentures refitted and also cut back on your indulgence in hot, spicy, mouth-igniting foods. You'll help speed healing of the lesions. Surgical removal of the patchy places is simple and will normally arrest the disease's development. Sometimes drug therapy is needed.

But don't try any treatment on your own. Leukoplakia has a dismal (though deserved) reputation for turning into oral cancer, and, as the National Institute of Dental Research warns, oral cancer has an equally dismal (though deserved) reputation for being dangerous—the mouth's rich blood supply and convenient location mean a tumor can disseminate to other parts of the body. You need to see your dentist or physician if you have any of the symptoms of leukoplakia.

Necrotizing ulcerative gingivitis. Commonly known as trench mouth, this is a painful infection and ulceration of the gums, usually between the teeth. The infection can result from any number of different mouth problems, including failure to clean the teeth and gums properly. Throat infections, smoking or gingivitis (gum disease) can also contribute to the development of this problem.

Poor nutrition and poor oral hygiene, though, are probably the disease's major catalysts, especially when combined with lack of rest and stress. The problem is consequently most common in young adults who live for junk food, stay up all night and can't be bothered with flossing. Though the disease is not thought to be contagious, it did rage like wildfire through soldiers in the trenches of World War I; hence its name.

Necrotizing ulcerative gingivitis requires dental treatment, says Norman Wood, D.D.S., M.S., Ph.D., professor and chairman of the Department of Oral Diagnosis at Loyola University School of Dentistry in Maywood, Illinois. See your dentist if your gums are sore, swollen, bleeding or sore-splotched, or if you have persistent foul breath.

In the meantime, hydrogen peroxide mouthwashes will help relieve any pain and inflammation. Scrupulous dental hygiene is also essential, and you'll probably need a prescription antibiotic to fully clear up the infection. "Later," Dr. Wood adds, "the underlying causes need to be corrected."

One of these "causes" that you can and probably should correct involves your life-style; you wouldn't develop trench mouth if you weren't worn down, overloaded and anxious. Try instead to worry a bit more about your general health and a bit less about whatever causes you stress. Good health and self-care should help to get your mouth out of the trenches and will probably help you out of the dumps as well.

Oral lichen planus. This disorder usually begins with the eruption of small, pale pimples in your mouth, most frequently on the inside of your cheeks or along the sides of your tongue. These tiny sores gradually join to form a fine, white, lacy network of slightly raised tissue. More rarely, the problem appears as shiny red patches sprouting along the lining of your mouth or side of your tongue.

Oral lichen planus is rare. It most typically develops in people who also have lichen planus in the skin. It sometimes causes discomfort, including a sore mouth or an unpleasant taste in the mouth. But it sometimes produces virtually no symptoms. And its cause remains obscure. It can be brought on by stress or irritation in the mouth, or by poor oral hygiene.

The best treatment and preventive for oral lichen planus is good, conscientious oral hygiene. Keep your mouth healthy by brushing your teeth and gums thoroughly twice a day. If you have dentures, ask your dentist to check them for proper fit and to correct any rough spots. These measures should ensure that your mouth will stay healthy and lichenless. Getting proper nutrition and plenty of rest couldn't hurt either.

Temporomandibular joint disorder. Nobody really knows what causes this condition, popularly known as TMJ, or what cures it. Ask five different doctors how they treat it and you'll get five different answers.

Some doctors believe that the way the jaw is structured at birth, combined with episodes of intense stress, causes the problem. Other doctors think that TMJ is caused by sudden or prolonged injury to the joint, infection or the onset of degenerative or inflammatory joint disease. Still others think it's caused by poor mouth habits, including grinding the teeth during sleep, chewing pens, pencils or pipes, resting the jaw on the hands. Also under suspicion are certain musical instruments, such as the violin, clarinet and trumpet, which stress the jaw or put it in an unnatural position.

Given this confusion, it should hardly be surprising that treatments are just as varied. Some doctors recommend biofeedback, transcendental meditation, yoga exercises and reshaping the teeth. Others suggest muscle tension awareness and relaxation therapies with tape-recorded reinforcement. Still others suggest hot compresses, ice massages and refrigerant sprays—none of which should be used if you have heart, circulatory or diabetic problems. Corticosteroid injections are another suggested treatment, although at least one doctor warns that multiple injections can tear apart the cartilage in the jaw joint. Surgery is mentioned occasionally, but generally by surgeons and only in very specific and very limited terms.

Any and all of these treatments may be correct for particular individuals who have TMJ. Different strokes for different folks, right? But as one group of researchers at the University of Georgia suggests, the best way to look at TMJ may be as a number of interlocking factors. Some of the theories they considered were joint and muscle dysfunction, faulty meeting of teeth and jaw and psychological stress.

Don't be discouraged if you need to see more than one doctor or dentist or therapist to eliminate your TMJ symptoms. Nobody, apparently, has all the answers. As David Fairbanks, M.D., suggests to his own patients: "Stubborn cases of TMJ may require several visits to your dentist and your ear, nose and throat specialist. But the team approach is usually quite successful."

Tetanus. Tetanus, also known as lockjaw, is a disease that comes from bacteria that have been lying around on the ground—particularly where animals have been—for centuries. (Yes, we do mean centuries.)

The bacteria usually enter the body through a deep wound—splinters, nails and tacks at home or in the garden are frequently the cause—that air cannot reach. A stiff feeling in the face and neck between 8 and 12 days after the wound usually marks the disease's onset. Later, difficulty opening the mouth and muscle spasms throughout the body will occur. And if you wait that long to go to the hospital emergency room, spasms may affect the muscles used for breathing, making it impossible to breathe.

Because there's a vaccine available that prevents the disease, nobody should die of tetanus. But people do, especially in the southeastern United States. Some people just can't seem to find the time or money to call their doctor or district health center and arrange for the shot. As a result, between 40 and 60 percent of those who contract tetanus will die—usually of sudden cardiac arrest. In developing nations such as Bangladesh, tetanus accounts for 26 percent of all infants who die.

Treatment for tetanus is generally aimed at maintaining life support until the body can eliminate the poisonous bacteria. Generally, doctors will open your throat to insert a tube that will keep your airway open. They may also provide a machine that can do your breathing for you. And another tube may be inserted into a vein in your neck. Sedatives, relaxants and anticonvulsant drugs may be given, as well as tetanus shots and antibiotics. The site of the wound may be given a special deep cleaning, and a tube that will provide fluids and nutrients will be passed through your nose to your stomach. Physiotherapy will be provided, and some doctors will also intravenously administer vitamin C.

But of all the treatments involved, several studies have found that one of the most important aspects of in-hospital tetanus care is the standard of nursing and monitoring. Keeping a sharp eye on someone for 48 days of hospital care—the average length of stay for tetanus—may be expensive. But it definitely seems to save lives.

If you get a deep puncture wound, see your doctor immediately. He or she may want to perform a special procedure that deep-cleans the wound, and to give you some antibiotics, a tetanus immune globulin and subsequent booster, or a primary tetanus shot.

Better yet, get a tetanus shot before you get hurt. The difference between hundreds of thousands of deaths due to tetanus during World War I and only seven tetanus deaths in World War II was one little shot called a tetanus toxoid immunization.

Tic douloureux. Tic douloureux—literally, "painful twitch"—is a syndrome in which a burning pain zips down a nerve in the face without warning. Its causes are generally unknown, but it's most likely to affect people over the age of 50. It can be triggered simply by shaving or washing your face or eating something very hot or cold. Even a cold draft has been known to bring it on.

Doctors frequently prescribe anticonvulsant drugs such as Tegretol, and an experimental form of an old drug—baclofen—may also prove helpful. But when drug therapies fail—or the side effects such as nausea, dizziness, fatigue and serious bone marrow problems can't be handled— it's time to consult a surgeon.

There are a number of surgical techniques that can relieve tic pain, says Russell H. Patterson, Jr., M.D., a professor of surgery and neurosurgery at Cornell Medical Center in New York City. But most involve trading off a degree of facial sensitivity for a degree of relief.

The most effective and least destructive technique, says Dr. Patterson, is microsurgical decompression, an operation in which a sponge is inserted between the trigeminal nerve, which controls facial sensation, and any neighboring vein, artery or bone that may be periodically putting pressure on the nerve.

If it sounds as though no one is really sure whether or not nerve compression causes tic, that's because they aren't. But they do know that the procedure relieves pain in 78 to 90 percent of the people who undergo it. Unfortunately, the chance that pain will recur—as it does with other tic procedures—is one in ten.

And microsurgical decompression *is* major surgery, emphasizes Dr. Patterson, which means it's only for those in good health. Tic douloureux victims who are not in the best health, however, have other options. Transcutaneous electrical nerve stimulation (TENS) and radiofrequency coagulation—a procedure that actually involves burning the trigeminal nerve's root—are helpful in almost half the people on whom they're performed. And surgical injections of glycerol can relieve pain in 67 percent of tic douloureux victims. Recurrent pain is not unusual with any of these procedures, however.

Some doctors also continue to recommend alcohol injections or freezing, although these treatments require expert administration and are rarely effective for any length of time. Of course, sometimes even a day free of pain is worth the risk. Especially when that pain is triggered by washing your face.

Chapter 9

Feet

SEE YOUR DOCTOR IMMEDIATELY IF:
- *A callused area becomes sore, red or hot or begins to ooze*
- *A sore on your foot doesn't heal*
- *You experience unexplained numbness, tingling or other unusual sensations in your feet*

Your feet have 52 bones, 38 muscles, 66 joints and 250,000 sweat glands between them—plus 214 ligaments to hold everything together. That's a lot to stuff into the fashionable styles of modern-day glass slippers. But it certainly doesn't stop you from trying.

Sharp toes, pointed toes, curled-up toes or no toes—if it looks cute we'll wear it. Whether it's Cinderella's pumps or Prince Charming's boots, we think nothing of balancing our bodies on three-inch stacks, four-inch stilettos or six-inch platforms.

The problem is that most of us have the feet of Cinderella's stepsisters rather than those of Cinderella herself. And in trying to make our feet look like what they're not, we sometimes crush a muscle here, stretch a ligament there or bend a joint over on the other side. Then we wonder why our feet ache!

Fortunately, many folks have discovered that wide toe boxes, one-inch heels, arch supports and heavy-duty shock absorbers between foot and pavement will prevent or slow down the development of bunions, blisters, corns, calluses, aches and most of the symptoms discussed in this chapter. And the shoes don't have to look like nineteenth-century orthopedic devices either. Zippy running shoes, flashy flats and cushy sandals can all provide a healthy podiatric environment with pizzazz— even if they aren't Cinderella's slippers.

But it takes some time for even enlightened feet to recover from the excess of fashion. So until they do, here's a guide to relieving the discomforts of life in—and on—the fast lane.

SYMPTOM: **Blisters.** *See* Symptom: Blisters in chapter 15

SYMPTOM: **Bunions**

COMMON CAUSE: Bunions are inherited, just like the color of your hair or the point on your chin, says Stephen Weinberg, D.P.M., director of podiatry at Columbus Hospital's Running and Sports Medicine Clinic in Chicago. They're caused when something in the way you walk encourages the big toe to turn toward the second toe. That in turn pushes one of the bones that form the arch out of alignment and makes it stick out like a big lump on the side of your foot. Bunions are aggravated by high-heeled and narrow-toed shoes.

BEST RESPONSE: "Your bones are programmed to grow at that angle," says Dr. Weinberg, "and there's no way you can stop them." A small percentage of people can slow down the development of bunions by using custom-designed arch supports prescribed by a podiatrist or orthopedist, but once the bunions have appeared—frequently around age 50 or 60—they need to be surgically removed. Afterward, says Dr. Weinberg, you should wear an arch support in your shoe to control foot movement while walking.

Warm foot soaks, aspirin and a special "bunion-last" shoe made with extra room in the toe may relieve your discomfort until you can get to the doctor.

SYMPTOM: **Burning**

COMMON CAUSES: Feet usually feel as though they're burning when there's not enough air circulating between the world inside your shoe and the one outside. When part or all of the shoe is made from a synthetic material—rubber soles, for example—heat generated by your foot is trapped inside until it roasts your piggies. Synthetic socks and stockings also contribute to the problem, as do ill-fitting shoes that rub your feet.

But sometimes it's just the gait with which you were born or, less frequently, vascular or circulatory diseases such as hardened arteries (see arteriosclerosis under Common Circulatory, Heart and Lung Conditions in chapter 5).

In rare instances, burning feet indicate heavy metal poisoning with compounds of lead, arsenic, mercury or lithium.

BEST RESPONSE: If you suspect your feet are on fire from hot shoes or the way you walk, pick up a pair of SPENCO insoles, says Stephen Weinberg, D.P.M. SPENCO insoles are an open-cell foam material that will reduce heat and friction inside your shoes.

But if you have any reason to suspect that neither heat nor gait is the problem, says Dr. Weinberg, see your podiatrist or physician.

SYMPTOM: **Corns and Calluses.** *See* Symptom: Thickening in chapter 15

SYMPTOM: **Heel, Black Marks on**

COMMON CAUSES: Tiny hemorrhages under your skin can produce brown or black dots on the back or bottom of your heel that make it look like you forgot to wash your feet. Sometimes the hemorrhages are caused by shoes that pinch the heel during athletic events such as basketball or tennis, but more often, says Stephen Weinberg, D.P.M., those little hemorrhages are caused by flat feet.

The heels of people with flat feet tend to roll inward when they walk, says Dr. Weinberg. Their rolling gait sets up push/pull forces on the sole of the shoe that—added to stiff leather or an uncushioned heel cup, for example—cause the shoe to pinch. Walk around with what amounts to a lobster claw in your shoe and black marks will appear in no time.

Black marks, however, can also mean that you have warts (see Symptom: Warts, Plantar), but, if this is the case, the marks most probably will be very painful.

BEST RESPONSE: Ignore them, doctors say. Your body will simply reabsorb the blood. If you don't like the way they look—when you wear sandals, for example—or your heel starts to hurt, ask your podiatrist to shave some of the accumulated dead skin off and the "marks" will go with it.

If you tend to develop these marks with any frequency, says Dr. Weinberg, make sure any new shoes you buy have reinforced heel backs—the kind that are found in hiking boots or running shoes.

SYMPTOM: **Heel, Bump on**

COMMON CAUSES: Heel bumps, which foot-weary women sometimes refer to as "pump bumps" in honor of that fashionable low-cut shoe style, can be caused by a prominence of the heel bone itself, says Stephen Weinberg, D.P.M. Or, particularly in people with high arches, the bumps can be caused by a heel bone that tends to roll inward and rub against your shoe as you walk.

If the bump seems to appear and disappear as though it's the result of swelling, however, two fluid-filled sacs under the skin in the heel area may be inflamed.

BEST RESPONSE: "Sometimes just raising the heel up out of the shoe by putting a heel lift underneath can alleviate pressure from the shoe," says Dr. Weinberg. But be sure to put a lift in both shoes, he cautions, so you don't trade a foot problem for a back problem.

An arch support prescribed by your podiatrist or orthopedist can control the roll of your foot if a high arch is causing your bump, and a butterfly pad—glued to the back of your shoe by a shoemaker—can reduce pressure on the fluid-filled sacs at the back of your heel.

SYMPTOM: **Itching**

COMMON CAUSES: Itchy feet are generally caused by athlete's foot (see Common Foot Conditions) or an allergy to the tanning chemicals used in leather shoes, says Stephen Weinberg, D.P.M.

The way to tell the difference is to check for the little blisters and peeling skin that also accompany athlete's foot. If there's only a generalized itching and some redness, says Dr. Weinberg, chances are the culprit is a new pair of shoes. Socks, he adds, are rarely a problem.

BEST RESPONSE: The first thing you can do, says Dr. Weinberg, is to take an over-the-counter antihistamine. That will relieve the itch until you've got the athlete's foot under control or have discovered and stopped wearing whatever pair of shoes is triggering an allergic response.

But once you've stopped scratching, says Dr. Weinberg, you can apply cool, wet compresses to the itchy area, then allow it to dry. Keep putting on fresh compresses, allowing the water to evaporate off your skin in between, for 15 minutes twice a day. If you have athlete's foot, follow the compresses with an antifungal powder. A nonprescription medication containing either tolnaftate or miconazole usually zaps the fungus into oblivion, doctors agree, although more severe cases may need a prescription medication from your physician.

The itching should begin to disappear within 48 to 72 hours, says Dr. Weinberg, but if it doesn't, check with your podiatrist or dermatologist. And in the future, remember that trying to keep the spaces between your toes dry is the best way to prevent a recurrence. Briefly soaking your feet once a day in warm salt water also helps. However, long and frequent soaks should be avoided. Also, don't wash your feet with soap more than once a day. Repeated washing with soap washes away an acid film that normally protects your body from bacterial invaders. Air dry your feet for five to ten minutes after cleansing and rub—don't sprinkle—a powder such as ZeaSORB into your feet, your socks and your shoes.

You should also wear 100 percent cotton socks, doctors advise, and leather shoes rather than shoes made of canvas or synthetics. Leather will absorb the half a pint of perspiration you excrete through your feet every day, and if you give each pair of shoes every other day off, the moisture will have a chance to evaporate instead of condense on your feet. You should also avoid shoes and boots treated with a water repellent, since repellents keep perspiration in as well as they keep water out.

SYMPTOM: **Odor**

COMMON CAUSE: Stinky feet are caused by the breakdown of bacteria that normally live on the skin, says Stephen Weinberg, D.P.M. Unfortunately, that process can be exacerbated by excessive perspiration, hot, humid weather and the lack of breathability of shoes and socks.

BEST RESPONSE: "Change your socks two or three times a day," advises Dr. Weinberg. Wear cotton socks and, for mild problems, use the charcoal-impregnated insoles available in drugstores.

If your feet perspire heavily, however, you may also want to lightly roll an underarm antiperspirant over the soles of your feet and the tips of your toes. But be sure you have no active athlete's foot lesions—the antiperspirant will burn if you do—and check to make sure the product contains an aluminum or zirconium compound, not just the stuff that makes you smell good. But don't bother with spray antiperspirants, says Dr. Weinberg. Most of their antiperspirant action is lost in the air when you use them.

Apply the antiperspirant two or three times a day for starters, he suggests, and gradually reduce the number of applications to once a day as your feet get dryer. If your feet still smell after two or three weeks, your podiatrist can prescribe a stronger antiperspirant to use at bedtime. Some people find, however, that soaking their feet in a strong solution of tea for 15 minutes each day can also reduce foot perspiration—as long as you don't mind tea-colored feet.

SYMPTOM: **Pain**

COMMON CAUSES: Pain can originate from anywhere in the foot: skin, nerves, blood vessels, muscles, ligaments, bones, joints, tendons or bursae—the body's internal cushions. It can be caused by arthritis (see Common Bone, Joint and Muscle Conditions in chapter 3), diabetes mellitus (see Common Whole Body Conditions in chapter 19), calluses and corns (see Symptom: Thickening in chapter 15), bunions (see Symptom: Bunions), fibrous growths, entrapped nerves, past injuries, current fractures and even tiny splinters. If the pain is confined to a toe or toes, the problem could be gout (see Common Bone, Joint and Muscle Conditions in chapter 3). If the pain is confined to the heel, it could be plantar fasciitis (see Common Foot Conditions).

But the major cause of pain is simply the way your foot is formed and the way you use it when you walk.

BEST RESPONSE: You need to see a doctor to help you sort out the causes, says Stephen Weinberg, D.P.M. Frequently, however, all that's necessary is a custom-designed arch support and a good pair of shoes.

Pain on the bottom of your foot between the heel and toes—especially on the ball of your foot—can frequently be relieved by switching to a shoe with a softer midsole and adding a cushioned arch support (available at your local drugstore), says Dr. Weinberg. Cutting down on your current level of activity is also helpful, as is icing the area if the pain is accompanied by any swelling.

Generally, says Dr. Weinberg, "icing should be done at least a couple of times a day—morning and night, but especially after any athletic activity. I like ice massage in particular, where the patient actually freezes up some Styrofoam cups of water, then peels back the Styrofoam and massages the ice over the area for 15 minutes—no longer.

"Doing that really helps a good bit, as does taking aspirin two to four times a day—as long as you have no aspirin allergy or history of stomach or bleeding problems—for five to seven days."

The treatment for heel pain is a custom-made arch support to correct the way you walk. Not only will it make walking more bearable during your recovery, while ice treatments and aspirin relieve the pain, but it will also *prevent* heel pain in the future. If the pain was caused by a direct injury to the foot, however, your doctor may suggest an injection of a steroid drug such as cortisone.

Generally, doctors agree, you should also switch to shoes that will help your arch supports control the way you walk. A stable shoe that doesn't allow your foot to wobble, good shock absorption and a flexible sole are the three qualities you should look for. And the shoe that is closest to meeting all three criteria, doctors say, is a running or walking shoe.

SYMPTOM: **Swelling.** *See also* Symptom: Swelling in chapter 19

COMMON CAUSES: "Everybody's feet are going to swell by the end of the day, just because gravity pulls fluid down into your legs," says Stephen Weinberg, D.P.M. And if you sit a lot, he adds, that restricts the flow of blood to the feet and causes swelling.

Pressurized aircraft cabins can also cause swollen feet, he says, as can arthritis (see Common Bone, Joint and Muscle Conditions in chapter 3) or a broken bone.

BEST RESPONSE: "Every tissue has its critical limits of stress," says Dr. Weinberg, "and what you've got to do is back off. Take a rest, change your shoes, elevate your feet—just give your feet a breather."

If your feet are actually so swollen that you see a line and indentation where your feet were in your shoes, says Dr. Weinberg, see your doctor. You could have a circulatory problem that requires further treatment.

SYMPTOM: **Toe, Blackened.** *See* Symptom: Bleeding in
        chapter 11

SYMPTOM: **Warts, Plantar**

COMMON CAUSE: Warts are not caused by an intimate encounter with a toad, doctors say, or manual abuse of a particular organ. They are caused by a virus that invades the skin, usually through a cut or abrasion on the bottom of the foot. They tend to nest in a non-weight-bearing area and multiply, but they never go any deeper than the skin. Tiny black dots, which are blood vessels that nourish the wart, form on the surface, and sometimes a callus develops, too. Unfortunately, plantar warts can become quite painful.

BEST RESPONSE: Some warts disappear without any treatment and others hang around for years despite every medical treatment available. Some disappear when rubbed with potatoes, saliva or cod-liver oil; others thrive and grow.

"You can also use commercial corn remover preparations on them," says Stephen Weinberg, D.P.M., who believes the acid in the corn remover will irritate the wart and cause it to go into remission. Diabetics and those with poor blood circulation should not use this product because serious complications could result.

"If it hurts and is causing limping and other walking problems," adds Dr. Weinberg, "go to your podiatrist. A lot of times these things can be scooped out of the skin and cauterized under a local anesthetic and that's it. No stitches, no nothing, and you're walking on it right away. All that's left is a little burn that fills in within a couple of weeks."

Soon, however, doctors may be trading in their cautery irons for lasers. Podiatrists have been vaporizing warts with a 95 percent success rate, researchers report, and the only thing holding up the widespread use of lasers is the cost.

Common Foot Conditions

Athlete's foot.   Athlete's foot is the name given to any one of 20 superficial fungus infections that can grow on the skin of the feet. The fungus thrives in the warm, moist environment provided by your shoes and socks and snuggles blissfully in the perpetual darkness between your toes.

It may seem to be little more than a minor irritation, but the cracked skin and popped blisters that usually accompany the condition make it possible for bacteria to enter the body and cause an infection. And just like any other bacterial infection, if left untreated it can spread throughout the bloodstream and attack virtually any organ of its choosing. Fortunately, with today's fungal repellents, it never has to get that far.

Plantar fasciitis.   The most common type of heel pain is caused by plantar fasciitis, an inflammation of the broad ligament that spreads out along the bottom of the foot from a point on the heel toward the big and little toes. The pain is not directly under the heel pad itself, but just in front. It's usually at its worst when you first get up in the morning or after any period when you've been off your feet.

The condition develops when you constantly walk in a way that pulls hard on the area where the fascia attaches to the heel bone. The bone eventually begins to grow in the direction of the pull—creating the distinctive shape on x-rays that causes doctors to call the condition a bone spur or heel spur—and the fascia itself shortens. At this point it becomes necessary for the fascia to overextend itself every time you take a step. The result is inflammation and pain. Fortunately, treatment is as easy as proper support for your arch.

Chapter 10
Hair and Scalp

SEE YOUR DOCTOR IMMEDIATELY IF:
- *You have a continuous or recurrent bleeding wound on the scalp*
- *You find a lump on your scalp following a blow and you feel drowsy, confused or nauseated*
- *You have a lump or sore on your scalp that does not go away within a month*

Are your tresses stressed? Are they frazzled or limp as a wet noodle? Does your 100-stroke-a-night habit appear to leave 100 strands in your brush? If so, you have troubles. Not life-threatening troubles, but definitely cosmetic or even psychological ones.

If the condition of your thatch is not all you'd like it to be, you've probably got no one to blame but yourself (or, in most cases of baldness, your ancestors). Abusing your hair with too much curling, straightening, dyeing or bleaching could be the cause of your frazzled look. Or you could be pulling your hair out by the roots every night with that 100-stroke brushing. Best to forget that old custom.

There are other self-inflicted factors that can threaten a healthy head of hair, according to Philip Kingsley, a renowned authority on hair care. Severe, unsupervised dieting and severe, sudden stress are two that may contribute to problem hair. Illness, hormonal changes and certain common drugs are other factors that affect hair health.

SYMPTOM: **Dandruff/Flaking**

COMMON CAUSES: Dandruff—"snow on the shoulders"—is an acceleration of the normal process of shedding dead cells to make way for new ones. This happens all over the body, but it is most noticeable on the scalp because the flakes of old cells get trapped in the hair shafts and can be seen as small white scales. The condition is more noticeable in some people than in others.

Dandruff is often an inherited problem, but it also can be aggravated by stress, hormonal changes and bad diet. What it's not is "catching" —you can't get it by using someone else's comb or brush. And it's one of life's few annoyances that gets less bothersome with age. Approximately 50 percent of those between 10 and 20 years of age have dandruff problems. After age 30, the percentage drops.

Flaking, however, doesn't always mean dandruff. If you've been out in the hot sun with no protection on your head and you later notice peeling and flaking of the skin, you probably have a sunburn. In the future, cover up with a sun hat.

BEST RESPONSE: Ordinary cases of dandruff require no medical treatment, doctors say, and daily shampooing will remove unsightly flakes. If regular shampooing is inadequate, an over-the-counter dandruff product that contains zinc pyrithione or selenium sulfide can be used. These medications work well and have few toxic effects, so they can be used daily. Coal tar products should be reserved for problem dandruff that fails to respond to lesser treatment, and they can be used intermittently with a zinc or selenium shampoo.

When using one of these products, follow the manufacturer's directions regarding duration of treatment and warnings. If none of these treatments is effective, you may then want to see your physician, who may prescribe a steroid lotion to suppress the underlying cause of the dandruff. Or, if bad diet is suspected, a sensible, well-balanced eating program may be the solution.

ACCOMPANYING SYMPTOMS: If your dandruff is large and coarse and is accompanied by redness and irritation of the scalp as well as patches of redness and scales on other parts of the body (such as the face, elbows, knees, chest, back and pubis), you probably have seborrheic dermatitis (see dermatitis/eczema under Common Skin Conditions in chapter 15) or psoriasis (see Common Skin Conditions in chapter 15). These are more complex problems that require treatment by a physician.

SYMPTOM: **Excess Hair**

COMMON CAUSE: Men don't usually mind being hairy. Women do. If you're a woman and excess hair appears on your face or body before age 20, and other women in the family have the same problem, the cause is usually hereditary. If you're pregnant, everything seems to grow more— including hair. It's merely a symptom of hormonal changes.

In a woman beyond age 40 or one who has had her ovaries removed, the decreased level of estrogen can cause excessive hair growth, especially on the face. Taking certain drugs, such as hormones, cortisone drugs or anticonvulsants, can also cause this problem.

BEST RESPONSE: If your excess hair growth is due to heredity or a temporary hormone imbalance, you can use an over-the-counter bleaching preparation to lighten facial hair, or consult a cosmetologist about permanently removing it by a method known as electrolysis. If your problem is brought on by pregnancy, it should go away after the baby's born.

ACCOMPANYING SYMPTOMS: If excessive hair growth is accompanied by unexplained weight gain, a deepening voice and menstrual changes (including absence of periods), you could have an abnormality of the ovaries. Another possibility is Cushing's disease, which is due to either a tumor of the adrenal glands or a problem with the pituitary gland. In either case, see your doctor.

SYMPTOM: **Graying**

COMMON CAUSES: Contrary to what mother may have told you, hair can't turn gray overnight because of some shock or terrible scare. Graying, unless it's done by chemical means, is a slow process that occurs because of a lack of pigment (melanin) produced by the cortex of the hair shaft. It's simply another sign of aging.

Periods of great stress, however, *can* cause alopecia areata, in which hair falls out in patches and new hairs grow in white. But this is not the usual case.

The age at which you start to gray (we *all* gray if we live long enough) is a question of heredity. So if you know someone up in years who has no sign of gray and claims not to have any artificial help (Ronald Reagan may come to mind), simply credit it to good genes.

BEST RESPONSE: There's no way to avoid the inevitable. You can only hide it. If you feel your youth is being stolen by gray locks, you can try temporary or permanent hair coloring.

SYMPTOM: **Ingrown Hair**

COMMON CAUSES: This is a problem reserved almost exclusively for dark-skinned men or men with coarse, curly hair. Stiff hairs on the face or neck penetrate the skin before leaving the follicle, or else they leave the follicle, then curve and reenter the skin. The result is a small, annoying pimple. Although less common, ingrown hairs can also occur in the armpit of an adult who shaves.

BEST RESPONSE: The best way to avoid ingrown hairs is to grow a beard. The second best solution is to adopt the Don Johnson (of "Miami Vice") look—take a rest from the razor for a day or two.
    But if neither solution is you (and it probably isn't), and you must shave every day, make sure you shave *properly.* Go with the grain of the hair, do not stretch the skin, use a light touch and always use a sharp blade. Sometimes changing to an electric razor helps. (For more tips on shaving, see Symptom: Irritation in chapter 15.)
    If ingrown hairs seem like a perpetual problem, you might want to consult a physician. Also, if an ingrown hair seems unusually sore or red, or even oozes, it could be a sign of infection. It's time to see the doctor.

SYMPTOM: **Itching.** *See also* Symptom: Itching in
                chapter 15

COMMON CAUSES: In young children and teenagers, an itchy scalp can be due to head lice or ringworm of the scalp (see Common Hair and Scalp Conditions), or to the fact that they haven't washed their hair in a while—again.
    In adults, the most common cause is an inflammatory dandruff condition called seborrheic dermatitis (see dermatitis/eczema under

Common Skin Conditions in chapter 15). Itching can also be a result of an allergy or sensitivity to an ingredient in hair products such as color rinses, dyes, permanent-wave solutions, setting lotions, hair sprays, conditioners or even shampoos.

An itchy scalp can also be a sign of psoriasis (see Common Skin Conditions in chapter 15).

BEST RESPONSE: The best and most effective way to get rid of head lice is with Kwell (lindane), a pediculide shampoo sold only by prescription, says E. Stanley Rodier, M.D., a La Jolla, California, dermatologist.

"One application, left on for five or ten minutes, is usually sufficient, but I frequently recommend repeating it the next night just to be sure," he says. "This product will kill the lice, but the nits, or eggs, will remain attached to the hair. The presence of these nits doesn't indicate active disease, but they can be removed with the fingers, tweezers or a fine-tooth comb."

Dr. Rodier doesn't automatically require that the entire family undergo the treatment if one child comes home with head lice. It depends how closely they've been in contact. "If an only child, for example, has head lice and the parents have no evidence of itching, there's no reason for them to undergo the treatment."

"Ringworm is not as common as it once was, and the fungi that cause the condition are different in different parts of the country," says Dr. Rodier. "Additionally, the severity of ringworm can vary from very mild and superficial to a serious condition that destroys hair follicles. For this reason, a dermatologist should diagnose and treat the condition."

The problem with seborrheic dermatitis is that the more you scratch, the worse the symptoms can get. Redness, swelling, weeping and crusting can occur. For a mild or moderate condition, says Dr. Rodier, over-the-counter dandruff shampoos are sufficient. If the problem persists, however, see a dermatologist, who will look for the underlying cause of the itching. In severe cases, says Dr. Rodier, prescription topical steroids may be needed.

Seborrheic dermatitis can occur in other parts of the body, particularly where oil glands are large and numerous.

If your itching problem is due to an allergy or sensitivity, and you can find the hair substance that's causing the problem, it's easy to eliminate the cause. But if that source can't be found and the itch persists, you should see your doctor.

As for psoriasis, diagnosis must be made by a physician. Although there is no cure for this disease, it can be treated with shampoos and PUVA, which is a therapy that combines the use of a medication, psoralen, with ultraviolet light treatments. In acute flare-ups, steroids sometimes are prescribed.

SYMPTOM: **Limp Hair**

COMMON CAUSES: Any veterinarian will tell you that one of the first signs of an unhealthy animal is a dull, lifeless coat. The truth is, what applies to Fido also applies to you. If *your* topknot is lifeless and lusterless, it could mean something is not right with your health. It can be a sign that you're not eating properly. It can even be a sign of anemia (see Common Whole Body Conditions in chapter 19). If you are sick or are recovering from an illness, dull, lifeless hair is just another symptom of the disease.

Also, think about where you've taken your hair lately. Has it been exposed to the sun or excess bottle bleaching? Have you been dunking it in the sea or a chlorinated pool? Has it been excessively lashed by the wind? Environment, too, can take its toll.

BEST RESPONSE: When your hair has lost its glow, look for other symptoms, such as pallor, fatigue, weakness, breathlessness or palpitations. If any of these are present, see your physician to find the source of your problem.

If you've recently been ill but are now on the road to recovery, be assured that proper nutrition and time will soon bring the shine back to your hair.

In the meantime, frequent shampooing with a low or neutral pH shampoo, followed by conditioning, will help restore lost sheen. The general rule of thumb is, the thicker the conditioner, the better it is for your hair. This, plus protecting your hair while outdoors, will also help if you suspect that it's the environment that is taking its toll on your hair.

SYMPTOM: **Loss of Hair**

COMMON CAUSES: On any given day, 90 percent of the hairs on your head are in an active growing state, which lasts from six months to two or three years. The other 10 percent are in a resting stage for a period of two to six months, then they fall out. All of this means that you can expect to lose 50 to 100 hairs a day. This is considered normal. If your hair loss consistently seems greater than that, it is not normal and you should look for a cause.

Poor diet—especially lack of protein—can cause growing hairs to shift into the resting phase. Severe hair loss will follow two to three months later. Iron deficiency anemia (see anemia under Common Whole Body Conditions in chapter 19) can also result in shedding.

Certain medications can also cause reversible hair loss, although this happens only in a relatively small percentage of people taking them. Some anticoagulants, antidepressants, antiarthritic and antigout drugs, as well as high blood pressure medicines and high doses of vitamin A, have all been implicated. You can also shed while you're taking birth control pills, or two to three months after you've stopped using them. Certain drugs used in cancer treatment can cause a loss of up to 90 percent of the patient's hair. The same goes for radiation therapy.

Any trauma in your life—such as major surgery, infection or high fever—can cause hair loss several months after the incident. A new mother may feel like pulling her hair out a few months after her baby is born, but it can fall out all on its own as a natural accompaniment to childbirth.

Thinning hair is also part of the package in thyroid disease (see Common Whole Body Conditions in chapter 19) and scleroderma, a relatively rare skin disease characterized by excessively hard, thickened skin.

The most common cause of thinning hair, however, is hereditary balding. And it can be inherited from either the mother's or the father's side of the family. It can also happen in both sexes. In men, the usual pattern is for the front hairline to recede as hair thins at the top of the head; eventually the balding areas join. Almost never are the sides or far back of the scalp affected. In women, thinning is gradual and occurs all over the head.

There is a specific but rare disease, alopecia areata, in which hair usually comes out in totally smooth, round patches about the size of a coin or larger. Occasionally it results in complete baldness and loss of some or all of the body hair. Both sexes can have this disease, and it occurs in all races and ages, although it's most common in people under 25.

BEST RESPONSE: Hair loss caused by a poor diet is reversible, says Thomas M. Krop, M.D., of Virginia Beach, Virginia. He advises eating a balanced diet supplemented with a daily multivitamin or B complex vitamin. If dietary indiscretion *was* the problem, he says, your hair shedding should cease in two to four months and then normal hair growth should resume.

If your hair loss is a result of illness, pregnancy or medication, time will usually restore the normal fullness. But it takes six months to a year for the normal hair-growth cycle to reestablish itself, says E. Stanley Rodier, M.D. So be patient.

"Recovery happens to a greater or lesser extent, depending on age, heredity or other factors," says Dr. Rodier. "Patience is most important in waiting for the normal hair rhythm to be reestablished. To make the hair seem fuller and more luxuriant, various high-protein, low or acid pH shampoos and conditioners are commercially available."

For some people, a medication called minoxidil may offer hope for baldness. Check with your doctor or dermatologist to see if it might work for you. Hair transplantation may also be an option; a dermatologist can tell you if you'd be a good candidate for this procedure. Otherwise, you'll simply have to get used to your new look. Or you may find comfort in wearing a wig or toupee.

In the majority of cases, the cause of alopecia areata is not known; occasionally an underlying illness, especially a hormonal condition, may be involved. "The future course in alopecia areata is unpredictable, and may get better or worse," says Dr. Rodier. "Treatment involves local surface application or injection of steroid drugs."

SYMPTOM: **Lump**

COMMON CAUSES: If you bang your head (or someone bangs it for you), a painful, tender lump may follow. The swelling usually occurs at the site of the encounter and the skin, if visible, becomes discolored.

You've got a bruise. If, however, the swelling is large and soft and not necessarily confined to the spot where head met foe, you could have a more serious problem, such as a skull fracture.

If you find a painless lump on your head and you haven't had a run-in with someone or something, it could be a wart or a sebaceous (pilar) cyst. A sebaceous cyst occurs when the gland that lubricates the hair becomes blocked. The secretions become trapped inside and turn solid.

The lump could also be a dermoid cyst. This uncommon developmental cyst found in early childhood occurs at the junctions of skull bones or the root of the nose or the corners of the eyebrow and is attached to underlying bone rather than skin. The cyst enlarges very slowly and may not be noticeable until a child reaches ten years of age.

BEST RESPONSE: To treat a painful lump that occurs at the site of an injury, doctors recommend applying cool compresses. It helps reduce the swelling.

Dermoid cysts are harmless growths that can be surgically removed. Sebaceous cysts, however, can usually be left alone. Although painless and benign, they sometimes grow larger and are prone to infection. When they become troublesome, doctors say, it's best to remove them.

ACCOMPANYING SYMPTOMS: If the blow on the head was hard, if you were knocked out or lost your memory or you feel drowsy, nauseated or confused, check with your doctor. See your doctor also if the swelling is not confined to the site of injury.

SYMPTOM: **Split Ends**

COMMON CAUSES: Split ends are the result of hair abuse. Too much dye or bleach, too many permanent waves and overuse of hot rollers, curling irons and blow dryers can all bring on a headful of split ends. So, too, can dry hair and too much brushing and teasing.

BEST RESPONSE: A quick fix for split ends is to cut them off and to continue trimming your locks every six to eight weeks. A more basic solution is to treat your hair more tenderly, condition it regularly and avoid those hair rituals that are known to cause damage.

Common Hair and Scalp Conditions

Head lice.   Pediculosis capitis, known to all mothers of school-age children as head lice, spreads quickly. *Any* child can bring it home. It's simply a matter of being in the wrong place at the wrong time.

Itching starts at the back of the scalp near the nape of the neck and around the ears. Later the whole head is itching. It can even involve the eyelashes. To diagnose the problem, look through your child's hair (or, heaven forbid, your own) for a gray-brown, shiny speck—about one-eighth inch long—crawling on the scalp. Remove it with tweezers and look at it under a magnifying glass. If the legs wiggle, you can bet it's a head louse. If you spot pearly gray lumps attached to the hair near the scalp, you've found the lice's eggs (nits).

An infestation of lice will often cause lymph nodes at the base of the skull to enlarge. To treat the problem, a physician can prescribe effective shampoos and lotions and will tell you other ways to kill both the lice and the nits. A very fine comb can be used for nit picking.

Ringworm of the scalp.   Tinea capitis, or ringworm of the scalp, is highly contagious and, fortunately, not the problem it used to be. "Probably, better hygiene—especially in children—is the reason we don't see it as often," says E. Stanley Rodier, M.D.

There are a number of different fungi that cause ringworm, and the appearance that each makes is slightly different. Grayish bald patches can occur with one kind and characteristic black dots (resulting from broken hairs) can occur with another. Itching and inflammation are common. This condition is best diagnosed and treated by a physician.

Chapter 11
Nails

SEE YOUR DOCTOR IMMEDIATELY IF:
- *Pus oozes from your nail*
- *Your nails turn white or take on a bluish tint*
- *Your nail or nails turn brown, black or green and the color won't go away*

Kids slam 'em in doors and adults hit 'em with hammers. And in between the doors and the hammers, they get torn, ripped, sliced, cracked and otherwise abused. They also do their own share of abusing—piercing, poking, stabbing and scratching.

Yet, what would you do without your nails?

For one thing, you wouldn't have a handy tool to scrape bubble gum off the bottom of your shoe or paint off the countertop. Nor could you scrape price stickers off gifts, pierce the cellophane around the supermarket cantaloupe or have something to gnaw on when the boss gets you nervous. And students couldn't torture their teachers in the time-honored fashion of screeching their nails across the blackboard.

Clearly, your nails have tons of useful purposes. But the truly most important one is the fact that your nails are a mirror to your health. Just by looking at your nails, your doctor can tell a lot about you—the kind of job you have, the chores you do at home, the way you've been eating, your general state of health.

Just what is it your doctor is "reading" by looking at your nails? Read on to find out.

SYMPTOM: **Bleeding**

COMMON CAUSES: This is usually a case of putting a finger or toe in the wrong place at the wrong time. A good slam on the nail will cause the small blood vessels (capillaries) under the nail to bleed. At first you'll see blood (in addition to stars, if you slam it hard enough), but what you'll probably end up with is an ugly, black-looking nail that will stay that way until it grows out.

Since the bleeding takes place under the nail, the blood has no room for escape. It stays put—trapped—and it will darken and eventually dry. If you bang the nail hard enough, it could even fall off.

If such an injury causes blood to ooze out around the nail, consider yourself lucky. This is helpful in relieving the pressure and pain.

Athletes, particularly runners and tennis players, can end up with black toenails as a result of the friction of a toe—usually the big one—rubbing against the front of the shoe. The friction causes blood to get trapped under the nail, which in turn causes pressure on the nerve endings and results in a very painful toe. It's almost always caused by poorly fitting shoes.

Another type of bleeding can occur under the nails, usually near the tips. Tiny hemorrhages in the capillaries may be seen as linear red or black streaks of blood, called splinters. This can occur after an injury. However, it also can be a symptom of such serious diseases as scurvy, which is a deficiency of vitamin C; trichinosis, which is a disease brought on by eating undercooked pork; and subacute endocarditis, an infection of the valves of the heart.

If you have a nervous habit of flicking your nails against your thumbnail (it's called nail-flicker's tic), you could also end up with these tiny red streaks, or splinters.

BEST RESPONSE: The best way to lessen the pain of a nail injury is to immediately run cold water over the injured nail or submerge the fingertip in a dish of cold water containing ice cubes for 20 to 30 minutes.

- If blood oozes out from under the nail, gently squeeze the nail and try to "milk" the blood out from under it. This will relieve pressure.

As healing occurs, doctors say, keep the area clean and trim away ragged pieces of nail to avoid getting it caught on something and pulled off. If pressure from the trapped blood is painful, see a doctor, who will drain it by piercing the surface of the nail.

If your problem is caused by your athletic shoe, the first thing you should do is go out and buy shoes that fit properly, suggest sports medicine experts. That means getting a shoe with plenty of room in the toebox. Immediate relief from the pain can be had by seeing a physician, who will drain the trapped blood. However, if left alone, the discoloration will go away by itself in a few months.

If you notice tiny red or black streaks under your nail and you haven't been injured, it's best to see your doctor. You could have one of the disorders described above. An exception to this, of course, are people who may be guilty of having nail-flicker's tic. In this case, you might want to switch to worry beads for relief of anxiety.

ACCOMPANYING SYMPTOMS: If your blackened nail is accompanied by considerable swelling, deformity and limitation of movement, the bone under the nail may be broken. See a doctor for diagnosis and treatment.

SYMPTOM: **Breaking**

COMMON CAUSES: Nails that break easily are caused by repeated wetting and drying. The in-and-out abuse of constant immersion in water, exposure to harsh soaps and detergents and overuse of nail polish removers are often the reason.

But there may be other causes, too. Sometimes kidney failure or any condition that impairs local circulation can affect the nails. So, too, can psoriasis (see Common Skin Conditions in chapter 15), athlete's foot (see Common Foot Conditions in chapter 9) and lichen planus, a form of dermatitis.

BEST RESPONSE: "One of the oldest, and wrongest, superstitions around is that you can make nails grow faster or stronger by eating gelatin (or various other products)," comments Kenneth A. Arndt, M.D., professor of dermatology at Harvard Medical School in Boston, in the *Harvard Medical School Health Letter.* No particular food or nutrient will help your nails grow stronger, he says. Malnourishment will affect your nails—along with the rest of your body—and proper diet will correct that problem.

However, say nail experts, there are a number of cosmetic measures you can take to help strengthen brittle nails caused by abuse or a medical condition.

Wear cotton-lined rubber gloves to do housework, and moisturize your nails with heavy cream two to three times a week. When applying nail polish, give your nails a protective edge by coating the polish over the tip of the nail, and use a basecoat and topcoat with each manicure. Use nail polish removers no more than once a week. Patch chips rather than completely redoing a manicure.

SYMPTOM: **Concave Nails.** *See* Symptom: Spooning

SYMPTOM: **Discoloration**

COMMON CAUSES: Even without polish, nails can change color. Nails can turn brown or black, for example, from using dark-colored hair dyes or photographic developer. However, a fungus infection, a vitamin B_{12} deficiency or even a cancerous tumor on the nail can cause it to turn black.

A red-brown tint will appear from frequent use of certain nail polishes. The color is a result of the pigments used in the products. Some acne products that contain resorcinol can do the same. Blue-brown nails may be a result of using certain antimalarial drugs.

Smokers often are plagued by yellow nails due to tar and nicotine stains. Those who work with special chemicals also display yellow-stained nails, as do those with fungus infections. Yellow nails are also associated with lymphedema (swelling caused by excess lymphatic fluid) and tumors of the chest cavity. Routine use of dark nail polish results in a yellow-orange stain.

Green nails are associated with a type of bacterial infection called pseudomonas. A ringworm infection (see Common Skin Conditions in chapter 15) can cause discolored, chalky and crumbly nails.

Nails with red half-moons may be seen in patients with heart failure. Blue (cyanotic) nails are a serious sign of lung or heart malfunction.

BEST RESPONSE: Take away the irritant and the unsightly color will eventually go away, say dermatologists. However, if you cannot pinpoint a reason—such as dyes, nicotine, etc.—for the cause of the discoloration, you should check with your physician. It could be a sign of an underlying medical problem that needs to be properly diagnosed.

ACCOMPANYING SYMPTOMS: If you notice your nail or nails turning yellow and thick, this could be a sign of ringworm or psoriasis (see Common Skin Conditions in chapter 15). You should see your doctor for diagnosis and treatment.

SYMPTOM: **Fragile Nails.** *See* Symptom: Breaking

SYMPTOM: **Grooves**

COMMON CAUSES: Horizontal (crosswise) grooves or ridges, often called Beau's lines, are the result of a temporary halt in nail growth that can happen during an illness. The list of conditions that can cause Beau's lines is long—heart attack, high fever, childbirth, drug reactions and emotional shock are among the most common. Sometimes the grooves can appear for no known reason.

BEST RESPONSE: Beau's lines can be compared to thunder and lightning. By the time you hear the thunder, the danger from the lightning is past. By the time you notice the crosswise grooves in your nails, the illness or trauma that caused them is a fading memory. The grooves will go away once the nails start growing again—often weeks or months later.

SYMPTOM: **Hangnail**

COMMON CAUSES: Those painful little slices of flesh that break away from the skin near the nails can show up if you're a nail biter or are continually exposing your fingers to irritating chemicals, solvents or detergents.

BEST RESPONSE: For immediate aid, dermatologists say you should trim the hangnail with sharp scissors as soon as it appears and frequently apply skin cream or lotion to the cuticle area. For long-term relief, try chewing gum instead of your fingernails, or try to find, then avoid, the irritant that's causing the problem.

ACCOMPANYING SYMPTOMS: If your hangnail results in a red and swollen cuticle and the cuticle separates from the nail (you may also see pus), you could have a bacterial or fungus infection known as paronychia (see Common Nail Conditions). You should see your physician, who may order antibiotic treatment.

SYMPTOM: **Loss of Nail**

COMMON CAUSES: Losing a nail can be a delayed reaction to an injury (see Symptom: Bleeding). It can also be the end result of allergies to solvents, nail polish basecoats, nail hardeners containing formaldehyde or artificial fingernails. Also, any condition that causes the nail to break away from the skin (see Symptom: Separating) can eventually result in its loss.

BEST RESPONSE: About the only thing you can do, say dermatologists, is to keep the area clean and dry to prevent infection while the new nail grows in. You should also keep the new nail trimmed during its growing process.

SYMPTOM: **Pitting**

COMMON CAUSES: Small pinpoint depressions on otherwise normal nails can be an early sign of psoriasis (see Common Skin Conditions in chapter 15), and are also part of the syndrome associated with alopecia areata, an uncommon disease in which hair falls out in clumps (see Symptom: Loss of Hair in chapter 10). Pits can also be a result of injury or infection. In some people, though, pitted fingernails have no causes.

BEST RESPONSE: If you suspect you might have psoriasis, you should see a dermatologist for diagnosis. If you feel otherwise healthy and there are no other symptoms that would indicate illness, then pitted nails are nothing to worry about.

Nevertheless, pitted nails should be treated gently during manicures, say dermatologists. Soak your hands and then massage cream into the cuticles with your fingers.

SYMPTOM: **Ridges**

COMMON CAUSE: Longitudinal ridges in the nail become more exaggerated with aging. Not everyone gets these ridges, of course, but if someone else in your family has them, chances are you will, too. The condition is common enough to have a name—aging nails.

BEST RESPONSE: Vertical ridges are harmless and require no treatment.

SYMPTOM: **Separating**

COMMON CAUSES: If the white color at the tip of your fingernail is receding toward your cuticle, it means your nail is separating from the nail bed. It is often a sign of disease.

The symptom is common in ringworm and psoriasis (see Common Skin Conditions in chapter 15), as well as in lichen planus, a type of dermatitis. It's also a symptom of thyroid problems (see thyroid disease under Common Whole Body Conditions in chapter 19). The antibiotic tetracycline combined with strong exposure to the sun can also cause the problem.

But the symptom isn't always the sign of some disease. Overzealous cleaning under the nails with a pointed file or other undesirable object could cause the nail to separate. So, too, could a good blow to the fingertips or a run-in with a splinter.

Also, don't rule out allergy or irritation. The problem could be a severe reaction to solvents, chemicals, detergents, drugs or nail preparations that come into contact with the hands.

BEST RESPONSE: A separated nail is an open invitation for bacteria to set in and cause even bigger problems. So the condition should not be ignored.

As the affected nail grows out, gently clip it away with manicure scissors and *always* keep the area clean and dry, say dermatologists. When immersing your hands in water, wear rubber gloves with a cotton lining.

If you suspect you might have an infection, you should see a doctor, who may order antibiotic treatments.

If you suspect that your nail separation is due to a drug sensitivity or allergy to nail products, discuss this with your physician. Most people don't have extreme reactions to such things, but if you're one of the unfortunate ones, a dermatologist can recommend alternative preparations.

ACCOMPANYING SYMPTOMS: If you see a buildup of a soft, yellowish white substance between your nail and skin, this could be a sign of a ringworm infection (see Common Skin Conditions in chapter 15). It's most common in toenails, but it can spread to the fingernails. The infection is usually spontaneous, but it may follow an injury.

Eventually, the entire nail pulls away and a partially destroyed, misshapen, discolored nail takes its place. Medical treatment is your best bet.

SYMPTOM: **Splitting**

COMMON CAUSES: Horizontal splitting and peeling of the nail are the final insults to fingertips that have been put through any variety of abuses (see Symptom: Breaking). You might notice that the problem becomes more prevalent as you age.

BEST RESPONSE: Nails that have gotten to the point of splitting and breaking need tender loving care, says Howard Baden, M.D., professor of dermatology at Harvard Medical School, in Boston.

"Cut your nails when they're wet to lessen the chance of breakage," he says. "Do yourself a favor and buy a new nail clipper that makes clean cuts, and file the edges of your nails with an emery board to eliminate defects that can become splits and breaks."

Nail hardeners, according to Dr. Baden, are of questionable benefit, but nail glue—*cyanoacrylate*—*can* be helpful in fixing breaks and cracks. When all else fails, you can treat yourself to a professional nail wrap to help restore strength to your nails.

Also, the same advice that was given for broken nails applies here—wear cotton-lined rubber gloves to do housework, and moisturize your nails two to three times a week. Be kind when manicuring. Always use a basecoat and topcoat with polishes, and use nail polish removers infrequently.

And remember to be kind to your nails—don't use them as tools to pry open bottles, pull out staples or pick locks.

SYMPTOM: **Spooning**

COMMON CAUSES: You know your nails are spooned if you can place a drop of water in the center of a nail and it doesn't roll off. The nails actually flip up to a concave curve, somewhat resembling the shape of a spoon.

Spooned nails may be hereditary or they may be caused by exposure to strong organic solvents such as kerosene, alcohol or acetone, says Howard Baden, M.D.

BEST RESPONSE: This is not the moon-on-a-night-in-June kind of spooning. If you have the symptom, you should see your doctor, who can diagnose the problem or find out if some external cause is to blame.

SYMPTOM: **Thickening**

COMMON CAUSES: Some people are naturally blessed with thick nails—they never have to worry about breaks or tears. But if normally not-so-thick nails suddenly start to gain weight, it could be a sign of a fungus infection or psoriasis (see Common Skin Conditions in chapter 15).

BEST RESPONSE: The nail problems associated with fungus infections and psoriasis are best treated by a doctor. Unless there is permanent damage to the nail production center or the nail matrix, which lies near the whitish half-moon at the base of each nail, thick nails will grow out and return to normal.

SYMPTOM: **Toenail, Black.** *See* Symptom: Bleeding

SYMPTOM: **White or Pale Nails**

COMMON CAUSES: Nails can display white in several ways. Small white spots or white stripes are usually nothing more than the result of an injury—from smacking your hand against your desk, for example.

White or pale nails may be hereditary, or they can be a symptom of kidney failure (see Common Urinary Tract Conditions in chapter 18), cirrhosis of the liver (see cirrhosis under Common Abdominal and Digestive System Conditions in chapter 1) or anemia (see Common Whole Body Conditions in chapter 19).

BEST RESPONSE: Excluding bumps and other injuries, it's difficult to find out on your own why your nails are turning white. You should see your doctor for proper diagnosis and treatment.

Common Nail Conditions

Ingrown toenail. This is a condition in which the sharp edge of the nail digs into the skin, causing irritation and tenderness. The big toe is the most common site, but other toes can be affected as well. If there is redness and swelling, the pain gets intense and you see pus, you know your problem's gotten even bigger—infection has set in.

The chief causes of an ingrown toenail are improper trimming of the nail (nails should be trimmed straight across the top) and ill-fitting shoes. But sometimes injury or disease can lead to ingrown nails.

If the ingrown nail has reached the point of infection, you should see a physician, who may recommend antibiotics and remove part of the nail. Moderately ingrown toenails can be treated by packing wisps of cotton under the affected corner to lift the nail up and protect the irritated area beneath.

Paronychia.   Your doctor may simply tell you that you have an infection, or he may more correctly say you have paronychia. What you'll already know is that you have soreness and pain around the skin at the base of the nail.

Infections are most often a problem for people who spend a lot of time with their hands in water, such as fishermen, household workers, bartenders and beauticians. Irritation and inflammation result. The infection can be caused by bacteria or yeast. Bacterial infections come on suddenly and severely; yeast infections are not as bad, but are harder to get rid of.

Antibiotics are the treatment of choice in acute (severe) paronychia. For chronic (long-term) paronychia, you must avoid immersing your hands in water. Antibiotics and antiyeast agents may help. Chronic cases may take some time to cure.

Chapter 12

Neurological System

SEE YOUR DOCTOR IMMEDIATELY IF:

- *You get a severe headache at any time following a head injury*
- *You have a headache and double vision*
- *You have a headache, eye pain and/or blurred vision*
- *Your headache feels worse when you bend your head forward, and you have a stiff neck, a fever and are sensitive to light*
- *Your headache is accompanied by vomiting and convulsions*
- *You black out*
- *You suddenly lose the ability to move part of your body*
- *You lose the ability to speak*
- *You are depressed and have suicidal thoughts*

Your brain is what makes you *you*.

A pretty face and a great body may make you *look* better than the rest, but it's what's inside your head—your thoughts, your emotions, your goals, your opinions, your prejudices, your interests and your intellect—that *really* sets you apart from everyone else.

Your brain is your living personal computer, controlling both conscious and unconscious actions. And just like the computer you might have in your home or office, it needs an electrical system to keep it running. In the human computer, that system is known as the central nervous system.

Your central nervous system contains millions of nerve cells and millions of tiny nerve fibers that radiate to every single part of your body. Considering the awesome complexity of this neurological network, it's a miracle that the system doesn't break down more often! Oh, sure, you may forget that loaf of bread at the store or your mother's birthday, or you can get a whopper of a headache that makes you want to hide under the covers for days. But for the most part, your brain is a smooth-running operation, matching input with output without a glitch.

But things can and do go awry. Usually, the problem is just minor—we all suffer headaches from time to time. Sometimes the trouble may *seem* major—like fainting—but turns out not to be that way at all. No matter what the problem, big or small, it deserves your personal attention.

The information in this chapter is to help you identify your source of aches or pains. But remember, if any symptom is truly plaguing you, don't play doctor—see one.

SYMPTOM: **Confusion**

COMMON CAUSES: If you are driving on the San Diego Freeway and are trying to find the Santa Ana Freeway, you have a right to feel confused. The same goes for asking directions from a Frenchman in Paris, trying to order from a menu in Chinatown or taking a calculus quiz.

But *real* confusion—a feeling of disorientation to time, place or person—is usually a reaction to a drug you've taken or to an illness. Numerous drugs, both the medicinal and the recreational kind, can cause confusion. These include antihistamines, appetite suppressants, muscle relaxants, painkillers, sedatives, tranquilizers, anticholinergics, nonsteroidal anti-inflammatory drugs and the ulcer medication cimetidine (Tagamet). Marijuana, cocaine, LSD, heroin—any mind-altering drug—can lead to complete disorientation.

Excessive dieting can be the problem, too. Just like any other organ of the body, the brain needs nutrients and can't function properly without them. A deficiency of any one of a number of vitamins can leave you feeling disoriented. And going without food for long periods of time could result in low blood sugar, which could also disorient you.

If you've recently suffered a fall or head injury, confusion could be a sign of a concussion (see Common Neurological System Conditions).

Confusion may be a side effect of these conditions: hypoglycemia (see Common Whole Body Conditions in chapter 19), kidney failure (see Common Urinary Tract Conditions in chapter 18), electrolyte and metabolic disturbances in the body's chemistry, endocrine gland disorders, any infection that is severe enough and dehydration.

Confusion also can sometimes signify a complication in those who suffer from diabetes mellitus, heart disease or lung disease.

BEST RESPONSE: If you suddenly become confused, sit down, relax and take stock of things. What could be going on? "You might find it helpful to write down your thoughts," says H. Randall Hicks, M.D., clinical instructor of psychiatry at the University of California at San Diego School of Medicine. "What are you feeling? What could be bothering you to make you confused?"

If you're guilty of not having eaten in a number of hours, the problem could be low blood sugar. "Get yourself something to eat," says Dr. Hicks. "If low blood sugar is the problem, you should begin to feel better after about ten minutes. If you still feel confused, you should call your doctor."

If the problem is an adverse reaction to a medication, your doctor can change it, or at least change the dosage. If the cause is diet pills, mood drugs or recreational drugs, it's likely that he or she will strongly advise you to stop using them. If medication can be ruled out, your doctor should examine you to see if there is a complication in a current disease, or to determine whether you are showing signs of a new one.

If you've been dieting excessively, your doctor can counsel you on the proper method of weight control. Dr. Hicks cautions that any diet that results in unwanted side effects, such as confusion, can lead to even more grave problems, such as eating disorders (see Common Whole Body Conditions in chapter 19).

Because any head injury has the potential to be serious, you should call your doctor at once at the first sign of this symptom after a fall or mishap, says Dr. Hicks. Routine treatment for a mild concussion is rest and quiet, with frequent monitoring of vital signs.

ACCOMPANYING SYMPTOMS: Confusion accompanied by slurred speech and weakness in the arms or legs can be a sign of a stroke or of a transient ischemic attack, or TIA (see Common Neurological System Conditions), sometimes known as a "little stroke."

Confusion with fever can be a sign of infection or of a present illness getting worse.

In all cases, a doctor should be called at once.

SYMPTOM: **Convulsions.** *See* Symptom: Seizures

SYMPTOM: **Delirium**

COMMON CAUSES: Delirium is a disordered state of mind that comes on suddenly and is usually fleeting. The mind wanders, speech is incoherent and there is usually continual aimless physical activity. A delirious person is also confused and disoriented and may even have hallucinations (see Symptom: Hallucinations).

Delirium can be caused by metabolic derangements resulting from such problems as kidney failure (see Common Urinary Tract Conditions in chapter 18), hypoglycemia (see Common Whole Body Conditions in chapter 19) and liver failure. And it's common in infections with high fevers, such as meningitis and encephalitis (see Common Neurological System Conditions), brain abscess, malaria and typhoid fever. Heart failure (see Common Circulatory, Heart and Lung Conditions in chapter 5), heatstroke (see Common Whole Body Conditions in chapter 19), any serious head injury or a brain tumor can also cause delirium. A person can also experience delirium when coming out of anesthesia.

Poisoning from substances such as arsenic, lead, belladonna and inedible wild mushrooms, or bites from poisonous insects, spiders and snakes, can also make a person delirious.

Perhaps the most common causes of delirium nowadays are related to drug and alcohol abuse. Withdrawal from a habit-forming medication, such as tranquilizers, or overdosing on any of the recreational drugs can cause a person to become delirious. So, too, can withdrawal from alcohol. And it doesn't just happen to tried-and-true alcoholics. It can happen to anyone who has been drinking heavily and long, even if the person were drinking just beer or wine.

BEST RESPONSE: Get in touch with your doctor immediately. In most cases, a delirious person must be seen by a doctor, since treatment of the problem or disease causing the symptom is what's most important. Persons suffering from delirium should be kept as comfortable as possible and should be protected from harming themselves. The doctor may immediately order a phenothiazine tranquilizer such as Thorazine, or a minor tranquilizer such as Valium, to quell the delirium.

ACCOMPANYING SYMPTOMS: If a child under 17 years old is delirious after vomiting for 24 to 48 hours, the problem could be Reye's syndrome, a sudden, severe disease that affects the liver and the brain. A doctor should be seen immediately. Reye's syndrome follows on the heels of a viral infection of the respiratory system. Its cause is unknown. Treatment is often carried out in an intensive care unit using such sophisticated equipment as monitors and ventilators, as well as intravenous solutions and medications.

A chronic alcoholic going through withdrawal (see alcoholism under Common Whole Body Conditions in chapter 19) can suffer from a syndrome known as delirium tremens—the DT's—which is characterized by delirium, fever, sweating and the shakes. Often the person will also hallucinate. Because of the severity of these symptoms, withdrawal is best undertaken in a hospital setting, where treatment also includes fluid replacement, vitamins and minerals and certain medications, as well as efforts to get the alcoholic to permanently give up the habit.

SYMPTOM: **Dizziness**

COMMON CAUSES: It's a strange sensation. Your body and the room around you are in a spin. You're lightheaded, unsteady. You want it to *stop*. Getting it to stop, however, usually means treating the cause. But treating the cause isn't always so easy. That's because dizziness is a very common symptom with many different causes, says Nagagopal Venna, M.D., assistant professor of neurology at Boston University School of Medicine.

"The most common cause of dizziness for all ages is hyperventilation," says Dr. Venna. Hyperventilation is abnormally rapid, deep breathing or overbreathing, usually due to anxiety (see Common Neurological System Conditions). What happens, explains Dr. Venna, is that when you overbreathe, you blow off large amounts of carbon dioxide, which results in a lower level of the chemical in your blood. "Carbon dioxide is a powerful stimulant for blood getting to the brain. Without it, blood flow is decreased and dizziness occurs."

But dizziness can also be a sign of disease, with ear disease the most likely suspect. Since the inner ear is responsible for balance, any disorder of the inner ear can cause dizziness. A middle ear infection (see Common Ear Conditions in chapter 6) and motion sickness are the most common, although any ear condition—even a buildup of earwax—has the potential for interfering with balance and causing dizziness.

If you get dizzy when you turn your head or when you get up in the morning, you could have benign positional vertigo, a degenerative inner ear disorder affecting older people. Most serious ear diseases, however, usually carry other symptoms, such as hearing disturbances and nausea.

Eyestrain can cause dizziness. And any disease or condition that causes infection, such as the flu, also has the potential for making you feel dizzy.

Severe coughing, especially in those suffering from chronic obstructive lung disease, or COLD (see Common Circulatory, Heart and Lung Conditions in chapter 5), can make you feel dizzy. That's because the hard hacking creates increased pressure on a chest that's already feeling pressure. This enormous pressure causes blood flow in the heart to decrease, cutting down on the blood supply to the brain.

Any heart or circulatory problem—all of which have the potential of slowing the supply of blood to the head—can cause dizziness. And if your dizziness is brought on by standing, is relieved by lying down and is especially noticeable on arising after prolonged bed rest, you have what is known as postural hypotension, meaning your blood pressure drops too low after a change in body position.

"This is especially common in older people, because the nervous system deteriorates and the reflexes change as you get older," says Dr. Venna. It's also a common side effect in those who suffer from Parkinson's disease and heart disease. And it can happen in those taking medication for high blood pressure, angina or depression, since these drugs can decrease the usual cardiovascular responses.

Nighttime dizziness is common in older men with an enlarged prostate. It usually occurs after an evening of drinking alcohol; the man feels dizzy just after he finishes urinating standing up. The condition is called micturition syncope.

BEST RESPONSE: "Dizziness is not a dangerous symptom by itself, so you don't have to do anything immediately—except protect yourself from falling," says Dr. Venna. "The most important thing you need to do is find out what's causing the problem, and an internist is probably the first person to see for evaluation. If necessary, the internist can refer you to another specialist."

It's also important to pay attention to any other symptoms, should they exist, since this will help the doctor make a diagnosis.

"If a doctor determines that hyperventilation is your problem, the immediate treatment is quite simple but effective—breathe into a paper bag for several minutes to restore the carbon dioxide to the lungs and blood," says Dr. Venna. "Hyperventilation, however, is often an indication of an underlying anxiety, and psychotherapy may be needed to make the breathing more normal.

"Dizziness caused by a drop in blood pressure that occurs when you sit or stand up can be managed by getting up slowly from a reclining position," says Dr. Venna. "First, sit on the edge of the bed for several minutes to allow time for the brain to readjust to the change in pressure. Then continue to get up slowly." In addition, Dr. Venna recommends wearing elastic stockings (Jobst stockings) to prevent blood from settling in the legs, and drinking more fluids to aid in replacing blood volume.

For severe cases of dizziness caused by postural hypotension, some doctors recommend increasing salt in the diet or using salt-retaining steroids. This should be done only under a doctor's supervision.

"If medication is the cause of your dizziness," says Dr. Venna, "the dosage may need to be modified or you may need to switch to another drug. But you should do this only under a doctor's supervision."

If your problem is an ear condition, treatment of the disease will stop the dizziness. The type of treatment, however, depends on the disease. Infections, for example, can usually be cleared up with antibiotics. Benign positional vertigo should go away by itself in six months to a year. Motion sickness can be alleviated by medications such as Bonine or Dramamine.

If your dizziness is brought on by a chronic cough, your doctor may suggest over-the-counter or prescription cough suppressants. If you're a man suffering from micturition syncope, Dr. Venna suggests avoiding alcohol or large intake of fluids in the evening and regularly emptying your bladder before retiring. In addition, a urologist may need to be consulted to treat the underlying problem of enlarged prostate.

ACCOMPANYING SYMPTOMS: If your dizziness is accompanied by nausea, vomiting or a headache, you could be suffering from a sudden disturbance in the inner ear such as labyrinthitis, bleeding inside the skull or a brain tumor. You should see your doctor.

If you're dizzy and also hearing a ringing in the ear, the problem is probably Meniere's disease (see Common Ear Conditions in chapter 6), a slowly developing disease that can result in hearing loss. You should see your doctor for treatment.

Dizziness accompanied by double vision, tingling or numbness of any part of the body can mean a stroke or a transient ischemic attack (see Common Neurological System Conditions) or some other disturbance of the brain. You should see your doctor immediately.

SYMPTOM: **Fainting**

COMMON CAUSES: You're a soldier standing at attention for a long time on a hot, muggy day; you're a student who works two jobs and stays up all night to study; you just hit the million-dollar lottery.

Any situation that brings on emotional stress can also bring on a fainting spell—a sudden but temporary loss of consciousness caused by insufficient blood getting to the brain. You can also faint as a result of overexertion due to too much exercise or if you've lost blood.

Certain medications can also bring on the reaction. These include injections of the local anesthetic procaine, which is often given for dental work or stitches; diuretics ("water pills") prescribed for fluid retention; certain cardiovascular drugs, such as nitroglycerin; high blood pressure medications or an overdose of insulin.

Fainting, however, can also signify a physical abnormality. Heart diseases that limit the amount of blood the organ pumps can cause fainting spells. These include a slow heartbeat, known as bradycardia, or a rapid heartbeat, known as tachycardia (see Symptom: Palpitations in chapter 5). Hypoglycemia and, in rare cases, anemia (see Whole Body Conditions in chapter 19) can also cause the problem.

BEST RESPONSE: Any unexplained fainting spell that happens even once should be evaluated by a doctor.

To treat a fainting spell, there really isn't much you have to do. Usually people just slump over a desk or slide down a wall, says Nagagopal Venna, M.D. "So just laying them out flat should send enough blood back to the brain to restore consciousness. In fact, had they taken a moment to lie down when they first felt faint, they would never have lost consciousness to begin with."

SYMPTOM: **Forgetfulness.** *See also* Symptom: Memory Loss

COMMON CAUSES: Yesterday you misplaced your car keys. Last week you couldn't think of your neighbor's name. Now today you left your wallet on the counter in the checkout line. It's all got you worried. Could you be getting senile before your time? Or could it be something worse—could you be losing your mind?

Not likely. Absentmindedness is often just another side affect of aging.

No one knows *for sure* what causes this, but scientists believe that it is due, at least in part, to a reduction in the amount of the chemical acetylcholine in the brain. Acetylcholine is a neurotransmitter responsible for sending messages back and forth from one cell to another.

Long-term memory—the permanent storage bank—isn't affected at all. For example, you don't forget the way home or the date you were married (even though you might like to). The greatest effect, say scientists, is on the short-term memory. For example, have you ever been introduced to someone at the beginning of a business meeting and then forgotten his or her name when it came time to address the person? Or how many times have you stood staring into the refrigerator wondering what it is you're looking for? Many people after the age of 35 or so start to complain of such things. The condition even has a name—benign senile forgetfulness.

But there are outside influences that can also cause memory to go on the blink now and then. Anxiety (see Common Neurological System Conditions) can put your mind—and memory—elsewhere. And almost any drug can be suspected of having some effect on brain function. The most frequent troublemakers are antidepressant drugs such as Tofranil and Elavil, drugs to lower blood pressure, drugs that calm or sedate the bowel and drugs used to treat Parkinson's disease. In addition, overuse or withdrawal from sedatives (such as Doriden, Placidyl or Valium), street drugs and even alcohol can affect memory.

BEST RESPONSE: Like cellulite and middle-age spread, benign senile forgetfulness is something you needn't give in to. Just as you exercise the body to keep it taut, you can also exercise the mind to keep it sharp.

One way to do so, say specialists, is to initiate a practice that you probably used in childhood when you were first building your memory bank—mnemonics, or associating unknown material with something familiar. For example, when your secretary introduces you to her sister, Fern, you can remember her by associating her with the plant hanging in your office window. Or, if you need milk, cereal, apple juice and bread from the grocery store and know you'll probably forget the list, try picturing milk cascading over the cereal onto the floor and out the door, where it will be stopped by the bread man, who is walking up the pavement eating an apple. The more ridiculous the association, the more likely you are to remember it, say the experts.

If you have to remember long numbers, break up the digits and attach them to something significant. For example, your 12 cousins, your husband's age, 42, and your house number, 619, may be your next door neighbor's telephone number.

To keep your mind fit, say the experts, you must exercise it. You could do this by memorizing something every day, learning a new language, reading or playing some thinking games like chess or bridge. They also advise that you make a habit of writing things down. Make a daily list of the things you must do and check them off as you go along. This, at least, will prevent you from forgetting what's most important—as long as you don't lose the list!

You should check with your doctor if you think that any medication you're taking could be slowing down your mind. He or she may be able to adjust the dosage or change the medication. You should also see your doctor if you're so anxious you can't keep your mind focused long enough to remember anything. Relaxation techniques, such as meditation and biofeedback, may be helpful. In some cases, psychotherapy may be in order.

SYMPTOM: **Hallucinations**

COMMON CAUSES: Hallucinations are strong mental images experienced as if they were part of reality. They can affect all the senses—sound, sight, touch, smell and taste.

Hallucinations can be caused by mental illness, physical illness or drug and alcohol abuse. Or they can be quite harmless and mean nothing at all.

Often young children, and sometimes adults, for example, experience a hallucination when falling in and out of sleep. It's considered a common experience and is associated with early rapid eye movement (REM) sleep, in which vivid dreams—similar to hallucinations—occur.

Total exhaustion can bring on hallucinations, and those who have dementia (see Common Neurological System Conditions) or those suffering from a severe illness like a brain tumor may see or hear the imaginary.

Hallucinations, however, tend to get more extreme when mind-altering drugs or mental illness are the cause. Street drugs and alcohol, for example, can induce feelings of bugs crawling under your skin, scary visual images and voices talking to you. Strong pain medication, such as morphine, can have the same effect. The hallucinations are the result of chemical somersaults taking place in the brain and creating interference with normal thought processes. Both drugs and alcohol "play" with the body's chemicals, and this subsequent bad reaction can occur while using them or withdrawing from them.

Those with the mental illness called schizophrenia, a complex and serious psychotic disorder, commonly hear voices talking to them, often telling them to do something ("God told me to do it.").

Hallucinations can also occur in those diagnosed as a "borderline personality," meaning they're mentally unstable. Victims cannot greet life normally; they may not be able to get along with others or even with themselves.

Hallucinations also occur in those who suffer a brief but serious mental collapse known as brief reactive psychosis, which is brought on by a sudden, severe stressor, such as a tragic death, and in those suffering from psychotic depression, a severe form of depression most commonly seen in middle-aged or older men.

BEST RESPONSE: Strange as it may seem, in most cases you *will* know that you're hallucinating. Even though you're seeing or hearing things, you'll know it's your imagination.

If it's associated with your sleep or dreams, you don't have to do anything, says H. Randall Hicks, M.D. If total exhaustion is the cause, a good, long sleep will restore you to normal.

But if you feel you or someone else is becoming mentally unhinged—be it from a drug or alcohol or from no apparent cause—get to a doctor or emergency room right away, says Dr. Hicks.

"If you're hallucinating, you should ask a friend to drive you there," he says. "Don't drive yourself." If alcohol or drug overdose or withdrawal is the cause of your hallucinations, the problem will gradually disappear after the drug leaves your body. However, if you're harming yourself or others or appear to have the potential to do so—no matter what the cause—the doctor may prescribe a tranquilizer, such as Thorazine or Librium, until the crisis passes.

To find the origin of your hallucinations, the doctor will ask you a number of questions concerning your psychological and physical health. He or she will also do a physical examination, which may include a neurological exam, and blood work to rule out physical causes.

If your illness is severe, hospitalization—either medical or psychiatric—may be necessary. If the illness is not as severe, medical or psychiatric treatment may be carried out on an outpatient basis, says Dr. Hicks. If you have a psychiatric problem, psychotherapy and/or antipsychotic or antidepressant medications may be necessary.

SYMPTOM: **Headache, Bandlike**

COMMON CAUSES: This is the common tension headache. Some sufferers complain that their "scalp is too tight," as if a band were being tightened around it. Others complain that their "whole head hurts." Such headaches are most often brought on by everyday stressors, such as traffic jams, board meetings or marital spats.

"Stress, in fact, plays a role in 80 to 85 percent of *all* headaches," says Robert Kunkel, M.D., head of the headache section, Department of Internal Medicine, at the Cleveland Clinic Foundation in Ohio. Sometimes they manifest themselves as a migraine (see Symptom: Headache, Migraine), but most stress headaches have bandlike symptoms.

The headache develops when muscles—especially those in the neck and shoulders—accumulate tension that gradually moves its way up to the head. But stress isn't the only thing that causes them.

Addicted gum chewers, for example, can complain of headaches. The constant chewing tires the jaw muscle and sends pain along both sides of the head. Poor posture can also tighten muscles in the neck, which in turn stresses the head muscles and causes pain.

Sleeping on the stomach and breathing through the mouth can cause tension headaches, says Lionel A. Walpin, M.D., medical director of the Walpin Physical Medicine and Pain Institute in Los Angeles. These are headaches related to posture and its effects on muscles, ligaments and joints.

When you sleep on your stomach, explains Dr. Walpin, your head is turned to one side, which can put too much pressure on the side of the jaw and upper neck, causing a headache. If you breathe through your nose instead of your mouth, you'll hold your head and shoulders in a better posture in relation to your body. You shouldn't use your upper chest and neck muscles to breathe. "They're not designed for that," says Dr. Walpin. "If you breathe through your mouth, they'll become sore and refer pain to your head and shoulders."

BEST RESPONSE: "A hot shower, a warm soaking bath, lying down with a warm pack to the head or a massage of the shoulders, neck and scalp can all help you to relax, and this is probably the best treatment for the occasional tension headache," says Dr. Kunkel. "In addition, the usual over-the-counter remedies—aspirin, acetaminophen (Tylenol) and ibuprofen (Advil or Nuprin)—offer the best relief."

In addition, Dr. Kunkel recommends exercise for relaxing tense muscles. "Rotation exercises of the neck are particularly helpful for tension headaches, but I'm also a believer in regular daily exercise— walking for example—as a way to reduce stress."

All these methods will help to soothe an aching head. But to help prevent the headaches from recurring, says Dr. Kunkel, you must identify the stresses in your life that are causing them. "A headache doesn't always come at the time of the stress, so you may have to do some investigating. Sometimes there are deeper worries that are causing the pain."

If you suspect bad posture is your problem, avoid slumping when sitting and avoid lying on your stomach when sleeping. In addition, you should breathe through your nose, not your mouth.

If none of these measures helps and your headaches are more than occasional—if you always seem to be reaching for your headache pills— then you should see your doctor, says Dr. Kunkel.

"One of the biggest problems that we physicians encounter with chronic headache is dependency on narcotics, sedatives or tranquilizers, and it's difficult to get off these medications," says Dr. Kunkel. "To make matters worse, some over-the-counter headache remedies that people take have caffeine in them, and when they take enough of these, they'll wake up in the morning with a caffeine withdrawal headache. The result? More pill popping. More headaches."

This is why plain aspirin or acetaminophen (Tylenol) is the best medication for those who suffer from chronic headaches, says Dr. Kunkel. They don't contain anything to perpetuate the problem. Dr. Kunkel suggests reading the labels on any headache preparation carefully.

ACCOMPANYING SYMPTOMS: If you're a heavy coffee drinker and suffer from headaches, nervousness and irritability, you could be addicted to caffeine. The symptoms redevelop when you've gone a number of hours without the stimulant. It's a withdrawal reaction. Gradually cutting back on caffeine in *all* food and drink will help wean you away from the habit.

If you suffer from tension headaches and notice that your jaw clicks when you open it, you probably have temporomandibular joint disorder, or TMJ (see Common Facial, Jaw and Mouth Conditions in chapter 8). You should see your dentist for proper diagnosis.

Headaches accompanied by fever are usually a sign of illness.

An overall or bandlike headache that is most severe in the morning is a sign of high blood pressure (see Common Circulatory, Heart and Lung Conditions in chapter 5). If you have not been diagnosed as having this disease, you should discuss your symptoms with your doctor.

SYMPTOM: **Headache, Cluster**

COMMON CAUSES: Cluster headaches are wicked. They cause agonizing pain on one side of the head that can last anywhere from half an hour to three hours. They're called cluster headaches because they're repeated—the attacks occur in groups or clusters. They most commonly strike men between the ages of 30 and 50.

"Patients often describe this pain as a dagger or poker through the eye," says Robert Kunkel, M.D. "Attacks occur two or three times a day every day for a month or two, then go away."

There is a definite personality type prone to this type of headache, says Dr. Kunkel. It's the hard-driven macho man who smokes heavily, drinks hard and pushes himself to achieve hard-to-attain goals. It all lets go in a siege of headaches.

When in the midst of a series of attacks, drinking alcohol or taking nitroglycerin (a heart medication) or anything else that dilates the blood vessels, can bring on an attack within minutes. At other times, however, drinking alcohol—even in large quantities—will not bring on an attack.

BEST RESPONSE: "An ice bag on the head can ease the pain of cluster headaches, as can certain prescription drugs," says Dr. Kunkel. "The usual medication for a sudden cluster headache is ergotamine tartrate (Cafergot), which can be given by inhalation, dissolved under the tongue or given in tablet form.

"Some people find relief from oxygen therapy. You can rent an oxygen tank from a supply house and use 100 percent oxygen at six to eight liters per minute. The oxygen usually gives relief in five to eight minutes, although the pain sometimes returns and inhalation has to be repeated." Dr. Kunkel warns, however, that such therapy requires certain cautions.

"Oxygen shouldn't be used for more than 12 minutes at one time, because it can damage the lungs and cause other problems," he says. "But oxygen therapy is harmless when used for short periods—like 8 to 10 minutes—then turned off and used later as needed." Also, he reminds, you shouldn't smoke near the oxygen.

He also warns against drinking alcohol or using nitroglycerin when in the throes of attacks. If you take nitroglycerin to relieve chest pain, you should check with your doctor about an alternative medication.

Because cluster headaches are so painful and debilitating, Dr. Kunkel says you should see your doctor, who will prescribe medication to prevent them from recurring. Such drugs as methysergide (Sansert), calcium channel blockers (Calan, Adalat), ergotamine tartrate (Cafergot), lithium and cortisone have been found to be effective, depending on the patient. "Your doctor may try each, one at a time, until your symptoms are relieved," says Dr. Kunkel.

SYMPTOM: **Headache, Hangover**

COMMON CAUSES: If you had a few drinks last night, you could have experienced an immediate headache. That's because alcohol has the unfortunate ability to dilate and irritate blood vessels in the brain and surrounding tissue. Worse still, if you drank too much last night, your head could feel even worse this morning, because the presence of the alcohol is still being felt. This headache, popularly known as a hangover, is due to the breakdown products of alcohol working on the body.

The reason your head is bearing the brunt of it all is because your brain rests in very tight quarters. The skull has no give (unlike your beer belly) and, as a result, when those blood vessels swell, they press hard against your crown, causing you pain and discomfort.

BEST RESPONSE: "Drinking a lot of fluids and eating some food—if it's tolerated—is the best way to treat a hangover," says Robert Kunkel, M.D. "This will speed up your metabolism, which will help get rid of the breakdown products of the alcohol." At the very least, it will help you to feel better.

But there really is no cure for a hangover except time, says Dr. Kunkel. Your body needs time to get rid of the effects of the alcohol in your system.

To prevent a hangover headache the next time, some doctors recommend drinking a glass of milk and eating a good meal—one that contains some fat, like cheese—beforehand. This will help your body absorb the alcohol more slowly. Also, limit your drinks to one every hour or half-hour (depending on your body size) so you can avoid getting drunk. And you might want to take a nonaspirin pain reliever such as acetaminophen (Tylenol) at bedtime to help soothe the inevitable hangover the next day. Aspirin isn't recommended because it may irritate an already overburdened stomach.

SYMPTOM: **Headache, Migraine**

COMMON CAUSES: Migraines cause throbbing and often debilitating pain on one side of the head that can go on for days. In some, the pain can be so severe that the victim can do nothing but lie in bed. Migraines are considered a hereditary disorder that most commonly occurs in women between the ages of 20 and 40.

There are two types of migraine: common and classic. The common type is the more prevalent and is often referred to as a "sick headache," because the pain is usually accompanied by nausea and often vomiting. A classic migraine is more complex. It is preceded by a characteristic "aura"—a period of mild confusion, lightheadedness, flashing lights, blind spots in the field of vision, sensitivity to sound, distorted speech and sometimes even partial paralysis.

Migraines typically last one to three days and then go away, only to return again . . . and again. If you suffer from migraines, your symptoms may be slightly different from those of the next person, but your own will usually follow the same pattern time after time.

"Migraine headaches are caused by arteries that first become narrowed and then swell," explains Robert Kunkel, M.D. "Although the problem tends to run in families, it can skip a generation. For years, migraine was called a blood vessel disease. Then some research suggested the problem might be related to a blood disorder or chemical change. Now we're looking at migraine sufferers with PET scans [positron emission tomography, a special x-ray of the brain], and what we see is hyperactivity within the brain, which may account for the swelling of the vessels."

Doctors have also found that certain foods or situations will trigger an attack. Cheese, chocolate and alcoholic beverages—particularly red wine—contain tyramine, a substance that can cause blood vessels to constrict (narrow), and can reduce the levels of serotonin, a chemical that acts on blood vessels in the body. "In some people, eating cheese or pizza can bring on a migraine," says Dr. Kunkel. "In children, the culprit is usually chocolate."

But there are other triggers, too, he says. Missing a meal, which can cause blood sugar to dive, can bring on an attack in some people. Environmental factors, such as weather changes—specifically, a falling barometer—and pollution are other causes. Even changes in sleeping or eating habits, travel and stressful events can bring on a migraine in some people. In women, menstrual periods or use of oral contraceptives can be the trigger.

BEST RESPONSE: For relief of migraine headaches, Dr. Kunkel suggests a cold pack on the head, which will help constrict the blood vessels. You should also lie down and relax. And, says Dr. Kunkel, many patients have found relief with biofeedback training, a method in which sensitive electronic equipment is used to help you regulate blood circulation and alleviate muscle tension, the basic cause of migraine headaches.

"Many migraine sufferers find, however, that drugs are the only effective remedy," says Dr. Kunkel. Most over-the-counter medications don't work for migraine. The one exception, he says, is ibuprofen (Advil or Nuprin), which should be taken as directed on the package. If this isn't effective, your doctor will probably prescribe ergotamine tartrate (Cafergot) or isometheptene (Midrin).

"If you suffer from migraines only once a month, you'll only need to take the medication at the time of the attack," says Dr. Kunkel."But if you have migraines once or twice a week, you should be under the care of a doctor, who will probably recommend preventive medication as well as medication when an attack comes on."

If you suffer from migraine headaches, the most important action you can take is to try to identify substances in your diet that may trigger an attack, says Dr. Kunkel. He suggests keeping a record of the foods you eat and when you eat them, and keeping a diary of your headache pain. By comparing the two, you eventually should be able to identify the foods that trigger an attack. "It's a trial-and-error thing, but it is the only effective way to find the source, since each person reacts to a migraine so differently," he says.

It's also a good idea to eat regularly, keep regular hours, avoid sleeping late and be aware of the effects that stress and weather changes have on your health.

ACCOMPANYING SYMPTOMS: If you are over 55 and for the first time you experience a dull, throbbing pain on one side of your head, and an artery at your temple is swollen, red and painful to the touch, you could be suffering from temporal arteritis. This is an inflammation of the temporal artery that causes thickening of the vessel lining and a reduction in the amount of blood it can carry. See your doctor, who will probably treat the condition with steroid drugs.

If you suffer from migraine headaches but also have symptoms that suggest tension headaches (see Symptom: Headache, Bandlike), you could be suffering from mixed headache syndrome, and you should see your doctor. This type of headache comes on if you're susceptible to migraines and also are a victim of stress. Treatment is carried out with prescription medications.

If your one-sided head pain is accompanied by severe jabs of pain in the face along the same side, you could be suffering from a type of nerve disorder called tic douloureux (see Common Facial, Jaw and Mouth Conditions in chapter 8) and should see your doctor. Treatment involves an anticonvulsant medication such as carbamazepine (Tegretol) or the drug baclofen (Lioresal).

SYMPTOM: **Headache, Sinus**

COMMON CAUSES: This is a dull and aching headache that is usually worse in the morning and intensifies when you move your head. It occurs when your sinuses, located in the front of your head, don't drain, usually as a result of a cold or allergy, but also possibly caused by a bacterial infection. Since the sinus is an enclosed cavity, inflammation and swelling of the mucous membranes result, blocking the nasal passages.

BEST RESPONSE: Anything that helps clear the sinuses will also get rid of the sinus headache pain, says Robert Kunkel, M.D.

"Over-the-counter cold tablets that contain an antihistamine and a decongestant are usually effective in relieving sinus pain," says Dr. Kunkel. "The antihistamine cuts down on secretions and the decongestant shrinks membranes. If infection is present, antibiotics will be needed."

Warm packs and steam inhalations are also helpful in opening up sinus passages, he says. You can prepare a warm pack by soaking a clean, thick washcloth in warm water, wringing it out and placing it over the eyes and cheekbones. When the pack cools off, warm it up and reapply. A hot steam vaporizer, available at drugstores, can offer relief to sinus sufferers. Or you can get the same effect by sitting in a bathroom that has been closed up tight and running hot water in the shower (you don't have to get in the shower).

SYMPTOM: **Memory Loss.** *See also* Symptom: Forgetfulness

COMMON CAUSES: This isn't the "Oops, I forgot" experience that everyone has from time to time, says Miriam Aronson, Ed.D., associate professor of neurology and psychiatry at Albert Einstein College of Medicine in New York.

"Severe memory loss is not that you go to a wedding and forget the names of a few people," she explains. "It's going to a wedding and forgetting you've been there. Or going to work the same way for 30 years and then one day going to work and getting lost."

This kind of severe memory loss is generally caused by dementia (see Common Neurological System Conditions), a condition in which the ability to think and reason is gradually lost. Although dementia comes in a variety of forms, Alzheimer's disease is the most common. Alzheimer's, however, isn't the only condition that can play games with the intellect.

Strokes (see Common Neurological System Conditions) and arteriosclerosis (see Common Circulatory, Heart and Lung Conditions in chapter 5), which are both characterized by a reduced flow of blood to the brain, can also impair memory, as can a severe head injury or a brain tumor. Also, hormone insufficiencies, particularly those that affect the thyroid and pituitary glands, and nutritional deficiencies, such as pernicious anemia (see anemia under Common Whole Body Conditions in chapter 19), can sometimes cause memory dysfunction. Severe infections, depression and overdosing on street drugs or medications also can sometimes cause memory loss.

BEST RESPONSE: Check with your family physician, says Dr. Aronson. Only a doctor can diagnose what's causing memory loss. If it's a side effect of a disease, such as pernicious anemia or a glandular problem, the symptom should go away once the disease is under control. Dementia can also be reversed in cases of overdose, depression and infection. If it's Alzheimer's, however, the symptom most likely will gradually get worse.

"It's best to go to a doctor who knows the person and can document any personality changes," says Dr. Aronson. "Your family physician can also run a number of tests to see if the problem is treatable. If necessary, a specialist can then be consulted."

Although Alzheimer's disease is not curable, there is a great amount of research going on and a sense of hope that an effective treatment will someday be found. In the meantime, doctors suggest, keep in mind that Alzheimer's victims mirror the emotional state of those around them. If you're tense, grouchy and hurried, the person with Alzheimer's with whom you're dealing will be, too.

Instead, remember to speak in a clear, low-pitched voice. Use short, simple words, sentences and questions and wait for a response before you continue. If there's no response, repeat your comment or question in exactly the same word order, without adding new words or explanations. If there's a way to demonstrate what you mean—gesturing toward the street you want to walk toward, for example—do so. Or if there's a way to break an activity down into steps—"Let's put on your coat and then your hat"—try it. Avoid arguing or reasoning. You'll only make the problem worse.

In the early stages, someone with Alzheimer's may merely need a little help in doing his or her job. In later stages, 24-hour nursing care may be necessary. But in between there are lots of ways to help someone with Alzheimer's function more normally. You can simplify discussions by talking about only one subject at a time, for example. You can avoid decision-making problems by asking questions that require only a yes or no answer.

You can tape typewritten operating instructions on stoves, washing machines, dryers, furnaces and other household items and provide safeguards such as alarms on doors to keep someone with Alzheimer's from wandering off. As a double safeguard, some families sew name and address labels in clothing in case wandering does occur.

A person with Alzheimer's should maintain a regular, structured routine, including exercise, proper hygiene and nutritious, easily chewable meals, say doctors. Support groups for patients and family members are also helpful, because people who have "been there" are frequently the only ones who truly understand the problems that are caused by the disease. They're also the ones who have a dozen little tricks up their sleeves for dealing with day-to-day situations, and they probably know where any adult day-care facilities are so that family caregivers can get a rest. For the support group nearest you, contact the Alzheimer's Disease and Related Disorders Association, 70 East Lake Street, Chicago, IL 60601.

SYMPTOM: **Nervousness**

COMMON CAUSES: You fidget. You tap your fingers on your desk endlessly. You can't sit still for more than five minutes without bolting out of your seat. You feel so shaky and nervous you want to jump right out of your skin to escape it.

There are a variety of causes that give people a case of nerves, and they can be both emotional and physical, says H. Randall Hicks, M.D.

One common cause is stress, says Dr. Hicks. "This could involve the death of a loved one, illness or injury, impending surgery, a move, a change in your work or economic status or even a change in mortgage.

"Another common cause of nervousness is the use, abuse or withdrawal of a number of drugs, such as diet pills; amphetamines, or 'speed'; pain pills; sleeping medications; antianxiety drugs and cold medications (both over-the-counter and prescription)," says Dr. Hicks. Too much caffeine can be a problem, especially for confirmed coffee or cola drinkers.

Certain conditions and diseases can also cause nervousness. It's a symptom in some women who suffer from premenstrual syndrome (see Common Reproductive System Conditions in chapter 14) and for those going through menopause. And chronic pain, such as backache and headache, can also make you feel strung out. Certain chronic diseases, such as chronic obstructive lung disease, or COLD (see Common Circulatory, Heart and Lung Conditions in chapter 5) can make a person nervous or anxious.

Nervousness is one of the first symptoms—and sometimes the only symptom—of hyperthyroidism (see thyroid disease under Common Whole Body Conditions in chapter 19), says Dr. Hicks.

There are also emotional illnesses that can cause nervousness, the most common being anxiety neurosis, a type of depression; mania, which is characterized by a mood of extreme elation; and psychosis, a severe form of mental illness.

BEST RESPONSE: "If you're feeling nervous as a result of anxiety or turmoil in your life, you can take some immediate steps to deal with the problem," says Dr. Hicks. "Find a quiet space in your home and sit down with your thoughts. Write down the things you think may be causing your nervousness. Put them in rank order and write down a plan of how you can effectively deal with them."

Some measures that might be effective in relieving stress-caused nervousness, says Dr. Hicks, include talking it out with someone you trust, taking a long, soothing bath, going for a walk, doing a physical workout or getting lost in a novel. "These activities can give you a sense of control," says Dr. Hicks. "They can dissipate some of your stress and they can divert your mind from troubling thoughts."

If you suspect you're suffering from the coffee jitters, the easy solution, says Dr. Hicks, is to cut down on caffeine consumption. This also means avoiding tea, cola and chocolate, which also contain caffeine. If you think a medication is causing your nervousness, you should discontinue over-the-counter drugs and consult your doctor about the necessity of taking prescription drugs.

"If your nervousness persists, you should see your family doctor to search for the cause of your problem," says Dr. Hicks. "When you see your doctor, you should explain what you're experiencing. He or she may do a number of tests to rule out physical problems or, based on observations, may refer you for psychotherapy."

What you should *avoid*, cautions Dr. Hicks, is going to a doctor who will prescribe a tranquilizer such as Valium as a treatment for your problem. A good physician will try to treat your nervousness at the root of the problem, he says. He also says you should avoid any over-the-counter medication designed to calm your nerves.

ACCOMPANYING SYMPTOMS: If your nervousness is accompanied by sweating, rapid heartbeat, headache or dizziness, you could be suffering from hypoglycemia (see Common Whole Body Conditions in chapter 19).

SYMPTOM: **Seizures**

COMMON CAUSES: They're sometimes described as "brain electrical storms." More accurately, they represent the uncontrolled activity of masses of brain cells, which usually show up as contractions of the muscles. Such seizures are termed convulsions.

In some cases, no one knows what causes the brain to act up like this or why it happens in some people and not in others—most people who suffer from seizures or convulsions show no signs of physical illness or brain abnormality. When seizures of any type are recurrent, they are called epilepsy (see Common Neurological System Conditions), meaning that not everyone who suffers from a single seizure would be classified as an epileptic.

"All human beings can suffer from a seizure," says Ira Sherwin, M.D., clinical professor of neurology at the University of Southern California School of Medicine. "If any person were to grab an electric wire with sufficient voltage, he or she would have a major motor seizure that would look the same as a convulsive seizure in a person with epilepsy."

There are many physical conditions that can trigger a seizure, says Dr. Sherwin. In children, high fever (see Symptom: Fever in chapter 19) can bring on a seizure. So, too, can an infection. Severe overheating can trigger one. Taking street drugs or withdrawing from overdoses of tranquilizers, sleeping pills or alcohol can cause a convulsion.

A seizure, however, can sometimes be a sign of a severe illness, says Dr. Sherwin. Meningitis and strokes (see Common Neurological System Conditions); tetanus (see Common Facial, Jaw and Mouth Conditions in chapter 8); acute kidney failure (see Common Urinary Tract Conditions in chapter 18); heart attack (see myocardial infarction under Common Circulatory, Heart and Lung Conditions in chapter 5); brain hemorrhage, infection or tumor; severe toxemia of pregnancy or anything that disturbs the balance of body chemistry can set off a seizure.

Recurring seizures—epilepsy—can usually be traced to a disturbance in the brain cells rather than an underlying bodily ailment. In addition to convulsive seizures, there are several types of epileptic seizures. These may range from a simple blank stare, almost as if the victim were daydreaming, to complex and purposeful but inappropriate activity, such as lip smacking. Sometimes the cause of these seizures can be traced to a birth defect, a severe head injury or an infection involving the brain. Most often, however, the cause remains unknown.

BEST RESPONSE: "Almost all seizures end by themselves," says Dr. Sherwin. "During an attack, it's most important that the person be kept as safe as possible to avoid injury. The person may lie on the floor, but any furniture or other objects should be removed from the immediate vicinity. Movements should not be restrained, and it's usually not necessary— and may even be dangerous—to try to force the person's mouth open and put something between the teeth. Instead, the person's clothing should be loosened to improve breathing. Turning the head to one side will allow saliva to run out of the mouth."

If a child has a convulsion because of a high fever, you should call your doctor, says Dr. Sherwin. In the meantime, you can attempt to bring the temperature down by wrapping the child in a wet sheet. This may prevent further convulsions and possible brain damage. If this is a recurring problem, your doctor may provide medication that can be given at home.

"A convulsion is such a serious symptom and can be caused by so many different problems that a person who has suffered one for the first time should always seek medical attention to determine the cause," says Dr. Sherwin.

Your doctor will probably give you a complete physical and neurological examination, and order laboratory tests of your blood and sometimes your spinal fluid. The spinal test is especially helpful in determining if an infection is at the root of this problem. Brain scans, which may determine the site of the seizure's origin, as well as the possible cause, will probably be ordered.

If epilepsy is diagnosed, medication can be prescribed to prevent seizures from recurring. The type of medication, however, will depend on the type of seizure. The most common drugs used are phenytoin (Dilantin), phenobarbital, primidone (Mysoline), carbamazepine (Tegretol), ethosuximide (Zarontin), valproic acid (Depakene) and clonazepam (Clonopin).

In many cases where epilepsy begins in childhood, medication can be stopped after several years, when the epilepsy is "outgrown," says Dr. Sherwin.

"If a diagnosed epileptic forgets to take his or her medication and a seizure occurs, there is usually no need to seek immediate medical help, although the doctor should be notified," says Dr. Sherwin. Resumption of medication should prevent a recurrence of the attack.

SYMPTOM: **Speaking Difficulties**

COMMON CAUSES: Problems with speech can be manifested in several forms. There's slowed or slurred speech, in which you may sound "thick-tongued" or drunk; stuttering, in which you may uncontrollably repeat words or syllables; muteness, in which you can't speak at all and aphasia, in which you have difficulty communicating coherently.

Slowed or slurred speech can occur as a reaction to or side effect of certain drugs, most commonly anticonvulsion medications such as phenytoin (Dilantin) or phenobarbital, and phenothiazine tranquilizers such as Thorazine, says Nagagopal Venna, M.D.

There are also a number of illnesses that affect speech in this manner. These include Parkinson's disease, multiple sclerosis, cerebral palsy and dementia (see Common Neurological System Conditions), all of which interfere with brain activity. However, Dr. Venna notes, slurred speech is usually a side effect rather than a sign of such diseases. Other, more serious, symptoms will usually have already taken place to signal the onset of such illnesses.

"Stuttering, muteness and aphasia are the forms of speaking difficulty that cause the greatest concern," says Ira Sherwin, M.D. Stuttering almost always begins in childhood. At one time it was considered an emotional problem; however, says Dr. Sherwin, later evidence suggests that it may result from a failure of the normal neuromuscular control of the larynx, the organ that houses the vocal chords and is responsible for speech.

Muteness is often the result of deafness, says Dr. Sherwin, but it can also be caused by autism, a complex disorder that may be related to childhood schizophrenia.

"Aphasia usually comes on suddenly and dramatically and results from damage to the language areas of the brain," states Dr. Sherwin. In adults, it's most commonly the result of a stroke (see Common Neurological System Conditions). However, it can sometimes occur in the course of another illness, such as an infection. It can even occur in women after pregnancy. In children, if aphasia occurs before age six, there's a good chance of recovery. After age six, that possibility is not as likely."

BEST RESPONSE: If you notice you're slurring your speech after starting a new medication, you should consult your doctor, who may change the dosage, switch you to another medication or discontinue the drug altogether.

"Stuttering that comes on gradually in childhood is usually not the result of a life-threatening condition," says Dr. Sherwin. "The parents of such a child would be wise to take the child to a neurologist for a full exam just to rule out the very few but serious disorders that could be present. Once it's been established that no serious illness is present, a speech therapist may be helpful.

"A child who is mute and autistic should be evaluated and treated by a pediatric neurologist and a psychiatrist," he says.

"*Anytime* aphasia occurs, the person should receive rapid medical care, since the cause is usually of a more serious nature, such as a stroke," Dr. Sherwin warns. Once the immediate problem is under control, a rehabilitation program can begin; this is often best carried out by a speech therapist.

SYMPTOM: **Vertigo.** *See* Symptom: Dizziness

Common Neurological System Conditions

Alzheimer's disease. *See* Dementia

Anxiety. Everyone has experienced anxiety at one time or another. It's a reaction to a danger—either physical or emotional—that causes a vague, uneasy sense of dread, nervousness or apprehension.

Anxiety that is brought on by something real—sickness, going for a job interview, taking an exam or getting on an airplane for the first time, for example—is *normal* anxiety. Anxiety that is brought on by an imaginary threat—an unfounded fear of cancer or someone stalking you, for example—is a *neurotic* anxiety.

Normal anxiety can actually be quite healthy for some people. They use creative outlets, such as art and music or other forms of "escape," as an antidote. There is nothing healthy about neurotic anxiety, however.

A person with neurotic anxiety suffers constantly with symptoms that range from mild tenseness, timidness, fatigue, apprehension and indecisiveness to the more serious discomforts of extreme nervousness. In addition, a person who is anxious has a greater need for reassurance, frequently shifts topics of conversation, asks lots of questions, has difficulty following directions and has a shortened attention span. Physical symptoms include restlessness, palpitations, shortness of breath, excessive perspiration, pale skin, nausea, vomiting, diarrhea, insomnia and loss of appetite. These symptoms are a result of the anxiety and are not caused by a physical problem.

Some persons suffer from short periods of intense anxiety that last from a few seconds to an hour or longer and vary in frequency from once a month to several times a day. These are called panic attacks or anxiety attacks, and the symptoms are similar to those of anxiety neurosis. An anxiety attack may cause dizziness, fainting, feelings of choking or smothering and a vague sense of impending death.

The main treatment of anxiety neurosis and anxiety attacks is psychotherapy to identify the stressors that are causing the problem. In extreme circumstances, medication—such as tranquilizers and sedatives—may be helpful for short periods of time. For best results, however, they should never be used alone but in combination with psychotherapy.

For mild cases, a good approach to treatment is practicing relaxation techniques, such as meditation and biofeedback. Phobic disorders—irrational fears of specific things, such as snakes or being closed in—can be treated with psychotherapy, family counseling and better understanding of the problem through education.

Attention deficit disorder. Attention deficit disorder (ADD), also known as hyperactivity, is the most common psychiatric disorder of childhood. With or without the busy-bee behavior most people associate with it, ADD affects at least 3 percent of America's children and accounts for almost half of all children's referrals to mental health clinics. Boys with ADD outnumber girls with the disorder nearly eight to one.

But hyperactive behavior is not a simple disease with a single cause and cure. It is, instead, a group of symptoms that may be triggered by one or a thousand different causes that may have one or a thousand different cures. Scientists suspect that the causes can range from anxiety, environmental stress, inadequate parenting and a genetic predisposition, to injury, infection, lead poisoning or lack of oxygen at birth. Nobody really knows.

That's why ADD's diagnosis and treatment are both complicated and controversial. Generally, doctors agree, a child can be diagnosed as having ADD if he or she is overactive, easily distracted, impulsive and excitable. What confuses things is that every "normal" child can act this way. In fact, 60 percent of all parents, at one time or another, will suspect that their children are hyperactive.

But a hyperactive child is something special. Even in the womb, mothers report, these children are restless. And when they're born, they often eat and sleep poorly. They resist cuddling and rocking. They destroy as soon as they can touch, climb as soon as they can stand and run as soon as they can walk. They cannot turn off their motors or their mouths and, by age three or four, they're often irritable, impatient and easily upset. And they usually drive their parents nuts.

The parents of hyperactive children, researchers report, frequently become hostile, critical, controlling and coercive to the point that the child's self-image is compromised.

Fortunately, many hyperactives can be helped by medication, a highly structured environment with one-on-one adult/child interaction and social skills training. Some, if they have a sensitivity to certain foods, may also find that eliminating those foods can be helpful.

Cerebral palsy. This disorder occurs at birth or in early childhood (usually before the age of five) and results in limited control over muscle movement because of permanent but nonprogressive damage to the motor centers of the brain.

The cause is not always known, but complications in the last part of pregnancy, premature birth, birth injury or severe diseases of infancy are frequently implicated.

There are three major types of cerebral palsy: spastic, characterized by stiffness and great difficulty in moving—often a "scissors gait" or toe walking is the result; athetoid, which causes slow, writhing, involuntary movements or abrupt jerky movements that increase with stress and disappear during sleep; and ataxic, characterized by poor balance, poor coordination and a staggering gait. It's possible to suffer from a mixed or combined form of cerebral palsy; spastic and athetoid most frequently occur together.

Convulsions, defects of vision and hearing, speech problems and mental retardation are other symptoms of the disease.

There is great variation in the degree of damage and disability with cerebral palsy. It's especially important—though sometimes difficult—to diagnose the disorder at an early age so that treatment can begin.

Although cerebral palsy is not curable, treatment is aimed at developing the greatest independence within the limits of the child's handicaps. Physical, occupational and speech therapies are helpful, as well as orthopedic surgery, wearing braces and taking medication to control seizures. Some children need special classes, whereas others can attend a regular school.

Concussion.   A concussion is defined as a state of temporary uncon-sciousness in which the brain's normal activity is interrupted. It's caused by a sharp, jarring injury to the head and can range from mild, where the person may feel momentarily dazed, to severe, where the victim can remain unconscious for a number of days and can experience perma-nent loss of memory about events just prior to the injury.

Treatment for a concussion includes bed rest for one to six weeks, depending on the severity of the injury. Symptoms should be closely watched during the time of recuperation.

Most concussions have no serious lasting effects, but repeated blows can cause permanent brain injury. Potentially dangerous situa-tions should be avoided by wearing protective headgear for contact sports and cycling and by wearing automobile seat belts.

Dementia.   Dementia is the deterioration of the ability to think and remember to the point that it interferes with your job, your family and your social life. It's usually divided into two categories, primary and secondary.

Primary dementias come on gradually, without apparent cause, and have no known treatment. Secondary dementias may appear more suddenly—there may be a triggering agent such as an operation, a diabetic coma or a recent hospitalization—and they are usually reversi-ble. About 20 percent of all dementias are thought to fall into the lat-ter category.

The most common type of primary dementia is Alzheimer's disease, which occurs severely in some 4 to 5 percent of those beyond age 65 and mildly to moderately in another 11 to 12 percent. The effects of multiple small strokes—multi-infarct dementia—is the second most common dementia, and it's also possible to suffer from a combination of Alzheimer's and multiple small strokes.

No one knows exactly what causes Alzheimer's, although medical researchers do know that having it means its victims will have tangled clumps of nerve fibers and patches of disintegrated nerve-cell branches in their brain. Medical researchers also know that there's a greater risk of developing the disease if you've previously had a serious head injury, if a close relative had the disease or if you have a genetic abnormality such as Down's syndrome. Interestingly, unusually large amounts of aluminum are found in the brains of Alzheimer's victims after death. Researchers aren't quite sure how it gets there or what effect it has on the brain, but they're investigating it as a possible cause of the disease.

Alzheimer's progresses through seven levels of brain deterioration, either quickly, over a span of 3 to 4 years, or slowly, over a period as long as 15 years. Each level of physical deterioration usually causes behavioral changes, although the changes are so slight in the first level that few people realize what's going on. But beginning at level two, there are usually slight complaints of forgetfulness (misplaced glasses or a slowness to come up with a name) that progress through level three (forgetting meetings or the names of important associates) to level four (forgetting how to do such routine activities as food shopping or balancing a checkbook).

At this point, most Alzheimer's victims need help in handling everyday activities. At least one-third can still function independently in their communities, although they may occasionally get lost or forget their address when under stress.

At level five, however, most Alzheimer's victims usually need daily supervision in choosing appropriate clothes and preparing meals. Driving a car also becomes hazardous at this stage. An Alzheimer's driver, for example, will suddenly speed up or slow down for no apparent reason, and may even absentmindedly zip through a stop sign.

At level six, driving is out of the question. Alzheimer's victims need help with such basic activities as dressing and going to the bathroom. They can't count backward from ten, have only a vague idea of where they live, begin to fear bathing and frequently don't recognize the people with whom they live. Near the end of this stage, they may become incontinent. The incontinence, however, is due to the fact that they forget the mechanics of sitting on a commode, wiping and so on, rather than to any physical problem.

At level seven, the ability of Alzheimer's victims to speak becomes reduced to grunts and screams. Eventually they also become bedridden and usually die of infections like pneumonia.

Although there's no known treatment for the victims of primary dementias such as Alzheimer's, secondary dementias are both treatable and reversible. They may be caused by blood vessel disease, hormone insufficiency, particularly an underactive thyroid or pituitary gland, depression, drug overdose, overmedication, head injuries, brain tumors, nutritional deficiencies such as pernicious anemia, and infectious diseases.

Because there is such a difference in outcome between primary and secondary dementias, making the proper diagnosis is crucial. Tests include a brain wave test (what doctors call an EEG, or electroencephalogram) and a special kind of x-ray called a CAT (computerized axial tomography) scan. A doctor will probably also do physical, neurologic and psychiatric exams, as well as laboratory studies.

These tests will rule out treatable dementias. If all tests are negative, the diagnosis is usually Alzheimer's. Unfortunately, at present the only way to confirm an Alzheimer's diagnosis is to examine the brain after death. Researchers feel that in the near future, specific laboratory tests will be able to confirm the diagnosis.

Depression. As part of the normal peaks and valleys of life, you may feel down for a day or two—like when a good time comes to an end or when life deals you a bad hand. You may even say you feel depressed.

But the *disease* of depression is more serious. It darkens everything in your life and casts a pall that lasts for weeks. Four or more of the following symptoms are usually present: recurrent thoughts of death or the wish to be dead; feelings of worthlessness or excessive guilt; impaired thinking or concentration; loss of energy or fatigue; reduced appetite and weight loss or sometimes the opposite, increased eating and weight gain; loss of sexual desire; sleep disturbance—either too much or too little; and a change in activity level—either nervously going on without end or the opposite, suddenly slowing down.

Some people suffer from depression that alternates with periods of mania, in which the person feels high on life and is incessantly active. This type of illness is called manic-depressive reaction.

Why some people suffer from depression and others don't is not fully understood, although depression is more common in those with a family history of the illness, in alcoholics and in those with chronic illnesses. The fact that antidepressant drugs are effective in many cases (except with alcoholism) suggests there's a chemical imbalance in the depressed person's brain.

Depression can be extremely painful for the person experiencing it and for those friends and relatives who are trying to be helpful. If the sufferer has strong suicidal tendencies or is seriously ill, hospitalization may be necessary.

Generally, though, treatment is carried out at home under the supervision of a doctor or therapist and includes psychotherapy or counseling combined with medication. Prescription drugs include tricyclics such as Sinequan, Elavil and Vivactil, MAO inhibitors such as Nardil and Marplan and, for the manic depressive, lithium. Persons who are depressed and psychotic require antipsychotic medications such as Thorazine or Mellaril.

Encephalitis. Encephalitis is an inflammation of brain cells usually caused by a viral infection. It is often acquired after being bitten by an infected mosquito. Sometimes it's a complication of other illnesses such as flu, measles, chickenpox, infectious mononucleosis, whooping cough or meningitis.

Encephalitis can range from a mild case, with headache, muscle ache and malaise as its chief symptoms, to a more severe form, with symptoms such as fever, delirium and convulsions. In severe cases, coma and death can result.

The most common form of encephalitis in the United States is due to herpes virus. Effective treatment for this form is now available in the antiviral drug acyclovir.

There is no specific treatment for other types of viral encephalitis except bed rest and adequate nutrition. Maintenance of fluid and electrolyte balance is important. Recovery from a severe attack is prolonged.

Epilepsy. This is a central nervous system disorder resulting from abnormal electrical activity in the brain. Most of those who have epilepsy suffer their first attack during childhood, young adulthood or after age 50.

In two-thirds of the cases, the cause of the seizures is not known; victims show no signs of physical illness or brain disorders. Outside of the seizures, they can lead a very normal life. One theory, however, being studied at Stanford University School of Medicine, in California, suggests that some forms of epilepsy are caused by abnormal brain cells that fire in bursts. "The unique ability of these 'bursting cells' to readily discharge a number of electrical impulses makes them possible initiators of epileptic seizures," says Barry Connors, Ph.D., assistant professor of neurology at Stanford University.

And in some cases, a physical cause can be found. An injury to the brain at birth, an injury due to a hard blow to the head, a brain tumor or an endocrine disorder can result in epilepsy.

All epileptic seizures are not the same, and treatment depends on the type of seizures suffered.

Those who suffer from the most common form of seizure, major muscular seizure, or grand mal, may experience a peculiar "aura" of smell, taste or sensation. They may see flashing lights or experience ringing in the ears. This aura is followed by sudden loss of consciousness and falling to the floor, with arms and legs held stiff. After about half a minute there is rhythmic jerking of the body, followed by incontinence. The seizure usually lasts about two to three minutes and is followed by a deep sleep. On waking, the victim may be dazed and have a headache or sore muscles but will have no recollection of the convulsion. Often, however, there is sudden loss of consciousness without any warning aura.

Minor muscular seizures, called petit mal, can occur as often as 20 times a day and may be mistaken for daydreaming. The victim becomes motionless and stares for a few seconds. He or she may lose balance and even fall. Petit mal convulsions are genetically determined and usually occur in children; they never begin after age 20.

Partial muscular seizures, called focal seizures, cause jerking movements that start in one part of the body, such as a twitching of the mouth or jerking of one arm, and may spread to other parts of the body.

Psychomotor seizures, or complex partial seizures, cause unprovoked behavior such as abnormal laughter, crying or violent acts brought on by fear. The victim doesn't fall but can't understand what is being said or what is going on around him or her. Typically, the victim may experience a peculiar smell or taste, a hallucination of sounds, or dizziness or memory lapse and appear dazed and dreamy for a few minutes in each spell. He or she may walk around aimlessly, fidget and appear confused. This type of convulsion may start in childhood or in adulthood.

Although there is no cure for epilepsy, there are over 20 medications—Dilantin, Tegretol, Zarontin and phenobarbital among them—that a doctor can prescribe to effectively keep the disease under control.

Most children with epilepsy can be taken off medication after two years without a recurrence of seizures.

Hyperactivity. *See* Attention deficit disorder

Meningitis.   This is an inflammation and infection of the meninges, the membranes that cover the brain and spinal cord. The cause can be viral, which is often spread from person to person through the air, or bacterial, which is caused by an organism that enters the body and spreads through the bloodstream. Meningitis can also be a complication from a head injury, an infected ear or an infected sinus.

The symptoms of meningitis are severe headache with a stiff neck, intolerance to light and sometimes sound, and nausea and vomiting. Sometimes there's a reddish or purplish rash all over the body. If meningitis is left untreated, drowsiness, delirium and unconsciousness can occur. Viral meningitis is less severe than meningitis caused by bacteria.

Diagnosis of meningitis and identification of the infectious organism is made through examination of the cerebrospinal fluid by means of a spinal tap. Treatment usually includes hospitalization and, in the case of bacterial meningitis, large doses of antibiotics. If proper treatment is carried out promptly, full recovery is expected.

Multiple sclerosis.   This long-term and gradually debilitating disease of the central nervous system, which is also known as MS, strikes young people, mostly between ages 20 and 40. It causes the gradual destruction of myelin, a substance that sheaths and insulates nerves. When the myelin is destroyed, scarring—sclerosis—occurs, resulting in slowed or blocked electrical signals between brain and body. Multiple sclerosis is so named because many scars eventually occur.

Although the exact cause of the disease is not known, it is believed that viral infections or the immune system's response to a virus play a role in its cause.

Symptoms of the disease and their severity vary from patient to patient. They include weakness, difficulty in walking, loss of bowel or bladder control, vision problems and speaking difficulties. Symptoms tend to come and go—when they are absent, the disease is said to be in remission.

Diagnosis of the disease is difficult, and there is no one specific test that can confirm its presence. Physical examination by a neurologist, laboratory studies of spinal fluid, a brain wave test known as an electro-encephalogram (EEG) and a special brain x-ray called a CAT (computerized axial tomography) scan are often performed when symptoms of the disease develop. A new test called magnetic resonance imaging (MRI), which uses magnetism and radio waves to view the inside of the body, has proven particularly useful in the diagnosis of multiple sclerosis.

MS is not curable and tends to get progressively worse. Physical and occupational therapy are helpful, however, as are muscle-relaxing drugs to reduce spasms. Cortisone-type medications can reduce swelling of myelin, but only for short periods of time. Prevention of urinary tract infections is important. Mobility and mental outlook can be improved by maintaining a regular exercise program and keeping socially active.

Parkinson's disease.   This is a slowly progressive disease of the central nervous system that strikes later in life—usually after age 40.

The disease is characterized by stiffness and rigidity of the muscles, slowness of movement and tremor or trembling of the arms and legs. At first the victim may only notice mild tremors or nodding of the head. Later, the loss of mobility results in a fixed facial stare. The victim can also experience balance problems and an awkward gait.

Studies show that the cause of the disease is related to a decrease of the neurotransmitter dopamine in the brain, creating a chemical imbalance. The drug levodopa (L-dopa), which synthetically replaces dopamine in the brain, is used to help control the symptoms. Use of the drug, however, requires close supervision.

For mild cases, less severe measures are generally taken. Physical, occupational and speech therapy can often be used to help the victim maintain independence. Anticholinergic agents, such as trihexyphenidyl (Artane), or antihistamines with anticholinergic properties, are often prescribed.

The disease, however, can only be controlled; there is no cure at present.

Senility.   *See* Dementia

Stroke.   A stroke, or cerebrovascular accident, is a sudden decrease in the blood supply to a part of the brain. When blood and oxygen cannot get to the brain, cells die, which can cause permanent paralysis and loss of speech and memory.

Strokes are caused either by a blockage of a blood vessel or a bleeding rupture of one. Older people are affected the most, especially those with high blood pressure or arteriosclerosis, hardening of the arteries. A stroke can also be caused by an aneurysm, which is a congenital weakening of a vessel wall. This can occur at any age.

Regardless of the cause of the stroke, immediate symptoms are the same: weakness or paralysis of, or loss of feeling in, an arm, a leg or both; visual disturbances; inability to speak; confusion; dizziness and, sometimes, unconsciousness.

Treatment of a stroke usually involves hospitalization, during which oxygen, if necessary, is given, and drugs, such as anticoagulants to thin the blood (if blood vessel blockage was the cause) and antihypertensives to reduce high blood pressure, are administered.

Adequate nutrition is important, and immediate rehabilitation is crucial. Exercises, taught by a physical therapist, can begin in the hospital and are absolutely necessary in achieving as full a recovery as possible. Speech therapy may also be necessary.

Transient ischemic attacks.   Often called TIAs or ministrokes, transient ischemic attacks are sudden, brief episodes of an abnormal sensation, such as dim vision, numbness and weakness on one side of the body, dizziness and thickened speech. They can last for minutes but are often fleeting. They always disappear without incident.

The attacks most commonly occur in the middle-aged and elderly and result when small blood vessels are blocked or go into spasm. Those with high blood pressure, heart disease, diabetes mellitus or polycythemia, a disease in which blood volume is enlarged, are often the victims.

Although TIAs are minor happenings, they should not go unchecked by a doctor. TIAs often recur and may herald the onset of a stroke. Besides treatment for the disease that's causing the problem, anticoagulant medication may be prescribed to thin the blood. For those who suffer only occasional TIAs, most doctors try aspirin therapy before starting anticoagulants.

In some instances, where the cause of TIAs is found to be a severely narrowed blood vessel in the neck that supplies blood to the brain, surgery is performed to decrease the risk of stroke. This procedure should be done only after very careful evaluation by specialists.

Chapter 13
Nose

Your nose does more than tell you when the chicken's burning, your mate's been drinking or you didn't make it home in time to let out the dog. It also acts as your first line of defense against viruses and bacteria that your friends, neighbors and countrymen have sprayed throughout your environment.

In less than the time it takes to sniff, your nose checks incoming air for germs and shoots down as many as its antibacterial cannons can handle. It then turns up its thermostat until the incoming air reaches 98.6°F—the same internal temperature as the rest of your body—and activates its humidistat until the incoming air is saturated with 75 percent humidity.

Sears couldn't make a better model.

SYMPTOM: **Bleeding**

COMMON CAUSES: Nosebleeds are rarely started by anything more serious than a cold or an inquisitive finger. They are uncommon in infancy but common in preadolescent children and adults who are between 50 and 70 years old.

Nosebleeds are usually caused by colds and allergies (see Common Nasal Conditions) that inflame the nasal passages, or by accidents, sneezes, violent nose blowing, nasal surgery that traumatizes delicate tissue, nose picking, dryness, or chemical vapors that can irritate the small blood vessels just inside the front of the nose.

Anticoagulant drugs that thin the blood can also cause nosebleeds, and an early sign of high blood pressure (see Common Circulatory, Heart and Lung Conditions in chapter 5) may very well be a nosebleed— especially if a headache precedes the bleeding, then recedes afterward. In rare instances, nosebleeds can also be caused by a tumor.

BEST RESPONSE:　Most doctors suggest you sit down, lean forward and pinch your nose tightly shut for 15 minutes. If your nose starts to bleed again, says Byron J. Bailey, M.D., Weifs professor and chairman of the Department of Otolaryngology at the University of Texas Medical Branch at Galveston, sprinkle a ¼ percent solution of Neo-Synephrine (available over the counter as children's-strength nose drops) on a little cotton ball, gently put the cotton ball inside the bleeding nostril, then pinch the nostril shut for another 15 minutes. Clotting time—the time it takes blood to plug up a wound and stop flowing—is somewhere between 5 and 10 minutes, says Dr. Bailey, so don't get impatient and pull out the cotton before your time is up.

Some doctors suggest you go to the nearest hospital emergency room if the bleeding doesn't stop within 30 minutes. The source of your nosebleed may be in the back of the nose—it more commonly is in adults—so pinching the front isn't going to help a bit. (Nor will applying a cold cloth to the back of your neck or constantly stroking your nose, which are two popular "home remedies.")

Instead, the emergency room doctor may pack your nostril with gauze, send up a tiny balloon inside it or cauterize the bleeding site with a drop of chemical or a tiny electrical charge. This latter procedure should be performed by an experienced specialist such as an otolaryngologist. Someone with less skill might injure your nose internally.

You might also give a thought to prevention, since garden-variety nosebleeds are common in dry climates or during winter months, when dry air parches the nasal membranes so that they crust, crack and bleed. To prevent this from happening, the American Academy of Otolaryngology—Head and Neck Surgery recommends that you rub *a bit* of cream or ointment inside the nose at the edge of the nostrils at bedtime. If needed, you can apply the lubricant up to three times a day. Over-the-counter lubricants recommended by the Academy include Borofax Ointment, A and D Ointment, Mentholatum Ointment, Vicks Vapo Rub and Vaseline.

SYMPTOM: **Dryness**

COMMON CAUSE: The nose produces roughly a quart of fluid every day. So if the back of it feels dry, you may suspect there's a problem. But the "problem" is actually a warning: It's the body's announcement that a cold (see Common Nasal Conditions) will attack—usually within 24 hours.

BEST RESPONSE: Add two tablespoons of salt to a quart of warm water, pour a small amount into your hand and snort it up your nose whenever the back of your nose feels parched, suggests Byron J. Bailey, M.D. If snorting isn't your thing, adds Dr. Bailey, fill an eyedropper with the solution and squirt it into your nose. It won't keep the cold at bay, but it will soothe your nose. Then grab a book, pull out an afghan and get ready for your cold.

SYMPTOM: **Itching**

COMMON CAUSES: If you're prone to furry nostrils, an itchy nose can very well be caused by excess hair. But it may be the first symptom of an allergic attack (see allergy under Common Nasal Conditions), to be followed shortly by a paroxysm of sneezing, rivers of mucus and a nasal blockade that could've stopped Sherman's march through Georgia.

BEST RESPONSE: Trim the hair in your nostrils if extra fur is tickling the inside of your nose, says Dr. Bailey. But be careful to trim, not pluck. If you pluck the hairs with tweezers, you have a good chance of starting an infection that can spread to your brain. And be sure to use blunt-edged scissors. Stabbing the inside of your nose with a sharp blade can set up the same infection as plucking with a pair of tweezers.

But if your itchy nose is really an allergic twitch from a dog, mold, dust or pollen, the best way to stop it is to get rid of the allergen. That can be pretty hard, of course—especially if your allergy is to pollen. A single ragweed plant, for example, can release as many as a million pollen grains a day, each of which can travel well over 200 miles. That's why some doctors recommend that you stay inside with the doors and windows shut during your allergy season's prime time.

Better yet, some doctors recommend an electrostatic air cleaner to remove pollen and dust. This device gives an electrical charge to the pollen particle, then attracts it to a collector plate inside the cleaner. Also, avoid tobacco smoke, which can aggravate the allergies you already have. In fact, smoke can cause allergic symptoms far more frequently than the allergens themselves.

But what can you do about household allergens? If you're allergic to molds, some doctors suggest you avoid spending time in damp places, such as basements and garages. If this is impossible, place a dehumidifier in the room to get rid of the moisture. And don't forget to clean it. Still water can breed disease.

Washing down bathrooms frequently—including fixtures—with soap and water (many common household cleaners can also aggravate allergies) and keeping the area well ventilated also seem to help eliminate molds, as does getting rid of your houseplants. Some doctors also suggest you avoid raking and burning leaves, and think twice about mowing the lawn. Isn't there somebody else in the family who can do it?

The most common allergen that's not tied to a seasonal appearance is house dust. But house dust is more than those curly little bunnies under your bed. It's actually made up of everything from plaster debris and flakes of skin to food remnants, bacteria and microscopic animals called mites. Clearly, there's something to be said for having a clean house. But if you're the one who has to clean it, you might want to wear a mask while you do.

Of course, if your allergy to dust is really severe, some doctors suggest you get rid of anything that collects or emits dust. Use only nylon, Dacron or Orlon fabrics in bedding materials, for example, and give away any cotton sheets or wool blankets, since these fabrics tend to attract and hold dust. You should get rid of your venetian blinds while you're at it, and wash your curtains or drapes—which should be made out of the same synthetics as your bedding—once a week. Dusting with a damp rag and mop every other day and using filters on your furnace and air conditioning vents are also helpful. If you do all this, your contact with allergens in the home will be reduced, and this lessened contact should lead to fewer symptoms as well.

If you don't want to spend the rest of your life wiping, washing and dusting, however, you might want to try keeping just your bedroom free of the allergen. After all, you spend at least 8 out of every 24 hours in that one room. And if it's free of dust and mites, so are you. For a while.

But what if your allergy is to animals? Actually, your allergy is not to the animal itself but to the animal's dander (flakes of skin) or feathers. And if you live with dogs, cats, birds or even feather pillows, there's no way to get away from it. And maybe you wouldn't want to. There are still folks in this world who will put up with an itchy, runny, stuffy nose in exchange for the love of a soft, four-legged bundle of fur or an exotic, silky-winged creature that rides on their shoulder.

So for those of you who can't—or won't—get away from your allergens, many doctors recommend that you use an over-the-counter antihistamine. The antihistamine should be taken regularly to be effective, but never take one if you intend to drive a car or truck or operate machinery, since antihistamines can make you sleepy. Nor should you let a child climb trees or ride a bike until you are certain that he or she will not be unsafe as a result of the drug's sedative effect.

Most people, however, find that antihistamines lose their effectiveness when they are continued longer than a month. It is better to use them only when you have symptoms, then try to stay off the medication for a month or two before using it again.

If the antihistamine doesn't give you as much relief as you need, you might want to talk with your doctor about prescription antihistamines or even about a series of injections designed to desensitize your body to the allergen.

Finally, if you don't know whether you have an allergy but your symptoms suggest that you might, see your doctor, who can give you a series of allergy tests.

SYMPTOM: **Redness**

COMMON CAUSES: At one extreme, a red nose can be caused by the cold, icy wind that just blew around the corner. At the other, it can be caused by cancer. And somewhere in the middle of this spectrum, a red nose can be caused by rosacea, which is sometimes called "whiskey nose" or "rum nose."

Years ago, many people apparently thought the red nose of rosacea was due to an overindulgence in whiskey or rum, an unfortunate assumption that probably turned the faces of many teetotalers red with embarrassment rather than disease. In some people, however, foods such as coffee, tea, nuts, chocolate, hot peppers, alcohol and spices do cause blood vessels to dilate, which in turn causes a flush.

BEST RESPONSE: If your nose flushes red every time you eat one of the foods listed above, avoiding the foods or ignoring your nose may well be your best response. But check with your doctor to make sure that's all it is. He or she might want to prescribe medications or topical preparations that will help you and, in severe cases, remove the skin growths that can accompany this condition. Your doctor can also detect if the redness is being caused by something more serious.

ACCOMPANYING SYMPTOMS: Rosacea is also characterized by pimples, an overgrowth of tissue, dandruff and, occasionally, ulceration of the eye.

SYMPTOM: **Runny Nose**

COMMON CAUSES: The mucus produced by your nose is actually a protective fluid generated by your body as a defense mechanism. Its job is to trap incoming bacteria, viruses and other irritants, then wash them out of the nose. Nasal secretions that are caused by allergy (see Common Nasal Conditions) are usually clear and watery. Secretions that are thick, colored or foul-tasting are usually caused by sinusitis (see Common Nasal Conditions).

Sometimes, however, a drippy nose has a more innocuous cause: it's simply overreacting to cold weather. Did you ever go outside on a snowy day and have your nose start to drip? The coldness and dryness of the air triggered your nose's natural heaters and humidifiers to produce as much warmth and humidity as possible. And they did. Since the outside air on that cold winter's day had so little natural humidity, your nose kept producing all the humidity it thought you needed until you had the good sense to go back inside.

But sometimes your runny nose is such a faucet that you're constantly wiping it with the back of your hand. Doctors call this gesture the "allergic salute" because it's such a tip-off to the cause of your misery. One warning: The constant rubbing of your nose may irritate and even infect the skin underneath. If the skin begins to take on a honey-crusted, scabbed appearance, see your doctor. You may need an antibiotic to clear up the infection.

Some drugs, such as aspirin and propranolol hydrochloride, a medication sometimes prescribed for high blood pressure, have also been known to cause a runny nose, as have colds (see Common Nasal Conditions) and common childhood viral diseases such as chickenpox and measles (see Common Skin Conditions in chapter 15). Less frequently, runny noses are caused by a deviated septum (see Common Nasal Conditions), cancer or cystic fibrosis, a hereditary disease that affects the pancreas.

BEST RESPONSE: "Your best response is to carry soft, clean tissues," says Byron J. Bailey, M.D. "I think it's a mistake to try and dry up every runny nose. If the nose is running, there's usually a reason. If it's an allergy, your nose may be trying to wash the pollen out. If it's a cold, it's trying to wash the viral products out. It's just a natural body defense mechanism that is annoying when it does too much."

ACCOMPANYING SYMPTOMS: If your runny nose is accompanied by a very high temperature and general body pains, it's more likely to be caused by influenza (see Common Whole Body Conditions in chapter 19) than anything else. Check with your doctor, particularly if your temperature goes above 102°F.

SYMPTOM: **Smell, Loss of**

COMMON CAUSES: Sometimes you only *think* you've lost your sense of smell. Actually, you've just gotten used to a particular odor, however delightful or disgusting. As *Working* author Studs Terkel's cleanup man in a factory where rotten meat, fat and bones are "rendered" into (preferably) anonymous substances puts it: "The odor was terrible, but I got used to it. It was less annoying when you stayed right in it. When you left for a week or so, a vacation, you had to come back and get used to the thing all over again."

An understandable phenomenon. So what really kills your sense of smell? Well, a cold (see Common Nasal Conditions), for example, can stuff up the nose so much that no gaseous odors reach the odor-detecting area at the top or roof of the nose. Or a tumor in the front of the head—a rare occurrence—can prevent the brain from interpreting the nose's signals. Chronic infections such as sinusitis (see Common Nasal Conditions) can damage the sense of smell, and swelling from allergy or polyps (see Common Nasal Conditions), injury or half a dozen other factors can deaden even the most sensitive proboscis.

Certainly one of the most common causes of a nose (and tongue) that no longer works well is old age. "Because the neurological functions that govern these senses decrease with age, the elderly can lose the intensity of taste and smell sensations they had when younger," reported Susan Schiffman, Ph.D., a Duke University professor, to a meeting of the American Aging Association.

In one study conducted by Dr. Schiffman, for example, only 55 percent of the older folks involved were able to recognize the taste of an apple when it was blended to the same consistency as other test foods. Eighty-one percent of the college students involved in the study could recognize the taste. The decrease in smell is even greater than the loss of taste, and this is why older folks may think that foods such as green pepper and chocolate taste bitter, says Dr. Schiffman. The strong odor is diminished in the elderly, and the bitter taste becomes more obvious.

BEST RESPONSE: If your loss of smell is due to a cold or sinus infection, there really isn't a whole lot you can do. Your sense of smell will return as your cold or infection diminishes.

If your lost or diminished sense of smell is due to an aging schnozzola, you can try adding extra seasonings such as minced onion, paprika, oregano, ginger, allspice, cinnamon, vinegar, lemon and dill seed to your food, suggests Dr. Schiffman. Since your sense of smell accounts for much of your ability to taste, the intensified smells will not only allow you to smell more, but to taste better, too.

But if you lose your sense of smell for more than 14 days, check with your doctor, says James B. Snow, Jr., M.D., chairman of the Otorhino-laryngology and Human Communication Department at the University of Pennsylvania in Philadelphia. Or make an appointment at one of the smell and taste research centers located mainly in the East. They include the Hospital of the University of Pennsylvania in Philadelphia, the S.U.N.Y. Health Science Center in Syracuse, New York, the University of Connecticut Health Center at Farmington and the University of Colorado Health Sciences Center in Denver. Many doctors still don't know the centers exist, says Dr. Snow, but if you happen to live within commuting distance, their expertise makes them worth a trip.

There are many different tests the centers or even your own doctor might use to measure your ability to smell, but one of the newest—and fastest—is The Smell Identification Test ("scratch 'n' sniff") developed by Richard L. Doty, Ph.D., director of the Smell and Taste Center at the University of Pennsylvania School of Medicine.

Neurologists and otolaryngologists in roughly 800 clinics around the country are using the ten-minute test to screen for more than 30 different disorders, says Dr. Doty. With such common odors as pizza, licorice, gasoline and pine to test your olfactory IQ, the $20 test can alert doctors to such uncommon diseases as Parkinson's disease and epilepsy (see Common Neurological System Conditions in chapter 12). All you have to do is scratch each of the 40 odor-bearing strips, take a whiff and guess what it might be.

SYMPTOM: **Sneezing**

COMMON CAUSES: Did you ever walk into a room and start sneezing? You may have just assumed that there was something in the room to which you were allergic. And you were probably right. But your sneezing might also have been due to a kind of pseudo-allergy triggered by a chemical irritant, especially if you already suffer from an allergy. A nonspecific irritant can partially paralyze the nasal cilia—the little hairs that sweep out the nose's secretions and accumulations—and provoke nose and eye watering as well as paroxysms of sneezing.

Some of the irritants that you are likely to encounter include room deodorizers, perfumed cosmetics, air-freshener sprays, floor and furniture waxes, soaps and other cleaning compounds, smoke, insecticides, turpentine, paint and indoor air pollutants such as ozone.

Sneezing can also be the body's attempt to dislodge cold germs, a foreign body or an insect that has just detoured up the nose. Or it might even be a complex reaction by the ultraviolet receptors in the nose to a fresh dose of sunlight.

BEST RESPONSE: Don't suppress your sneeze. In some cases suppressing a sneeze has led to a stroke.

"If it's from a cold, you wait for the cold to go away, usually three to ten days," says Byron J. Bailey, M.D. "If it's from a foreign body, you get it out. And there's nothing practical that you can do about sunlight."

When the sneezing seems overwhelming, however, some doctors recommend that you lie down with your head tilted back and let the nasal waterfall flow down the back of your throat. Then swallow. At least you'll get five minutes of peace.

And consider yourself fortunate. Centuries ago a sneeze was taken as a popular indication that you were going to drop dead from pestilence. In fact, that's where the customary "God bless you!" or "Zum gesund!" ("to health") or "Gesundheit!" got started. During a particularly violent seventh-century plague in Italy, when people would sneeze a few times and then die, Pope Gregory VII suggested that when someone sneezed, neighbors should immediately bless the person.

SYMPTOM: **Snoring**

COMMON CAUSES: "Laugh and the world laughs with you. Snore and you sleep alone." Almost one-quarter of us understand all too well this old wag's saying every night, because that many of us snore every time we succumb to the sandman's dust. Maybe that's why there are more than 300 devices on the market that purport to cure snoring: everything from chin straps and mouth inserts to head binders, neck collars and electrical gadgets. The problem is that few of them—if any—work.

Flabby muscle tone can cause snoring by allowing the throat muscles to be drawn into the airway when muscular control is overly relaxed by alcohol, drugs or deep sleep. Or a long soft palate can narrow the opening from nose to throat, and a part of it—the uvula—which usually sticks down into the throat where you can see it, may act as a flutter valve during relaxed sleep.

Excessive bulkiness of throat tissue can also cause snoring, whether the bulkiness is due to large tonsils and adenoids or simply to a fat throat. And there are few of us who haven't snored during a cold or other infection when the nose was so stuffed that we had to pull hard to inhale any air at all. Unfortunately, while we were trying so hard to breathe, we created a vacuum in the throat and pulled all the floppy tissues together for an ensemble performance.

But when snoring becomes disruptive, or when another member of the household notices that your snoring is interspersed with seven- to ten-second periods of totally obstructed breathing, you may have a condition called sleep apnea, says Byron J. Bailey, M.D.

"Snoring is something that people kid about a lot," says Dr. Bailey, "but it's also something that indicates a condition that can be fatal. Breathing pauses during sleep plus chronic daytime drowsiness are strong indications of a serious sleep apnea problem."

During obstructive episodes, for example, the body is so starved for oxygen that the heart must pump harder to circulate the blood faster. Unfortunately, this condition can cause irregular heartbeats and—over time—high blood pressure and an enlarged heart.

A child who is experiencing sleep apnea may find it easy to go to bed at night but hard to wake up in the morning. He or she may also have either academic or behavioral problems in school, or bed-wetting at night. And anyone who breathes through the mouth during sleep may well be experiencing an obstruction in the nose.

BEST RESPONSE: For adults who are mild or occasional snorers, the American Academy of Otolaryngology—Head and Neck Surgery recommends that you exercise daily to tighten muscle tone. You should also lose weight, avoid alcoholic beverages within two hours of retiring, avoid tranquilizers, sleeping pills and antihistamines before bed and sleep on your side rather than on your back. Sewing a pocket on the back of your pajama top to hold a tennis ball is one uncomfortable but effective way to make sure of the latter.

If you suspect you have sleep apnea, see your doctor. It's a condition that requires medical attention, says Dr. Bailey. Your doctor may recommend a laboratory sleep study to evaluate your problem (for more on sleep laboratories, see Best Response under Symptom: Drowsiness in chapter 19). Then treatment is as simple as an exercise program or—in life-threatening cases—as complex as a trip to the operating room for removal of the excess palate and throat tissue.

SYMPTOM: **Stuffiness**

COMMON CAUSES: Most of the time your stuffy nose is going to be caused by a short-term cold or allergy (see Common Nasal Conditions). But occasionally it's going to come from an underactive thyroid gland (see thyroid disease under Common Whole Body Conditions in chapter 19); enlarged adenoids, polyps, sinusitis or a nasal deformity such as a deviated septum (see Common Nasal Conditions); an overactive hormone, triggered either by pregnancy or birth control pills; high blood pressure medications that contain a drug called reserpine; a tumor or even getting angry. Actually, any strong emotion can have a physical effect on the lining of the nose. Sexual stimuli cause nasal congestion in some people, resulting in a series of sneezes during intercourse. Gesundheit!

BEST RESPONSE: Three thousand years ago the Chinese inhaled vapors from a plant called "horsetail" to relieve a stuffy nose. Today you can buy its equivalent over the counter of a modern American drugstore in nasal decongestants such as Actifed or Sudafed. However, Byron J. Bailey, M.D., notes that these medicines can cause high blood pressure, and their use should be limited. If you already have high blood pressure or a heart condition, says Dr. Bailey, you should *never* take any drugs without consulting your physician.

Nose drops and sprays such as Neo-Synephrine are also helpful decongestants, says Dr. Bailey, but buy the ones that indicate they're ¼ percent. This small solution is so mild that it can be used for up to 30 days without the "rebound" effect of stronger sprays and drops.

And that's a serious consideration. If used for more than three or four days, nose drops and nasal sprays with a stronger solution will *cause* the very nasal swelling and stuffiness that you're trying to eliminate.

Of course, adds Dr. Bailey, a pregnant woman should not take decongestants, since any drug can harm her developing child. Fortunately, however, the hormonal condition that causes her stuffiness will only last for a month. The stuffiness caused by birth control pills may be stopped by switching to a different pill.

One nondrug way to decongest your nose is, of course, to add moisture to the air you breathe, either through a vaporizer or humidifier or even a hot shower. But Irwin Ziment, M.D., a professor of medicine at the University of California at Los Angeles School of Medicine, likes to take the historical approach to naturally relieving a stuffy nose. He believes that "a hot remedy for a cold disease" is the way to go—just as mama always told you.

Actually, the old folk remedies such as mustard plasters and chicken soup have a physiological basis in fact, says Dr. Ziment. They really do work—by helping to liquefy nasal secretions. With the mustard-plaster-on-the-chest routine, for example, the heat from the plaster stimulates blood flow to the upper part of the respiratory tract and may lead to an increase in secretions.

An alternative treatment popular in Russia, says Dr. Ziment, is to combine one teaspoon of freshly ground horseradish with eight ounces of water and one teaspoon of honey, then gargle with it. This stimulates a reflex that increases secretions in the nose and increases the effectiveness of the fumes.

But his favorite stuffy nose recipe, says Dr. Ziment, is adding several mashed cloves of garlic to a pot of chicken soup. As you eat the concoction, it will relieve your stuffy nose, the good doctor says, and you should add "as much garlic as friends, lovers and neighbors will tolerate."

Common Nasal Conditions

Adenoiditis.   Adenoiditis is an inflammation of the adenoids, which are nothing more than bits of tissue located at the very back of the nasal passages. They start to develop when children are around three years old to help the body fight infections. They begin to shrink around the age of five and are completely gone by the time a child reaches puberty.

But until they disappear, the adenoids themselves can become infected, swell, and plug up the back of the nose—particularly during a bout of sinusitis or tonsillitis. Infected secretions may drip out of the nose by day and drip down the throat by night, causing a cough. Your child may also breathe through the mouth, speak with a nasal twang and bring the house down with snores.

If you suspect your child has adenoiditis, see your doctor. Treatment will probably include an antibiotic to kill the infection and prevent it from spreading to the ear. Doctors remove adenoids when they trigger repeated earaches and ear infections that interfere with school or threaten hearing, or when they cause obstruction to breathing.

Allergy. Allergy is the simple name given to a very unsimple condition. It means that your body responds to something that is harmless—dog dander, tree pollen or eggs, to name just a few—with great sensitivity. Tiny amounts that do not produce symptoms in others produce symptoms in you.

The most common allergens are mold spores (for example, the yellow and green molds commonly found in bathrooms), animal dander (the flaky white "sand" that appears on your dog or cat's coat when you scratch its back or chest) and pollens from various plants. Food allergens are not all that common and are more likely to affect infants than children or adults.

If you suspect you have an allergy, check with your doctor. He or she may be able to determine what the allergy is with a special diet or a series of skin tests in which a minute amount of the suspected allergen is injected just under the skin of your arm. If your suspicions are confirmed, allergy relief is as simple—or as complicated—as avoiding the allergen. Eliminating citrus fruit from your diet is a lot easier than banning Whiskers or Spot or Rover from your heart.

Cold. "Cold" is the common name given to over 200 relatively minor viral infections that are transmitted primarily through hand contact.

You may feel, for example, that covering your mouth with a hand when you sneeze is a thoughtful effort to contain your germs and keep them away from others. But not if you then extend that same germ-laden paw to other people and shake hands. All they have to do is rub their eye or touch their nose and they've got your cold.

Most people are primarily susceptible to nasal viral infections between the ages of one and three, then again at the start of kindergarten.

You gain some degree of immunity as you get older, so colds become less frequent and less severe. And it has nothing to do with learning to put on your galoshes. Generations of mothers have forced their children into shoes, slippers, boots, sweaters, mufflers, mittens and snow pants in the mistaken belief that getting a chill causes a cold. It does not. But don't feel uncomfortable if you have trouble believing that. A group of nurses in the nursery at a Philadelphia hospital do, too. At one point, they kept turning up the nursery thermostat even though the hospital's chief of pediatrics, Patrick S. Pasquariello, Jr., M.D., kept telling them to turn it down. They knew that colds are caused by viruses, says Dr. Pasquariello, now a senior pediatrician at Children's Hospital of Philadelphia, but they just couldn't believe that temperature didn't affect the viruses. Actually, he adds, *higher* temperatures do affect cold viruses. They make them grow.

Deviated septum. A deviated septum is nothing more than an internal part of your nose that is crooked. You might have been born with it, or maybe your sister gave it to you in third grade when she flattened it over your smart mouth.

The septum itself is a long wall—bone at the top and cartilage at the bottom—that divides the nose into two compartments (left and right) of roughly equal proportions. When it's crooked, the compartments are unequal and one side doesn't breathe as well as the other.

Most people just live with it, but if it causes problems, check with your doctor. He or she may suggest an operation, which is usually done under local anesthesia, to straighten out the septum. The operation usually requires an overnight stay in the hospital.

Polyps. If you're between 25 and 50 years old, any unilateral nasal obstruction is likely to be caused by nasal polyps. The polyps themselves are soft, grapelike growths that hang down into the nasal cavity.

Polyps are usually caused by repeated infections, inflammations that heal by scarring the nasal cavity, allergies or aspirin "idiosyncracy" —which means that your nose drips when you take aspirin or other anti-inflammatory drugs such as ibuprofen (Advil or Nuprin) or in-domethacin (Indocin). Yellow food coloring (F. D. & C. No. 5), which is frequently found in foods such as margarine and hot dogs, may also be a triggering agent.

If you suspect you have nasal polyps, see your doctor. Treatment is usually surgical removal of the polyps under local anesthesia, either in your doctor's office or a hospital.

Sinusitis.   Sinusitis—whether experienced as a sudden attack or a chronic, ongoing problem—is due to an inflammation of the sinuses, which are nothing more than air spaces inside the skull around the nose and eyes. The problem is that inflammation can block a sinus's drainage holes and cause a mucus backup. The mucus-stuffed sinus then becomes the perfect growth medium for any viruses or bacteria generated by a cold or other infection. In fact, doctors estimate that 90 percent of all cases of sinusitis are the result of a nasal infection fighting its way up the nose and into the nurturing curves of a stuffed sinus.

That's why you should give your doctor a call if the symptoms of sinusitis continue for more than three or four days. He or she may want to prescribe an antibiotic to clear up the infection.

In extreme cases, when the infection persists and threatens to spread into the brain, lungs or ears, your doctor may want to pierce the bone between your nose and sinus to open an extra drain, then wash out the sinus cavity with sterile water. This procedure is performed under local anesthesia and—properly done—should not be painful. In about 1 out of 20 people, the procedure must be repeated.

Fortunately, sinusitis is relatively rare. Only 10 percent of those who go to an ear, nose and throat specialist complaining of sinusitis actually have it.

Chapter 14
Reproductive System

SEE YOUR DOCTOR IMMEDIATELY IF:
- *You experience vaginal bleeding during pregnancy*
- *You're not sexually aroused and you have a painful erection that just won't stop*
- *You get a sudden, severe pain in your testicles and your scrotum becomes swollen, red and tender*
- *You get hit in the testicles and the pain lasts for more than an hour*

Your reproductive system may be a lot of fun to operate, but in between, and even after, making and having babies, it can cause a lot of trouble.

Discharges, odors, drips and occasional malfunctions—not to mention misfirings—along with the usual infections and inflammations seem destined to send most of us to the doctor at one time or another. But for all the trouble our plumbing gives us, most of the problems are easily solved.

Don't believe it? Read on and see for yourself.

WOMEN
SYMPTOM: **Bleeding, after Intercourse**

COMMON CAUSES: Most women bleed at least a little after their first intercourse, or when their partner is simply too rough. But some women bleed because they have an eroded cervix, a condition in which the inner lining of the cervix migrates to the outside and makes the uterus more susceptible to infection or polyps, which are small, tubelike protrusions from the mucous membranes that line the uterus or cervical canal.

Bleeding can also be caused by abrasions from fingernails and tampons, cervical cancer or infections such as syphilis, herpes and chlamydia (see sexually transmitted disease under Common Reproductive System Conditions). In postmenopausal women, the cause is most likely a lack of estrogen (see Symptom: Bleeding, after Menopause). And sometimes the bleeding may not even be from you: It may be in the ejaculate of your sexual partner.

BEST RESPONSE: "Generally the bleeding will stop on its own," says Michael R. Spence, M.D., chairman of the Department of Obstetrics and Gynecology at Hahnemann University Medical School in Philadelphia. "It'll ooze a little bit and you'll want to wear pads, but it won't be as heavy as a menstrual period."

Nevertheless, you should check with your gynecologist, adds Dr. Spence. "If a woman is pregnant," he cautions, "she should come in and see us right away, just to be sure that she doesn't have a low-lying placenta," a condition in which the structure of the uterus that nourishes the fetus could tear and bleed.

If you're not pregnant, however, your gynecologist will probably give you a routine pelvic exam, take a Pap smear and check the area around your genitals for lumps, sores, inflammation and anything else that doesn't look right. He or she will separate the folds of skin around your vagina to expose the urinary and vaginal openings and probably ask you to "bear down" in order to check that the muscles supporting your vagina are doing their job.

Usually your gynecologist will also insert a speculum—a metal instrument that looks like two medieval shoe horns hinged together— into the vagina. The speculum, which will feel cold unless your gynecologist warms it under a lamp, holds the vaginal walls apart so your doctor can clearly see the vagina and the cervix, a small mound of skin that is actually the opening into the uterus.

In a routine exam, your gynecologist will check for inflammation or infection, scars, growths or any other abnormalities. He or she will push down on the outside of your pelvis with one hand and up on your cervix from the inside with the other to check the size, shape, consistency and tenderness of the uterus and ovaries. This usually causes a twinge of discomfort, not because there's anything wrong but because your ovaries are like the rest of you—they don't like being pushed around.

Your doctor will also painlessly scrape a few cells from the cervix and vagina (a Pap smear), then send them to a lab that can identify any infections or tumors that might be causing your problem. If an infection is responsible for the bleeding, your gynecologist will prescribe an antibiotic or other drug specifically designed to cure it.

If your pelvic exam reveals that the bleeding is caused by cervical polyps, however, your doctor will probably remove them—quickly and painlessly—right in the office. Your gynecologist can also handle bleeding caused by an eroding cervix in the office, by destroying the droopy lining of the cervix with heat or chemicals. This procedure is also painless, although it's usually followed by two or three weeks of a heavy, watery discharge as your cervix heals.

SYMPTOM: **Bleeding, after Menopause**

COMMON CAUSES: "Bleeding after menopause is considered cancer until proven otherwise," says Michael R. Spence, M.D. "All doctors, all gynecologists, when they have a postmenopausal bleeder, must rule out cancer before they can call it anything else."

Frequently, however, postmenopausal bleeding is caused by cervical polyps or by the lowered estrogen levels that trigger menopause. A lack of estrogen, explains Dr. Spence, can thin vaginal walls, which makes them susceptible to cracking and bleeding—particularly during intercourse.

BEST RESPONSE: Check with your doctor immediately, advises Dr. Spence. The incidence of cervical cancer is increasing, and the average age of onset is 48, although women both older and younger can get it. The only women who seem to escape the threat are nuns—an interesting observation that seems to support a theory that women may get cervical cancer from a virus in their partner's sperm. Fortunately, a simple Pap test can reveal cervical cancer. It is curable in almost every case where it is detected early.

If a lack of estrogen is causing postmenopausal bleeding, however, many doctors will suggest that you simply replace your diminished supply of estrogen with a synthetic form of the hormone—usually a pill. You should know that estrogen replacement therapy (ERT), as it is called, has been linked to an increased incidence of cancer, but only if it is taken continuously, says Dr. Spence.

He says doctors can administer ERT safely in two ways—three weeks on estrogen followed by one week off, or five days on progesterone followed by estrogen the rest of the month. You may want to read up on the subject before you make any decisions, get more than one medical opinion or contact a local women's health group.

When postmenopausal bleeding occurs after intercourse, the application of an estrogen *cream*—which contains minimal amounts of the hormone—or even a nonpetrolatum lubricant such as K-Y Lubricating Jelly or vegetable oil prior to intercourse may solve the problem without further ado. Dr. Spence warns that estrogen creams, if used continuously, carry the same risks as ERT.

SYMPTOM: **Bleeding, between Periods**

COMMON CAUSES: Bleeding between periods, or, as it has been termed at one time or another, "spotting" or "breakthrough bleeding," can be caused by endometriosis (see Common Reproductive System Conditions), benign growths called fibroid tumors, pelvic infections, ovarian cysts, cervical polyps, cancer, miscarriage or normal hormonal fluctuations. It can also be caused by an intrauterine device (IUD) or birth control pills.

BEST RESPONSE: In most cases, bleeding between periods is usually due to normal hormonal fluctuations, explains Michael R. Spence, M.D., and nothing needs to be done. Just check with your gynecologist to make sure there's no other problem.

And even if there is, the problem may not be serious. The right antibiotic can clear up pelvic infections, for example, and nearly one-third of all women beyond age 35 will find they have fibroids on their uterus.

Fibroids are solid, bumpy growths in an elastic kind of tissue (connective tissue) that holds your uterus in place. Generally, doctors will simply monitor their growth. But if the fibroids cause too much bleeding or perhaps some pain, your gynecologist may suggest that they be removed with a D and C (dilation and curettage), a relatively simple surgical procedure in which your doctor scrapes the lining of your uterus with a curved surgical instrument called a curette.

Occasionally, however, bleeding between periods is caused by an ovarian cyst, a small fluid-filled sac that develops when an egg is not released during ovulation. It usually disappears after a period or two, and your doctor can monitor it through regular internal exams. If it persists or seems unusually large, your gynecologist may suggest an ultrasound scan, a procedure that uses high-frequency sound waves to identify the size and location of the growth and to determine whether it is a fluid-filled cyst or a solid-mass tumor.

Some individuals claim that supplementing their diet with vitamin E and reducing caffeine may help. (You should take supplements only with the approval and supervision of your doctor, however.) Or your doctor may suggest you temporarily take a hormone pill. If necessary, it's possible to drain or surgically remove the cyst and repair the ovary.

If the problem is polyps, which are small, tubelike protrusions from the mucous membranes that line the uterus or cervical canal, the solution is usually relatively simple. Your doctor can remove them painlessly and quickly right in the office.

SYMPTOM: **Blisters**

COMMON CAUSES: Perfumes, toilet tissue, feminine "hygiene" sprays, the deodorants added to maxipads or minipads, even the detergent in which you washed your panties can all cause blisters around the vagina, says Michael R. Spence, M.D. Unfortunately, so can infections and sexually transmitted diseases, or STDs (see Common Reproductive System Conditions).

BEST RESPONSE: "If you just recently switched to some new toiletry product or you started using one of the hygiene sprays," says Dr. Spence, "that's a clue." You can discontinue using whatever it is you started and see if the blisters clear up.

If they don't, he adds, you need to visit your doctor. You may have an infection or sexually transmitted disease that will require further tests and medication.

If the blisters become uncomfortable while you're waiting for an appointment, says Dr. Spence, try soaking your bottom in a tub of cool water. And throw in a handful of Epsom salts. You may even want to soak a washcloth in the solution, add some crushed ice and drape it directly over your blisters. Or you could soak some tea bags in cold water and apply those. Plain tea is best, says Dr. Spence, since herb teas can be irritating.

And just in case you have a sexually transmitted disease such as herpes, you might want to take the precaution of placing your towel where others will not be tempted to borrow it. Disinfecting the tub—or even the toilet seat—is unnecessary, doctors say, but keeping others away from your towels and washcloths is a good idea.

If your blisters sting as you urinate, get into a tub full of water and urinate in the bathtub, suggests Dr. Spence. "Acid in the urine often goes across the blister, making it hurt like hell. Urinating in the bath water avoids the problem."

SYMPTOM: **Bulge, Vaginal**

COMMON CAUSES: Vaginal cysts or a prolapsed uterus can both cause what may appear to be a bulge of skin hanging down into—or even out of—the vagina.

A prolapsed uterus is the medical term for a condition in which the muscles that hold the uterus in place have been weakened—usually by having carried and borne children—and are no longer doing their job. It can sometimes cause pain when you walk.

BEST RESPONSE: Cysts can frequently be treated by sitz baths, in which you soak your bottom in warm water, says Michael R. Spence, M.D., although sometimes your doctor will have to open them up so they'll drain.

A prolapsed uterus can easily be pushed back into place. You can even shove it back up yourself, says Dr. Spence, although the first time you cough it'll come back down. That's why your doctor probably will insert a device called a pessary.

"A pessary is a fancy doorstop that fits in the vagina and wedges the uterus up," explains Dr. Spence. "It's usually rubber or plastic. It's a short-term solution for younger women who are physically fit and want to undergo surgery to permanently correct the problem.

"But if the patient is older," adds Dr. Spence, "it's a long-term solution as well. The risk of the surgery just outweighs the benefits you're going to reap."

Fortunately, the pessary is comfortable. But tell your gynecologist if you're sexually active, warns Dr. Spence. Otherwise, your doctor may use a big rubber block that fills the entire vagina. "And then," adds Dr. Spence, "nothing goes in except the pessary."

SYMPTOM: **Burning**

COMMON CAUSES: A burning sensation around the entrance of your vagina is usually caused by vaginitis, which is an irritation and inflammation of the outer opening, the vagina itself and the cervix.

Vaginitis is frequently triggered by chemical irritants, hormone imbalances or one of half a dozen common infections, including herpes (see sexually transmitted disease under Common Reproductive System Conditions). Some doctors feel that postmenopausal women are particularly vulnerable because a lack of estrogen reduces the vaginal moisture necessary for the vagina to wash itself clean.

BEST RESPONSE: Generally, doctors say, you should bathe daily and rinse the genital area well. You should avoid unnecessary antibiotics, which kill both good and bad germs; tight or synthetic panties and panty hose, which keep you so damp that bacteria are invited to set up housekeeping; and perfumed sprays, soaps or bubble baths, colored toilet tissue, tampons, hot tubs and douching, which can be irritants.

You should also avoid sex until you and your sexual partner have been treated with medication designed to kill the infection. That means you need to see your gynecologist.

Your doctor will rub a few cells off the walls of your vagina and cervix and examine them under a microscope. Then, depending on which of several little bugs is causing your problem, he or she will prescribe an appropriate medication. Just make sure you don't douche within 24 hours of your exam, doctors say. Although douching may seem like an effective form of first aid, it can interfere with your exam, both on the table and under the scope.

After you've seen your doctor, however, a sitz bath, in which you soak your bottom in warm water, can help you feel more comfortable. Add half a cup of salt or white vinegar to warm, shallow bath water and sit in it. If you place your legs on either side of the tub and open the vagina with your finger, the solution can enter and may help soothe the burning.

ACCOMPANYING SYMPTOM: If the entrance to your vagina burns for hours after intercourse and hurts when your partner inserts his penis, you may have vestibular adenitis, which is the inflammation of a mucus-producing gland near the entrance to the vagina, says Michael R. Spence, M.D. It's a condition that is missed by most doctors, he adds, so if you suspect it's causing your problem, you might want to ask your doctor to specifically check for it.

SYMPTOM: **Cramps, Menstrual**

COMMON CAUSES: Described as spasmodic or a dull, constant ache in the lower abdomen, cramps plague nearly half of all menstruating women. They're often the main event in a ring of premenstrual side effects (see premenstrual syndrome under Common Reproductive System Conditions) that can include nausea, vomiting, fatigue, diarrhea, lower backache and headache.

Although the exact cause of cramps is not known, hormonelike substances called prostaglandins are believed to play a part. According to medical reports, prostaglandins have been found in increased amounts in the menstrual blood and uterine wall of women who complain of monthly discomfort. And prostaglandins have been implicated in stimulating excessive uterine contractions. When the uterus contracts, the blood supply to the uterus is temporarily cut off, which creates a cramping feeling in the lower abdomen.

Medically, painful periods, especially menstrual cramps, go by the term dysmenorrhea and are classified as primary or secondary. The primary kind is not a symptom of any health problem. It is simply related to the normal hormonal changes that occur during menstruation. Secondary dysmenorrhea, however, is more likely to signify that there's something wrong somewhere in the reproductive system. Actually, any number of conditions affecting the female reproductive system can cause uncomfortable cramping. Pelvic inflammatory disease and endometriosis (see Common Reproductive System Conditions) and benign uterine growths known as fibroids all can produce menstrual cramps.

The question, however, is, how do you know if your cramps are of the primary or secondary kind? According to gynecologists, primary dysmenorrhea most often occurs in young women within the first three years of menstruation and can last for several years, often into the childbearing years. Secondary dysmenorrhea usually occurs in women who have had little or no cramping in their first three years of menstruation.

Another common cause for cramping, especially in women who have never had children, is the intrauterine device (IUD), a small object usually shaped like a coil or a loop that's designed to prevent conception. Cramping after insertion of an IUD is normal, say gynecologists, but persistent cramping is not. It indicates that something is wrong somewhere, and the IUD should be removed.

BEST RESPONSE: For menstrual cramps, doctors recommend nonsteroidal anti-inflammatory drugs such as ibuprofen (Advil or Nuprin), which is available over the counter, or naproxen (Anaprox), which is available by prescription.

One ibuprofen tablet (200 milligrams) is equal to two aspirin tablets (650 milligrams) in effectiveness, says Neta A. Hodge, Pharm.D., of the Philadelphia College of Pharmacy and Science. But, cautions Dr. Hodge, ibuprofen is not for everyone. If you've ever had a bad reaction to aspirin, you shouldn't take ibuprofen, she says. Nor should you use it if you have a kidney problem, asthma, high blood pressure or heart disease, or if you are pregnant or nursing. Since ibuprofen can cause stomach bleeding, as aspirin can, you should not use it if you are on anticoagulant drugs or if you have an ulcer.

Most doctors strongly recommend that sexually active women not take *any* medication for cramps until after their period has started each month, in case of undetected pregnancy. In the meantime, however, there are a number of self-help measures that can be used. These may be especially useful for those women who do not want to take or cannot take medication.

Wearing warm clothes, making love and exercising are all believed by many to help relieve cramps naturally. Also, the old standby, snuggling up with a heating pad or hot water bottle, can bring relief. All of these measures help relieve pain by improving blood flow. Some women also have reported relief from taking vitamin E and calcium tablets.

Some women, however, get cramps so badly that *nothing* seems to help. In such cases, doctors will sometimes prescribe low-dose estrogen/progesterone birth control pills to suppress ovulation, thus relieving pain.

If neither medication nor self-help measures help relieve your cramps, then a trip to your gynecologist is in order. Probably, a procedure called laparoscopy will be done to check for abnormalities, such as cysts or endometriosis.

If cramps hit in the middle of the night, there are a few positions that can ease the pain, say doctors. Lie down with a pillow under your knees to elevate your legs. Or, if you sleep on your side, pull your knees close to your chest. Both positions will help relieve pain by taking pressure off your abdomen.

This, however, does not mean that bed rest is called for when menstrual cramps hit. Bed rest may have been the doctor's orders a generation or two ago. Nowadays, however, you may be told to keep active.

SYMPTOM: **Discharge**

COMMON CAUSES: A healthy vagina is *supposed* to produce a discharge. That's how it cleans itself out. The normal, everyday hormonal activity in the vagina stimulates the production of moisture, which flushes assorted microscopic flora and fauna out of the body. Otherwise they might cause an infection.

You may notice that this natural discharge is thick and profuse about the time you ovulate, doctors say, usually 14 days after your period starts. You may also notice an increase in vaginal moisture whenever you're sexually aroused.

But occasionally you may notice that the discharge either significantly increases or changes in color or odor. When this happens, chances are the natural balance of the vagina's ecosystem has been disturbed and one of half a dozen infections has begun.

Any number of bacterial infections can cause discharge. The most common cause of a discharge is bacterial vaginosis, an infection that produces a pasty gray fluid that looks like mucus and smells like rotten fish. Roughly 10 to 20 percent of all sexually active women have this problem, and up to 40 percent of them may not notice any symptoms.

Discharges are also frequently caused by a fungus *(Candida)* which produces a white, cheesy fluid that can drive you crazy from the itching (see Symptom: Itching).

In postmenopausal women, a sticky brown discharge is likely to be caused by decreasing estrogen.

Less frequently, an abnormal discharge can be caused by cancer or an eroded cervix, a condition in which the inner lining of the cervix migrates to the outside, making the uterus more susceptible to infection.

BEST RESPONSE: "If the discharge only lasts for two or three days at midcycle and then goes away," says Michael R. Spence, M.D., "it's probably a normal physiological discharge. If it doesn't go away, it should be checked out."

Generally, your gynecologist will give you an internal exam and scrape a few cells from the vagina and cervix to view under a microscope. If your problem is bacterial vaginosis, it can be cleared up with antibiotics, as can most infections. Depending on the type of infection, your sexual partner may have to be treated, too, even though he may not show any symptoms.

Fungus infections are a little more stubborn. Your gynecologist can prescribe an antifungal cream to combat the condition. But researchers at Cornell University Medical Center in New York have discovered that, for a large number of women, traditional treatments such as antifungal creams not only may not work but cannot be expected to work.

In a study of 65 women with recurrent vaginal infections, says Steven Witkin, Ph.D., director of the immunology division in the Department of Obstetrics and Gynecology, 75 percent of the women had a major yeast-specific defect in their body's defense systems. Their white blood cells—which are essentially the armed guards of your body—simply were inhibited from responding to the yeast-causing flora as something harmful. So the cells failed to build up the troops as they normally would when faced with an invasion. They simply turned their cellular backs and let the fungus take over.

Further work, says Dr. Witkin, led him to suspect that this entire process was caused by allergies to things like contraceptive jelly, semen and, in some cases, the *Candida* organisms themselves. And the solution, he adds, seems to be finding your allergen and eliminating it, or, when that's not possible, using antihistamines to suppress your body's response.

The sticky brown discharge that troubles those in menopause can be discouraged with topical estrogen creams. They should be used daily for two weeks, then two to three times a week as needed. On occasion, small doses of estrogen in pill form may be temporarily needed to relieve the problem. Estrogen cream or pills should not be used continuously, however, because frequent use carries some risk of cancer.

ACCOMPANYING SYMPTOMS: If you've recently been pregnant and have a vaginal discharge, chills, very high fever, fast pulse, abdominal distress and vomiting, see your doctor immediately. You may have childbed fever, a rare but life-threatening condition that can easily be cured with an antibiotic.

SYMPTOM: **Dry Vagina**

COMMON CAUSES: Usually a dry vagina is caused by the lowered estrogen levels of menopause, although it can also be caused by psychological factors.

"A lot of women won't lubricate adequately prior to intercourse," says Michael R. Spence, M.D. "One of the reasons is inadequate stimulation or plain old boredom. Another is inadequate foreplay. One more is friction in the family.

"Let's say, for example, that a woman found out that her husband's been seeing someone else. They can foreplay until the cows come home and she just isn't going to lubricate. So when I talk to a woman who says she isn't lubricating adequately, we spend a fair amount of time talking about the relationship between her and her sexual partner. He may have seen someone several months ago, and she may think 'We're over that now,' but she's really not. And we need to take some time with that."

BEST RESPONSE: Vaginal dryness can easily be alleviated with a nonpetrolatum lubricant such as K-Y Lubricating Jelly, says Dr. Spence. "But one of the things you'll find with K-Y Jelly is that it's only good for one time. If you have sex the second or third time the same night, it becomes very irritating and it loses its lubricating ability. Then you have to use the jelly over and over again. Otherwise it dries and causes friction."

Another way to prevent a dry vagina, researchers say, is to keep sexually active. In a study of 54 women over age 60, the famous research team, Masters and Johnson, found that the 3 women in the study who remained sexually active throughout menopause were the only women who responded to sexual stimulation with a flood of vaginal lubrication.

And a study of 52 postmenopausal women at the New Jersey-Rutgers Medical School revealed that women aged 50 through 65 who had intercourse three or more times a month did not experience the vaginal shrinkage of menopause that usually accompanies dryness. "Some support for the adage 'use it or lose it' was obtained in this research," was the understated conclusion of the Rutgers investigators.

SYMPTOM: **Hot Flashes.** *See* Symptom: Flushing in
chapter 8

SYMPTOM: **Itching**

COMMON CAUSES: A fungus infection is the most common cause of vaginal itching in younger women, while a low level of estrogen is the most frequent cause in women over the age of 45.

Other causes are diabetes mellitus (see Common Whole Body Conditions in chapter 19), poor hygiene, scented toilet paper and bacterial infection.

BEST RESPONSE: "The one thing you *don't* want to do," emphasizes Michael R. Spence, M.D., "is go down to the local pharmacy and buy an over-the-counter anti-itch drug. All you're doing is treating the symptom and not the cause." And if the cause is a serious one such as diabetes, he points out, your health can be seriously affected.

Instead, says Dr. Spence, if the itching persists for two weeks, check with your gynecologist to see what you've got. If it's a bacterial infection, your doctor will probably prescribe an antibiotic. If it's a fungus, he'll probably advise an antifungal cream.

In any case, you can help prevent the itch by keeping your genitals clean and dry, avoiding tight synthetic clothing such as nylon panties, panty hose and exercise tights, reducing your sugar intake, getting extra rest and eating a balanced diet. You should also avoid cornstarch (it's actually used to *grow* fungus in the lab), talcum powder, feminine hygiene sprays, bubble bath, scented soaps and colored toilet paper, since they are all likely to increase any irritation.

And check your hygiene habits. Wipe away from the vagina to prevent intestinal bacteria from entering it. Change tampons often and alternate them with sanitary napkins to allow your vagina to clean itself out.

ACCOMPANYING SYMPTOM: Itching accompanied by pain or swelling in the genital area may mean herpes (see sexually transmitted disease under Common Reproductive System Conditions). Check with your doctor as soon as possible.

SYMPTOM: **Loss of Sexual Desire**

COMMON CAUSES: Boredom, excessive physical training, emotional problems, diabetes, drugs for high blood pressure or anxiety can all cause a loss of interest in sex. So can fear and anxiety about disease, pregnancy and children, as well as a long period of chastity, virginity or not being loved.

Some doctors even think that anger at the opposite sex or a bad sexual experience can also kill your libido. For some women, the constant frustration from a partner who is either impotent or who prematurely ejaculates can zap sexual appetite.

Menopause can trigger a loss of interest in some women. In a Stanford University study of menopausal women, 48 percent of the women involved reported a noticeable decline in sexual desire. Unfortunately, no one knows why—although researchers suspect that there's an as yet undiscovered relationship between hormones and sexual desire. To confuse the issue even further, the same study revealed that 23 percent of the women reported a definite *increase* in sexual desire.

BEST RESPONSE: If you're just too tired or too bored, you might try setting aside a specific time for you and your mate to make love, suggests Lonnie Barbach, Ph.D., assistant clinical professor of medical psychology at the University of California at San Francisco School of Medicine. If that sounds a little planned, well, so what? It's definitely better than leaving sex for the last thing at night when you're so exhausted you can hardly crawl into bed.

Why not take an afternoon nap one Sunday? Or take the beach blanket along on a wilderness hike? Whatever you do, spend a little time thinking about it first, suggests Dr. Barbach, and be willing to take a few risks. Create a special mood or atmosphere with clothes or settings, and don't become preoccupied with techniques or achieving orgasm. Instead, concentrate on closeness, touching and relaxation. Everything else just naturally falls into place.

If you suspect your loss of sexual desire is a drug side effect, your doctor may be able to change the type or dosage, says Michael R. Spence, M.D. But if you suspect your problem is caused by fear, anxiety or sexual dysfunction, you should see a therapist or family planning clinic that specializes in sexual problems. Check the Yellow Pages of your local telephone directory, suggests Dr. Spence, or ask your family doctor for a referral.

SYMPTOM: **Menstrual Periods, Absent**

COMMON CAUSES: Pregnancy and menopause are natural occurrences that are supposed to make periods stop. But there are other body conditions that can cause periods to cease unnaturally. These include diabetes mellitus (see Common Whole Body Conditions in chapter 19), rapid weight change, excessive physical training, malnutrition, stress, tumors, a change of environment, going off birth control pills, and drugs such as morphine and nitroglycerin.

Sometimes menstruation never even gets a chance to get going.

Young girls usually begin to develop sexually by age 14 and begin to menstruate by age 16½. But sometimes this is delayed by chronic disease, a low proportion of body fat, too much weight, too little weight or even intense athletic training.

One study of young athletes undergoing intensive training, for example, demonstrated that almost 50 percent of the girls had hormonal abnormalities that altered their menstrual periods. And in a study of young ballet dancers, researchers found that instead of progressing through puberty within the normal two-year period, the girls would make no progress at all while dancing, then would go through the whole process in the four to six months during which they were resting or on vacation.

BEST RESPONSE: Check with your doctor to make sure that you're not pregnant or that there's no undetected disease such as diabetes. Otherwise, doctors say, a return to normal eating patterns, a break from rigorous physical training or the successful management of stress may be all the treatment that's necessary.

If you're between the ages of 40 and 50, however, you may be experiencing menopause, a time in which your ovaries stop producing the hormone estrogen. Absent menstruation is the only symptom of menopause for many women, although roughly half of all women have uncomfortable symptoms such as hot flashes (see Symptom: Flushing in chapter 8), skin tingling, a change in desire for intercourse (see Symptom: Loss of Sexual Desire) or a dry vagina (see Symptom: Dry Vagina).

Like many other life changes, however, menopause requires some psychological adjustments, doctors say. But how successfully you make those adjustments depends more on how well you have met other changes in your life than on what your body is doing. Those who are generally unsatisfied with themselves and their lives will remain so. Those who are generally satisfied will also remain so.

Contrary to public opinion, researchers say, there are no emotional problems associated with menopause that weren't there before it started. In fact, a study at New Haven, Connecticut, revealed that women suffer from symptoms of depression less often as they get older.

ACCOMPANYING SYMPTOMS: If your period is late and accompanied by irregular spotting and pain in your lower abdomen, see your doctor at once. You may have an ectopic pregnancy, a situation in which the fertilized egg is implanted somewhere in the reproductive system other than in the uterus—usually the fallopian tube. This condition is frequently caused by chronic pelvic infection. Almost 50 percent of all tubal specimens removed because of an ectopic pregnancy show evidence of pelvic infection, usually caused by such things as douching, intrauterine devices (IUDs), hormone-stimulating drugs, tubal defects or previous abortions. Ectopic pregnancies almost always result in the death of the fetus.

SYMPTOM: **Menstrual Periods, Heavy**

COMMON CAUSES: Close to a quarter of all women are heavy bleeders at some point in their lives, says Michael R. Spence, M.D. Some may even alternate light and heavy bleeding within the same period. And a study at Stanford University revealed that 20 percent of women approaching menopause will bleed so heavily or so continuously that fastidious dressing may become difficult.

Occasionally, however, heavy periods can be caused by a hormone imbalance, an intrauterine device (IUD), benign uterine growths known as fibroids or a pelvic infection. More rarely, the cause is endometriosis (see Common Reproductive System Conditions) or cancer.

BEST RESPONSE: A "normal" period will last three to seven days and amount to 10 to 15 moderately soaked tampons or pads.

"The average woman loses about three shot glassfuls of blood during her menstrual period," says Dr. Spence, "even though it looks like a lot. So if you think your period is heavier than that, you should see your doctor." Ask him or her to do a blood count just to make sure you're not anemic. If you are, adds Dr. Spence, your doctor may suggest iron supplements.

But some women, particularly around their first or last period, keep menstruating for days and weeks without pause. If this happens, you should see your doctor to make sure there is no problem that needs treatment. He or she may suggest that you take hormone tablets for a few months. Hormone therapy usually controls excessive bleeding within 24 to 36 hours, doctors say, but if it doesn't, a D and C—dilation of the cervix and scraping out of the uterus with a curette—will usually do the trick.

ACCOMPANYING SYMPTOM: If your period is late as well as unusually heavy, you may be having an early miscarriage. See your doctor as soon as possible.

SYMPTOM: **Menstrual Periods, Irregular**

COMMON CAUSES: For some women, the menstrual cycle runs like clockwork. Their period begins at the same time every month (somewhere between 28 and 35 days), just as nature intended. Others are not so lucky. Their menstrual cycle could use a good set of training wheels.

The cause of irregular periods is usually failure to ovulate. You menstruate only if the ovary has produced an egg. That sets in motion a chain of chemicals speaking to glands and glands speaking to eggs and eggs relaying messages back to glands again. The bottom line is that the uterus sheds its lining when this line of chemical messengers is fully informed that you're not pregnant and there's no need for it to hang around any longer.

But what if your body doesn't ovulate? What if there's no egg? When ovulation doesn't occur, doctors say, a thick, ragged lining often forms in the uterus that can slough off irregularly and incompletely. Since the body's chemical messengers aren't really sure whether to build up the uterine lining for pregnancy or tear it down for menstruation, neither is the body.

Usually, irregular bleeding is most likely to occur at puberty, when the ovaries are setting up shop, or at menopause when they're shutting things down.

BEST RESPONSE: Every woman has irregular menstruation once in a while, says Michael R. Spence, M.D. But if you have three or more periods in a row that are late or early, check with your gynecologist. You may need to do nothing, but chances are the doctor will suggest a short course of hormones that will help your body stabilize its cycle.

If you are approaching menopause, your gynecologist may suggest a D and C—dilation of the cervix and scraping of the lining of the uterus—or an endometrial biopsy to sample tissue. Both measures are intended to help your doctor figure out what's causing the problem rather than to solve it.

SYMPTOM: **Odor.** *See also* Symptom: Discharge

COMMON CAUSES: Your vagina is supposed to generate its own identifiable scent—not like "mountain herbs" or "country flowers," as some television advertisements say it should, but an odor all its own. The odor comes largely from glands associated with pubic hair follicles and increases when you are angry, afraid or sexually stimulated.

If the odor increases to the point that it's highly offensive, however, you may have an infection or, in some cases, a tumor.

BEST RESPONSE: Any offensive smell should be evaluated by your gynecologist, doctors say, but the normal, everyday "woman" smell should be accepted and ignored. The only cleaning required is a mild soap and water wash or an occasional warm water soak. *All* douches and feminine hygiene sprays—including the so-called medicated ones—should be avoided.

ACCOMPANYING SYMPTOMS: If you have a foul-smelling, watery and bloody discharge as well as bleeding from the vagina between periods, after intercourse or after menopause, you may have cancer of the cervix. Check with your doctor as soon as possible.

SYMPTOM: **Pain, Pelvic**

COMMON CAUSES: Gynecologists hear more about pelvic ache or pain than almost any other symptom, even though the nature of the pain varies from person to person, as does its intensity.

It's frequently caused by endometriosis (see Common Reproductive System Conditions), stress, inflammation, infection, pelvic adhesions or ovarian cysts. Less frequently it's caused by a tumor. In 90 to 95 percent of women it's related to a specific, organic cause.

BEST RESPONSE: "We all have pains once in a while, and it's no big deal," says Michael R. Spence, M.D. "But if the pain is something that's persistent, bothersome and distressing, it should be checked out."

Sometimes biofeedback, biofeedback-assisted relaxation training, desensitization methods or any combination of these techniques is helpful in reducing pain, doctors say. Birth control pills and ibuprofen (Advil or Nuprin) have also been helpful. If the problem is infection, antibiotics are used.

Occasionally, ovarian cysts that do not shrink require surgery, as does a bacterial infection that does not respond to antibiotics. Some doctors feel that surgery, such as dilation and curettage (D and C), is also justified when they can't figure out what's causing the pain or why it doesn't respond to medical therapy, but other doctors disagree. As one doctor notes, "Rarely does surgical treatment produce long-lasting relief."

SYMPTOM: **Painful Intercourse**

COMMON CAUSES: Painful intercourse can be caused by pelvic inflammatory disease or endometriosis (see Common Reproductive System Conditions); a vaginal infection; a prolapsed or tipped uterus; ovarian cysts; vestibular adenitis, an inflammation of the mucus-producing gland near the entrance of the vagina; vaginismus, which causes vaginal muscle spasms; cervical polyps; a dry vagina due to menopause; tumors or pelvic adhesions. Moreover, anticipating the pain may prevent vaginal lubrication and compound the problem.

BEST RESPONSE: "If you've had comfortable intercourse for many years and then all of a sudden it becomes painful, you ought to be checked by your gynecologist," says Michael R. Spence, M.D.

You may simply need a temporary hormone supplement or vaginal lubricant or, if infection is causing your pain, an antibiotic. Or maybe you just need to change positions when you have intercourse.

A tipped uterus, for example, can be painful when it's hit by a thrusting penis, says Dr. Spence. But if you flip over and have intercourse on your hands and knees or on your back with a big pillow under your bottom, the uterus "tips" back into a less painful position. If painful intercourse continues despite treatment or a change of positions, your doctor may suggest surgery.

But pain caused by an involuntary tightening of your vaginal muscles—one that may even make penetration impossible—may respond to "retraining." One way, experts suggest, is to insert one finger at a time into the vagina until you can insert several fingers. If you do this exercise daily, intercourse with pleasure—and not pain—may well be your just reward.

SYMPTOM: **Warts**

COMMON CAUSE: Warts around the vagina are no different from warts on the finger. They're caused by a virus that may have spread from anywhere else on the body or even from your mate. They seem to proliferate in moist and unhygienic conditions, and occasionally they sprout during an infection or during pregnancy, when there's a natural increase in vaginal moisture.

BEST RESPONSE: Warts neglected for many years may become malignant. So see your doctor as soon as you get the chance. He or she will check for any vaginal infection that could be causing the warts, and treat the infection with the appropriate drug. The warts may then disappear along with the infection.

Frequently, however, your doctor will simply paint the warts with an antiviral chemical that kills the virus, or shoot them down with lasers.

MEN
SYMPTOM: **Blisters.** *See* Symptom: Blisters under women's symptoms

---

SYMPTOM: **Discharge**

COMMON CAUSES: A discharge from the penis usually means infection or inflammation. But it can also mean you have a sexually transmitted disease, or STD (see Common Reproductive System Conditions).

There are many kinds of STDs that can cause a discharge, say doctors. A chlamydial infection may cause a mild discharge, or none at all. An inflammation of the urethra (the passageway for urine) called urethritis, which is often caused by gonorrhea, causes a copious, thick, yellow discharge.

BEST RESPONSE: See your physician. Doctors say you need to have a sample of the discharge checked out under a microscope and cultured to see what it is. In most cases your doctor will suggest an antibiotic to kill the bugs that are causing the discharge.

If there's a persistent problem, doctors add, have your partner treated and use a condom. You could be playing hot potato with a bug.

ACCOMPANYING SYMPTOM: Redness at the opening of the penis accompanied by a copious, white, creamy discharge is a sign of gonorrhea (see Sexually transmitted disease under Common Reproductive System Conditions). See your doctor right away for treatment.

SYMPTOM: **Foreskin, Pale and Shriveled**

COMMON CAUSES: A pale, shriveled foreskin can be caused by diabetes mellitus (see Common Whole Body Conditions in chapter 19), a localized infection, poor hygiene or balanitis, which is an inflammation of the foreskin and the underlying glans penis (tip of the penis).

BEST RESPONSE: Pull the foreskin back and wash your penis with regular soap and water, doctors say. Most important, dry yourself completely before dressing. If the foreskin won't retract, see your doctor.

SYMPTOM: **Impotence**

COMMON CAUSES: "Male potency is one of the last sexual topics in America left in the closet," asserts Richard Berger, M.D., chief of urology at Harborview Medical Center in Seattle and coauthor, with his wife, Deborah, of *BioPotency.* But despite men's fears, sexual function is one of the last things to decline with age.

Almost two-thirds of married men under age 70 and one-third over

75 engage in regular sexual activity, researchers say, although most of the older men take more time to reach orgasm and have shorter orgasms. Erections may also be slower and softer, they report, and older men may not feel like having intercourse as often as they used to. This, however, does not mean they are impotent.

Impotence is defined as the inability to get and maintain an erection sufficient for sexual intercourse. And there are about 10 million impotent men of all ages in the United States who fit that description. Most of them are over age 55.

Years ago doctors thought that the majority of impotence was caused by emotional hang-ups. Today they know that 75 percent of the time the problem is physical—frequently triggered by drugs prescribed for colds, stomachaches, ulcers, depression, high blood pressure, epilepsy, pain and hormones that are out of whack.

Surgery can also cause impotence, doctors say. Removal of the prostate gland, for example, frequently triggers impotence, even though the surgery is required by two out of every ten men beyond age 60. Until recently, the cause of impotence after prostate surgery was likely to be described as psychological, because scientists couldn't figure out what was happening. Now, however, they've begun to suspect that a particular group of nerves is damaged during surgery, and many urologists are using a nerve-sparing technique that is reported to prevent the problem.

Disease is also a major instigator of impotence, doctors say. Up to 60 percent of all diabetics are impotent, for example, because of the disease's destructive effects on penile nerves and blood vessels.

Men who have had heart attacks can also become impotent, but the cause is attributed to fear of death (from the exertion of sex), not heart disease. Generally, doctors say, any man who has had a heart attack who can walk several blocks at a brisk pace or climb two flights of stairs without chest pain, shortness of breath or palpitations can be reassured that the chance of sudden death due to intercourse is minute—about 1 in 10,000.

Other causes of impotence include fatigue, all sorts of stress and even watching your wife have a baby. A survey of 400 men who witnessed natural childbirth revealed that 30 percent became impotent for months and years afterward.

"An important cause," says Richard J. Macchia, M.D., acting chairman of the Department of Urology at the State University of New York

Health Science Center at Brooklyn, "is decrease in libido due to lack of an erotic partner."

BEST RESPONSE: "An occasional erection failure is nothing to be concerned about," says Bruce Forman, Ph.D., director of marriage and family therapy training at the University of Miami. "If you are having chronic problems—and by that I mean a pattern of total inability or multiple misfires over a period of six months—then I would get a physical exam and a psychological life-style check to determine if the problem is physical or mental."

The best way to differentiate between physical and psychological impotence, explains E. Douglas Whitehead, M.D., a urologist with the Association for Male Sexual Dysfunction in New York, is this: If you can become erect any time other than during attempts at intercourse—including while asleep—that strongly suggests that the problem is psychological.

But what do you do if it is? The answer, suggests Dr. Berger, is probably simple. Learn to communicate with your mate—to tell her how you really feel—and set some time aside for some nongenital touching. Get to know the kinds of touching that are pleasurable for both of you, advises Dr. Berger, then, after a few sessions, you can attempt to have intercourse. He says it usually takes about ten weeks to achieve success.

"Be sure you discuss what you want to do and why with your partner before beginning," writes Dr. Berger in *BioPotency*. "Take things very slowly. Don't push yourself to do something you feel unready to do. Make sure you have a private, comfortable environment in which to practice your (touching) exercises, and set aside a special time for this purpose."

And don't hesitate to seek professional counseling, adds Dr. Berger. "There are professionals who can teach you to relax and be a better, more confident public speaker. A sex therapist can offer the same kind of help with erection problems."

Sometimes, however, even counseling won't help impotence. And in that case, doctors say, penile implants may provide an answer. There are several different kinds of rod-shaped implants available, both semi-rigid and inflatable, and most studies report sexual satisfaction in 93 to 98 percent of the men who try them. Doctors point out that once you have them inserted, however, you'll never be able to have a "natural" erection again. The semirigid devices apparently are more reliable, but newer inflatable models may eliminate this difference.

But what if the cause is physical? Implants may also provide an answer to physical impairment, doctors suggest, as may injections of drugs that dilate the arteries in your penis. Although studies on the long-term effectiveness of these shots have not yet been completed, in at least one study, 59 of 62 impotent men were able to have erections and, subsequently, intercourse.

Moreover, an experimental device—the Male Electronic Genital Stimulator, or MEGS, as it is known to its inventors—may soon join the anti-impotence arsenal. If early reports are to be believed, MEGS—a suppository-like cylinder that can be inserted into the rectum just before intercourse and be activated by a tiny remote control mechanism that fits into a piece of jewelry—may make push-button erections a reality.

If you're not quite ready for push-button sex, however, you may want to talk with your doctor about suction devices and cock rings. And by suction devices we do *not* mean vacuum cleaners. Vacuum cleaners may produce erections, warns Dr. Berger, but they can also strip the skin off your penis. Moreover, some machines have blades in places you wouldn't expect.

Suction devices, available from your doctor or by prescription, work by creating a vacuum around your penis that sucks blood into it the same way you sip a cocktail through a straw. The only difference is that you slip a constricting band similar to a cock ring—a thick, rubberlike ring—over your penis and down to the base, where it will keep your penis engorged and erect.

But you've got to be careful with these devices, cautions Dr. Berger. Restrict your use of both suction device and cock ring to 30 minutes, or the time period recommended by your doctor, and discuss their use with him or her. An overzealous application of either can leave you with gangrene—a condition that requires amputation.

SYMPTOM: **Itching**

COMMON CAUSES: Itching around the genital region is usually a dermatologic problem, because occasionally men can have a local allergic reaction to such things as underwear. It's rarely a plumbing problem.

But itching *inside* the urethra—the eight-inch tube that carries urine from the bladder to the opening in the penis—can be caused by trichomoniasis (see sexually transmitted disease under Common Reproductive System Conditions) that can irritate the urethra.

BEST RESPONSE: Ignore it, and if it goes away in a day or two, you're OK, say doctors. Wear cotton underwear if you suspect the cause was a superficial irritation.

If the itching doesn't go away, however, check with your doctor. You may have a sexually transmitted disease. Your doctor may prescribe an antibiotic and suggest that your mate be treated as well. To reduce the inflammation, you can get cortisone creams at the drugstore. Use them sparingly, suggests Stephen B. Webster, M.D., a Wisconsin dermatologist, and quit when the rash goes away.

ACCOMPANYING SYMPTOMS: If your itch is accompanied by a bright red, nonscaly rash with sharply defined borders, says Dr. Webster, you may find that wearing loose-fitting clothes that don't bind in the groin, keeping the area cool and dry (using fluffy talc or ZeaSORB powder helps) and bathing the area with antibacterial soap and then carefully drying may clear up the problem.

If your itch is accompanied by a dull red rash that extends outward in a ringlike pattern, you may have a fungus infection. The border of the rash is scaly, and the scrotum, the skin covering the testicles, is often unaffected in these kinds of infections, says Dr. Webster. An over-the-counter antifungal medication such as Micatin is often effective.

One other localized infection that causes both redness and itching is a yeast infection, which is usually distinguished by a bright red, scaly area on the inner thigh, with an irregular, serrated border, and a bright red, shiny scrotum. Micatin can often clear this up, too, says Dr. Webster, but if it doesn't, check with your doctor.

SYMPTOM: **Loss of Sexual Desire.** *See* Symptom: Loss of Sexual Desire under women's symptoms

---

SYMPTOM: **Lump**

COMMON CAUSE: Any hard lump or spot on the testicle can be cancer, doctors say. A warty lump, sore spot or draining sore that slowly spreads across the skin of the penis can be, too. Fortunately, both types of cancer are rare.

BEST RESPONSE: See your doctor at once. Cancer of either the penis or testicle can spread to other parts of the body.

SYMPTOM: **Pain**

COMMON CAUSE: If you're feeling pain between the scrotum and the anus, you could have prostatitis (see Common Reproductive System Conditions). It most often affects younger men.

BEST RESPONSE: Sit in a tub of warm water to relieve the pain, say doctors. But don't worry about it unless you develop other symptoms. If you develop a high fever, chills and painful or difficult urination, check with your doctor. You may need an antibiotic.

SYMPTOM: **Painful Erection**

COMMON CAUSES: A painful erection can be caused by a too-tight foreskin or by Peyronie's disease, a condition in which scar tissue forms within the penis.

Nobody knows what causes Peyronie's disease. The penis looks normal when it's flaccid, but the scarred area is unable to expand as it becomes engorged during an erection. The uprushing blood is halted in its tracks, pain sets in and the penis frequently bends over at the site of the scar tissue. The condition is fairly common and most often occurs in men around age 50.

BEST RESPONSE: A too-tight foreskin is easily treated by removing it, doctors say. And Peyronie's disease goes away by itself in roughly half the people it affects. If the condition persists, however, you may want to consider surgery. The scarred tissue can sometimes be removed or cut to allow normal sexual activity, doctors say, and when it can't, a prosthetic device can be implanted (for more on penile implants, see Best Response under Symptom: Impotence).

Your doctor may, however, prescribe potassium aminobenzoic acid (Potaba) to treat the fibrosis and inflammation. Large doses of the medication are needed, and it takes time to work. "Sometimes patients tire of swallowing six pills a day and stop taking the medication before it can be determined if it would have helped or not," says Richard J. Macchia, M.D.

Another common way some doctors treat the condition is with vitamin E. "But this method of treatment has not been scientifically proven effective, and should be tried only under the supervision of your doctor," says Dr. Macchia.

Currently, there is no consistently effective drug for Peyronie's disease, although a study at the University of California at Los Angeles offers some hope. In that study, 31 men aged 22 to 67 with Peyronie's disease were injected with collagenase, a purified enzyme. Within four weeks, the researchers report, pain was eliminated in 93 percent of the men who experienced it, and deformities were improved in 65 percent of the patients.

ACCOMPANYING SYMPTOMS: If you have pain in your penis, testicles or groin, or itching and pain between the scrotum and anus, see your doctor. You may have an infection that requires antibiotics.

SYMPTOM: **Premature Ejaculation**

COMMON CAUSES: Premature ejaculation—the emission of semen during penetration or immediately after penetration has taken place—is usually psychologically caused, doctors say. That's because your penis is a barometer for the anxiety, frustration and resentment you experience both inside and outside the bedroom. It's a common sexual problem in men.

Frequently, men who ejaculate prematurely have a history of recurrent nervous tension and stress, doctors say, or a history of hurried masturbation or intercourse due to fear of discovery. And some men apparently use premature ejaculation as a way to express a deep-seated fear of or anger toward women. But no matter what the initial cause of the problem, the *fear* that it will occur almost ensures that it will.

BEST RESPONSE: Between 50 and 100 percent of those who try sex therapy are able to eliminate the problem, doctors say. And at least one study suggests that couples can teach themselves to avoid premature ejaculation without much more than written instructions and telephone conversations with a therapist.

It's the job of your therapist to help you sort out all your feelings about life, your mate and the world. But because a continued problem with premature ejaculation can lead to impotence, your therapist may also suggest one or two exercises you and your partner can do right away to stop early ejaculation: the stop-start method developed by Dr. James Semans, and the squeeze method of famed sex researchers Masters and Johnson.

The stop-start method starts with masturbation. You should stimulate yourself up and down the length of your penis, suggests Richard Berger, M.D., concentrating on how you feel. When you sense you're going to ejaculate, but before it becomes inevitable, stop and wait until the feeling passes. Repeat the entire procedure four times, and don't allow yourself to ejaculate until the end of the last exercise. Then teach your partner to manually stimulate you as described above.

Once you can delay your ejaculation with masturbation and your partner's stimulation, Dr. Berger advises, you're ready to try intercourse. It's best to start with your mate on top. You'll have less body tension in this position, says Dr. Berger, and with your hands on her hips you can control the amount of stimulation you receive. When you're ready to let your mate control her own movements, do so—but ask her to stop if you feel you're going to ejaculate sooner than you would like. And remember, adds Dr. Berger, you can expect premature ejaculation to continue until you have mastered the method.

The squeeze method also starts with masturbation and, when successful, also progresses to intercourse. The difference between the stop-start exercise and squeezing is that when you sense you're going to ejaculate, put your first and second fingers on top of the head of your penis—with the thumb just below—and squeeze until the feeling goes away. But if you start ejaculating, let go.

The squeezing can be done by your partner, and you can progress to intercourse as soon as you can control your ejaculations.

Some couples don't like intercourse using the squeeze technique, however, because removing your penis abruptly from your mate's vagina for a squeeze is annoying. An alternative, suggests Dr. Berger, is to squeeze the *base* of your penis for about 15 seconds. If your mate is on top, this allows you to stop your ejaculation while your penis remains in her vagina.

And don't forget your partner's needs. If these exercises become frustrating, suggests Dr. Berger, explore other ways of satisfying her.

SYMPTOM: **Semen, Bloody**

COMMON CAUSES: Bloody semen is one of the few conditions where the symptoms usually seem a lot worse than they are, say urologists.

Generally, bloody semen is caused by prostatitis (see Common Reproductive System Conditions) or infection of the prostate or seminal vesicles, which are the two organs that provide most of the penile ejaculate.

In an older man, there's a slight potential for cancer, and in the old days tuberculosis or syphilis (see sexually transmitted disease under Common Reproductive System Conditions) might have been additional causes. Fortunately, syphilis and tuberculosis are rare today.

BEST RESPONSE: Some doctors say you should ejaculate more frequently than usual. Others say you should ejaculate less. Still others don't think it makes a whole lot of difference. Just check with a urologist to be sure of what's causing the problem.

The odds are it's an infection, and your doctor will treat it with an antibiotic. The problem will probably heal itself, although if you look closely, you may see blood in your semen for several days.

ACCOMPANYING SYMPTOMS: If you find blood in your semen and also experience high fever, chills and pain in and around the base of your penis, you probably have prostatitis. These symptoms sometimes, but not always, accompany the disease.

SYMPTOM: **Swelling, Penile**

COMMON CAUSES: A swollen penis is usually caused by infections such as herpes (see sexually transmitted disease under Common Reproductive System Conditions), friction from damp briefs or irritation from chemical substances in clothing, condoms or creams. Diabetics are especially vulnerable to this type of problem because their sugary urine permits infection to flourish.

BEST RESPONSE: Most conditions that trigger a swollen penis will clear up if you rub a soothing ointment over the area. If your problem is caused by an irritation or friction, you'll also have to avoid the irritant.

If the swelling persists, however, check with your doctor. He or she may want to prescribe an antibiotic or antiviral cream or tablets, and, in cases where it's painful or difficult to draw back your foreskin, circumcision or a surgical "loosening" may be suggested.

SYMPTOM: **Swelling, Testicular**

COMMON CAUSES: Any inflammation can cause swelling, but there is something called a hydrocele, which is a fluid-filled sac in the scrotum (the skin covering the testicles), that may reflect an earlier inflammation. Even though there's nothing wrong now, the hydrocele remains. It could be a sign of cancer.

BEST RESPONSE: Any swelling should be checked by a urologist, doctors say. Any mass in a testicle is considered a tumor until proven otherwise. However, most doctors will leave small swellings and cysts alone unless they prove troublesome.

ACCOMPANYING SYMPTOM: A swollen testicle plus infertility may suggest a varicocele, which is a collection of congested veins.

A swollen scrotum, sickening pain, a fever and chills may indicate either epididymitis or orchitis (see Common Reproductive System Conditions). See your doctor immediately. With epididymitis, prompt treatment can reduce your convalescence by half. With orchitis, it can reduce your chances of sterility by a third.

SYMPTOM: **Warts**

COMMON CAUSES: Warts on the penis are similar to warts anywhere else on the body and are just as contagious. Occasionally, however, a growth that *resembles* a wart either on the penis or just inside the penis's opening may be an early symptom of cancer or syphilis (see sexually transmitted disease under Common Reproductive System Conditions).

BEST RESPONSE: Check with your doctor. If the diagnosis is warts, he or she can prescribe a specific antiwart "paint" to get rid of them. Do *not* try and save a buck by treating your warts with an over-the-counter preparation designed for warts elsewhere on your body. The skin on your penis is far more sensitive than the skin on your foot, doctors say, and easily damaged by ordinary watch-your-wart-disappear ointments.

Common Reproductive System Conditions

Endometriosis. Endometriosis is a condition in which tissue lining the uterus (endometrial tissue) occurs in places outside the uterus. This tissue bleeds during a regular menstrual period and can cause severe pain depending on the location of the tissue.

Scientists still aren't sure why and how it happens, but they do know that it's a leading cause of pelvic pain and infertility. It occurs in 10 to 15 percent of all women of childbearing age—particularly those between ages 30 and 40 who have never had children—although at least one study from the Mayo Clinic indicates that it may occur in as many as half of all women.

Endometriosis is generally handled in one of three ways, doctors say. Your gynecologist may just keep a sharp watch on the disease and treat symptoms as they occur, or suggest you take anti-inflammatory agents such as ibuprofen (Advil or Nuprin). Or your doctor may recommend that drugs be used to fool your body into thinking you're either pregnant or menopausal—in which case the decrease or absence of menstrual flow decreases your symptoms.

A third alternative, usually reserved for severe endometriosis or for women who have tried to get pregnant and failed, is surgery. Your doctor can remove small growths of tissue by electrical current, by laser or during laparoscopy, a procedure in which a stiff tube (the laparoscope) equipped with lenses is inserted through a small incision in your abdomen. Larger growths can be removed through abdominal surgery.

Generally, doctors say, one-third of those with severe endometriosis can become pregnant if they undergo abdominal surgery, and three out of four women with mild to moderate endometriosis can become pregnant within two years of treatment. Interestingly, 65 to 75 percent of women with mild endometriosis are likely to achieve pregnancy no matter what their doctor does.

Epididymitis. Epididymitis is an inflammation of the epididymis, a long, tightly coiled tube that lies along the back of each testicle. The epididymis is a holding area for new sperm—nurturing them as they mature prior to launch—and the inflammation is usually caused by an infection that spreads from the urinary tract.

The first indication of its arrival is often a sausage-shaped swelling along the back of the testicle that becomes hot, tender and painful. It develops over the course of a few hours and is followed by a painful stiffening and swelling of the scrotum, the skin covering the testicles.

Your doctor will probably want to run a few tests on your urine and prostate gland secretions to identify the bug that's causing your infection. He or she may also suggest checking your mate, since you can swap this type of organism back and forth. Once the bug is identified, however, your doctor can prescribe an antibiotic to kill the infection. Bed rest, ice packs and scrotal support can relieve your pain.

Infertility. Approximately one out of every six couples is infertile—meaning they've engaged in unprotected intercourse for at least a year without causing pregnancy. And, according to at least one researcher, the incidence of infertility is on the rise.

Generally, doctors agree, studies reveal that infertility may be caused by defective sperm or an ovary that doesn't know when and how to produce an egg. In one study of 708 couples at the University of Bristol in England, for example, defective sperm caused infertility in 24 percent of the couples. Women failed to produce an egg in 21 percent of the couples, while another 14 percent had damaged fallopian tubes—those hollow strands of tissue through which the egg passes on its way from the ovary to the uterus. The cause of infertility was undetermined—not an infrequent occurrence with this type of study—for 28 percent of the couples.

At least part of the increase in infertility is due to an epidemic of pelvic inflammatory disease, or PID (see Common Reproductive System Conditions). PID, which puts more than 250,000 women in the hospital each year, is an infection that can spread throughout a woman's reproductive system. It's generally caused by a sexually transmitted bacterial infection called chlamydia (see sexually transmitted disease under Common Reproductive System Conditions). Some researchers believe that an intrauterine device (IUD) used for birth control may also encourage the bacterial organisms that trigger it. Left untreated, PID can cause damaged reproductive organs and infertility.

The most common problem affecting male fertility, however, is a kind of varicose vein near the testicles. This enlarged vein, called a varicocele, is thought to damage sperm production because it overheats the temperature-sensitive testicles by supplying too much blood.

Another problem, though uncommon, may be overexposure to such factors as lead, nicotine and marijuana, and to environmental chemicals such as DDT, PCBs, hexachlorobenzene and pentachlorophenol. Some of these chemicals, however, have been banned or restricted in recent times, and consumer awareness is reducing the use of others.

But there are other causes of infertility that, lumped together, make figuring out how to get pregnant something of a challenge: endometriosis, prostatitis, an undescended testicle, diabetes mellitus, acidic vagina, cervical polyps, fibroid tumors, internal scars from previous infection or surgery, x-rays, incompatible sperm, excessive weight loss, excessive weight gain, alcohol, premature ejaculation, atrophy of the testes from mumps or other causes, malnutrition, tight briefs and drugs such as arsenic, carbon disulfide, cocaine and stilbestrol.

Before you head for a fertility specialist, doctors say, there are a few commonsense things you can do yourself.

If you're a man, for example, you should avoid overexposure to pesticides, marijuana, tobacco and other unnecessary drugs. You should pass up jockstraps, tight pants, frequent and prolonged baths or anything else that might overheat your testicles.

If you're a woman, doctors say, you should also avoid exposure to chemicals and drugs and make sure that you're not exercising or dieting so much that you stop menstruating. You can use a mild baking soda douche (a tablespoon or two of baking soda to one quart of water) before intercourse if you suspect your husband's semen is too acidic. You should avoid using lubricating jelly before intercourse and leaping out of bed afterward. In fact, you might just snuggle back under the covers for another 30 minutes and give your husband's sperm an extra chance to play peek-a-boo with your egg. And don't douche when you get up. Even Olympic-class sperm have a hard time swimming upstream.

There are also a few things you can do together, doctors say. You can abstain from intercourse for the first four to seven days of your cycle to increase sperm concentration (the first day you bleed is day one), and you can make sure that ejaculation occurs deep in the vagina by keeping the man on top during intercourse. It also helps if you can make love during your most fertile period—usually around the fourteenth day of your cycle.

If you're still not pregnant after a year of effort, doctors agree, it's time to get professional advice. But it's not always an easy process. To overcome infertility, you need to open the most private part of your private life to probing, testing and analysis.

After a battery of tests, treatment can begin. Sometimes it is as simple as having your mate wear a condom for several months, a practice that can drive down your concentrations of antibodies so your vagina won't treat his sperm as the enemy. Then, when you do have unprotected intercourse, your vagina won't bring on the antisperm artillery.

But the most successful treatments, doctors claim, are drugs, surgery and artificial insemination. A varicocele, for example, can frequently be corrected by snipping the veins leading from the penis. Physical causes such as diabetes mellitus and bacterial infections can be treated with drugs, and oral decongestants can also "decongest" cervical mucus that may be blocking the sperm's passage like a natural diaphragm. A small pump can even dispense a synthetic version of the hormone that stimulates ovulation. *In vitro* fertilization techniques—removing the mother's eggs and fertilizing them in a glass tube or dish outside her body, then placing them in her uterus—is becoming more certain and more sophisticated by the year.

But *in vitro* fertilization is not perfect, and it's not for everyone. It is most useful, doctors suggest, when they can't figure out why a woman can't get pregnant or when they find a woman with damaged fallopian tubes—roughly a fifth of all couples who are infertile.

The procedure is expensive—$4,000 to $8,000 each time fertilization is tried—and it doesn't always work. In one of the few follow-up studies done, for example, Australian researchers found that 244 *in vitro* pregnancies resulted in only 135 live births. Of course, that may not be terribly impressive from a win/lose point of view, but that's 135 children who wouldn't be here if their parents hadn't been willing to take some financial and emotional risks.

Orchitis.   Orchitis is an inflammation of a testicle that is usually caused by mumps, but it can also be triggered by infection or an accidental blow. Bed rest, scrotal support and ice bags are usually helpful, doctors say, and an antibiotic or mumps serum, depending on the cause, will help clear up the problem.

Pelvic inflammatory disease.   Pelvic inflammatory disease, commonly known as PID, is an inflammation of the reproductive system. It's triggered by one of several bacterial infections ascending through the vagina into the uterus, and even extending up further, into the ovaries.

The major attackers seem to be the sexually transmitted diseases chlamydia and gonorrhea, but it's not unusual for them to join forces with other infections and launch a multibug attack. One study indicated that one in seven women developed PID during their reproductive years. Risk factors include intrauterine devices (IUDs) or an infected partner. Nearly 10 percent of all women who get the disease may become infertile from the damage done by a single episode.

Birth control pills are known to create a particularly appealing vaginal environment for chlamydia. Most doctors recommend diaphragms and condoms for sexually active men and women, since they protect against both gonorrhea and chlamydia.

At one time, treatment for PID involved surgery. Today, however, most doctors fight the infections triggering the disease with a combination of antibiotics. Only a very few women—those who have ruptured abscesses in pelvic organs, for example—require surgery.

Premenstrual syndrome.   Premenstrual syndrome, or PMS, is the name given to a group of symptoms that generally include headache, breast swelling and tenderness, abdominal bloating, swelling of the hands and feet, fatigue, depression, tension, irritability and increased appetite—especially for sweet or salty foods.

PMS affects up to 90 percent of all women at one time or another, and usually begins at or after ovulation, peaks in severity just before a period starts and disappears as soon as it does. Between 20 and 40 percent of those with PMS may experience some interruption in their normal functioning, while 5 percent may be truly incapacitated.

Perhaps that's why many doctors suggest that the majority of women with PMS don't need treatment. Only those whose symptoms disrupt their life need help, doctors say. And for most of them, dietary changes— limited alcohol, caffeine and salt, plus six small meals a day that are rich in complex carbohydrates and protein and low in simple sugars—and exercise—at least three times a week—will alleviate the problem.

High doses of vitamin B_6 at levels determined by each woman's physician, may be effective for women with symptoms that disrupt their life. In one study that compared vitamin B_6 with a placebo (fake pill), for example, 21 of 25 women taking B_6 showed significant improvement in all their symptoms.

For the few women with more severe symptoms, some doctors say that a drug to reduce excess water in the body, preferably spironolactone, or natural progesterone, should be added to the treatment.

Prostatitis.   Prostatitis is an inflammation of the prostate gland, a doughnut-shaped organ that sits just below a man's bladder, next to the rectum, with a tube that provides a conduit for urine running through a hole in its center. Its main purpose is to produce the milky ejaculatory fluid that nurtures semen, although some men might claim that its only purpose is to give its owner trouble.

Rarely does a man escape some kind of prostate problem at some point in life. That's because every time the "doughnut" swells, it pinches off the tube sliding through its middle and obstructs the flow of urine. And it swells whenever there's an inflammation. An inflammation can be triggered by bacteria, and it should be treated with antibiotics.

Sexually transmitted disease.   Sexually transmitted diseases, or STDs, are a group of at least 22 genital infections that are transmitted from one person to another through sexual contact. They include chlamydia, herpes, and yeast infections, as well as the old standbys, syphilis and gonorrhea. They are most likely to occur in sexually active people with multiple partners, as well as in the poor and uneducated.

Chlamydia, a bacterial infection that affects 4.5 to 10 million men and women every year, is probably the most common STD. It causes one-quarter to one-half of all cases of pelvic inflammatory disease (PID) and sterilizes 11,000 women annually. It also causes nearly half of the estimated 500,000 cases of acute epididymitis.

Men infected by the bacteria may notice a discharge from their penis and feel a constant urge to urinate even though it hurts when they do, says Donald Kaye, M.D., an infectious disease specialist and chairman of the Department of Medicine at the Medical College of Pennsylvania in Philadelphia. Women may have a vaginal discharge and a burning feeling when they urinate. But, "chlamydia does not always manifest warning symptoms," cautions Dr. Kaye, "and often couples 'ping-pong' the infection back and forth, making treatment difficult." Once discovered, however, chlamydia can be killed by a ten-day course of tetracycline—for both partners.

Another common vaginal infection is caused by *Candida albicans,* a fungus that can be treated either with antifungal drugs such as clotrimazole or 10-grain vaginal capsules of boric acid. *Trichomonas vaginalis,* the parasite that causes trichomoniasis, requires treatment with the drug metronidazole (Flagyl). Since both of these diseases are sexually transmitted, both partners need to be treated.

Another well-known STD is herpes, a viral infection that is closely related to chickenpox, shingles and the common cold sore. Five to 20 million Americans have it, and another 260,000 to 500,000 get it every year. It is generally transmitted by close body contact—kissing, intercourse, oral or anal sex—although researchers have found that it can live on a plastic toilet seat for 1½ hours. Fortunately, it can't penetrate your skin unless there's a cut. So you might want to think twice about scratching any mosquito bites on the back of your thighs.

The first herpes attack feels a lot like the flu, with fever, aching muscles and swollen glands in the groin. Blisters or lumps soon erupt, usually accompanied by itching and burning. The first attack can take as long as two to three weeks to run its course, although—fortunately—recurrent episodes are usually shorter and milder. Recurrence is usually signaled by the "prodome," a set of symptoms that includes tingling, itching or burning in the perineal or genital area, twitches, pain or tenderness of the groin and general weakness, like the onset of flu.

You're contagious as soon as the blisters appear, doctors warn, which may be why at least one study indicates that two-thirds of those with herpes experience sexual problems, a loss of self-esteem and a feeling of isolation.

Generally, your doctor will prescribe a drug called acyclovir either orally, topically or—should you have a complication such as meningitis—intravenously in the hospital. But that's only for the first episode. For recurrent episodes, topical acyclovir has only a slight effect in men and none at all in women. But there is a new over-the-counter ointment that can ease the pain and send herpes packing—for a long time, in some cases.

In a recent clinical trial, patients using a new substance called Intervir experienced almost immediate relief from the pain, itching and burning of herpes outbreaks. Complete symptom relief was obtained within 30 to 60 minutes of the first use, compared with four days in patients using a placebo (fake) ointment without the active ingredient.

The duration of outbreaks averaged 2½ days less, too, and the patients using Intervir reported longer periods of time between recurrences. In one out of every five patients, early use of Intervir aborted the outbreaks altogether.

Fortunately, half of all those who get herpes will never have a second attack.

The same can't be said for syphilis, a bacterial disease that can continue to grow and invade new tissue. It can destroy the heart, aorta, brain, eyes, central nervous system, spine and trachea. No vital organ is safe. Doctors estimate that close to 25,000 new cases occur every year, but fortunately syphilis can usually be shot down with a single injection of antibiotics. Its major symptom is usually a hard lump around the genitals that turns into a running ulcer or sore, although occasionally the lump is so small it can be mistaken for a pimple.

Gonorrhea, which is usually vulnerable to antibiotics, may indicate its presence with a heavy, creamy discharge of whitish or yellowish pus from the vagina and from the urinary opening of both sexes. The discharge will usually cloud your urine and stain your underwear. Urination is frequent, urgent and painful. Gonorrhea causes infertility and—left untreated—can also cause arthritis or infections of the heart and brain. Fortunately, gonorrhea has been on the decline in the United States since 1975.

Toxic shock syndrome.   Toxic shock syndrome, often called TSS, is a potentially fatal illness caused by poisonous bacteria. It usually occurs when bacteria normally found on the skin invade the vagina and begin to grow, although it has been known to occur in men. It apparently thrives on tampons with synthetic fibers—particularly the superabsorbent kind—when they are left in the vagina for longer than 6 hours. Contraceptive sponges left in the vagina for more than 24 hours have also been linked to TSS.

A recent study at the Kaiser-Permanente Medical Care Program in Oakland, California, revealed that the incidence of toxic shock increased when tampon manufacturers added synthetic materials to their product in an effort to make the tampons more absorbent. The incidence decreased when, in the wake of several deaths and headlines across the country, at least one of those manufacturers removed its product from the market and the number of women who used tampons rapidly declined.

But TSS is once again increasing. And although scientists are groping for a reason, researchers at New York University Medical Center have noted that a synthetic fiber is once again being added to tampons.

The symptoms of toxic shock syndrome include vomiting, high fever, dizziness, faintness, severe muscle aches, red eyes, sore throat, headache, rash and diarrhea. But as Michael R. Spence, M.D., points out, "A lot of people get toxic shock syndrome who don't get the full-blown syndrome. Anytime a woman gets a fever or gets fainty (during menstruation), then she has to be concerned that she might be seeing one of the minor varieties of toxic shock."

To be safe, Dr. Spence suggests, "Go ahead and wear tampons, but don't wear the super tampons, don't wear the ones that have artificial fibers and change your tampons a minimum of four times a day."

Undescended testicle.   Occasionally, a testicle can't be found in the scrotum at all after birth. It gets stuck somewhere between the abdomen and the scrotum. If it doesn't eventually descend, your doctor may suggest either surgery or hormone treatments to force it down. Otherwise, doctors say, your child will be susceptible to a high incidence of pain, hernias, tumors and infertility as an adult.

Chapter 15
Skin

SEE YOUR DOCTOR IMMEDIATELY IF:

- *Your skin feels numb*
- *Your skin turns yellow*
- *You have a red line or lines moving up your arms or legs*
- *Your skin has been broken as a result of a bite from an animal or a person*
- *You're bleeding profusely*
- *You've been severely burned*
- *You notice pus oozing from a cut*
- *You develop a flat, red rash on your palms, wrists, ankles and soles of your feet after being bitten by a tick*
- *Your skin is pale, moist and cold, and this is accompanied by faintness, nausea, panting and rapid pulse rate*
- *Your skin turns blue*
- *Your skin turns black*
- *You have a swollen, tender bite that is accompanied by fever and swollen glands*

Your skin, the largest organ of the body, can give away a lot of information you would rather keep to yourself—like the condition you were in when you crawled into bed too late last night. It can also tell a great deal about your state of health (or lack of it), since it often shows the first outward signs that something inside has gone wrong.

But if the skin is an informant, it's also a bodyguard. And the epidermis, the outer layer, bears the brunt of it all. It suffers abrasive washings, slatherings with cosmetics, burns in the summer sun, cuts, scrapes and a number of other abuses. But the epidermis is mighty strong, and it adjusts and adapts as needed to such insults, though it's most sensitive where it's thinnest—on the eyelids—and toughest where it's thickest—on the soles of the feet.

The second layer of skin, the dermis, is where all the action takes place. It contains the sebaceous glands (which manufacture the skin's oil, or sebum), the sweat glands and the hair follicles. This is also where the nerve endings are located that tell you when you've stepped on a nail, burned a finger or been stung by a bee. The elasticity of the dermis provides the firm, youthful skin that we all admire, especially when we're 50.

Just below the dermis is the subdermis, also known as body fat. This provides the "padding" for the bones and muscles and rounds out the contours of your body.

It's the quality of your skin that lays claim to your beauty—but in truth, beautiful skin is much more than the lack of wrinkles, blemishes and other flaws. Truly beautiful skin exudes health.

When you don't look good, chances are you don't feel good. So pay attention to your skin's signals and symptoms. The information below will help you translate what your skin may be telling you.

SYMPTOM: **Birthmarks**

COMMON CAUSES: Port-wine stain, strawberry hemangioma, cavernous hemangioma. These are accurately called vascular birthmarks, meaning they are caused by a concentration of tiny blood vessels in the skin. They are fairly common.

Although it's not precisely known what causes birthmarks to occur, evidence does not support the belief that they are caused during pregnancy by some event in the mother's life such as a fright, a bad dream, a bad injury, medication or even a mishap during childbirth. But, as their name suggests, they are almost always something we are presented with at birth.

Birthmarks go by the three names mentioned above because they have three distinct characteristics. According to the American Academy of Dermatology, this is the lowdown on birthmarks.

Port-wine stain is the most common and appears as a red, blue or purplish discoloration of the skin on the face, neck, trunk or limbs. Less often it occurs in the mouth, nose or other body openings. At birth, the surface of the port-wine stain is usually flat and not elevated above the surrounding normal skin. Later in life, the birthmark may appear thicker and develop small bumps and ridges. Port-wine stains often bleed after injury and the bleeding is sometimes difficult to control.

A strawberry hemangioma, as you might guess, resembles the color and contour of a strawberry. This type of birthmark is elevated above the surface of the skin and is usually one to two inches in diameter, although it can cover an entire arm or leg. Strawberry hemangiomas can appear at birth or during the first few months of life. Unlike port-wine stains, which are usually permanent, most strawberry birthmarks disappear by early childhood—50 percent are gone by age five and 70 percent by age seven. Of the birthmarks that don't disappear, only about 6 percent are so cosmetically disturbing that they require treatment to remove them or prevent further growth.

A cavernous hemangioma is the least common type of vascular birthmark. It is elevated and bluish in color, and usually no larger than three inches in diameter. Its growth and disappearance are similar to a strawberry hemangioma except that, in some cases, a cosmetic flaw will remain.

Pigmented spots and moles are also considered birthmarks. (For more on moles, see Symptom: Mole, Change in.)

BEST RESPONSE: It's very important that birthmarks be examined by a physician as early as possible so that a correct diagnosis and a decision about treatment can be made. Many authorities recommend waiting for at least four years before treating the ordinary strawberry or cavernous hemangioma. By that time, it will be evident if improvement is going to occur naturally.

In the past, people with port-wine hemangiomas had only two choices for treatment—covering the area with cosmetics or having plastic surgery. Now they can be removed by laser beam, says David Apfelberg, M.D., a plastic surgeon at the Palo Alto Medical Foundation in California. With this method, about 50 to 70 percent of a birthmark can be faded out. A deep blue port-wine stain will become light violet, and a red one will pale to pink after five or six half-hour treatments.

The procedure can be done in a doctor's office, and the patient needs only a local anesthetic. Occasional possible side effects include scarring or changes in skin pigmentation or texture.

SYMPTOM: **Bites and Stings**

COMMON CAUSES: When it comes to sting operations, Mother Nature outdoes the FBI. A bee, wasp or hornet stabs the skin, and that sharp pinprick sensation is quickly followed by pain that can sometimes be pretty intense. Pain isn't the end of it, though. A red dot surrounded by a pale area appears, followed by a red ring. The area may itch and sting for a few hours.

That's if you're stung *once*. But if you're attacked by a gang, the pain can be torturous, and multiple stings can cause headache, muscle cramps, fever, drowsiness or even unconsciousness. If you receive several hundred stings, death can occur.

But for a person who's *allergic* to an insect's venom, even *one* sting can kill. Fortunately, allergic reactions are rare. Most result in localized swelling and itching at the site of the sting and may produce hives and itching all over the body.

A moderate reaction is accompanied by generalized swelling, wheezing, dizziness, nausea and abdominal pain. The most severe reaction—anaphylactic shock—causes breathing difficulty as the throat swells. Total collapse can occur in a matter of minutes.

Allergies to stings are not uncommon. About 1 million people develop extreme reactions to stings each year, although less than 50 people die as a result. If you have allergies, make sure your doctor tests for this possibility.

But bees, wasps and hornets aren't the only pests. There are plenty of other critters that can leave you red and scratching.

Among them are chiggers, which are sometimes called red bugs or harvest mites. They like to attack at such damp, moist places as the ankle, groin, beltline or wherever clothing is tight. The skin reacts to a chigger bite with hives or with an itchy, red, pimplelike bump. Occasionally blisters, swelling or larger red patches develop.

Fleas can leap from dog to master in a single bound. The little red bumps they leave cause irritation for up to several days and leave you scratching along with little Snappy. Fleas can cause more serious problems. In the western states, particularly the Southwest, fleas from wild animals can carry plague. Keep this in mind if you go camping in the Southwest and come in contact with wild rodents like squirrels or chipmunks, or their nests.

Mosquitoes cause a pimplelike lesion and itching when they bite, even if you manage to slap and destroy at the first sound of their buzzing. The discomfort they leave as a remembrance seems to last forever. For some, the itching can lead to an infection, and for a small number of hypersensitive individuals, a severe local reaction can occur, causing hives in other parts of the body, severe swelling and small areas of bleeding under the skin, as well as nausea, dizziness and lethargy. Mosquitoes also can be blamed for spreading such diseases as yellow fever, malaria and equine encephalitis.

Ticks are nasty little bloodsuckers that burrow their head into the skin, then swell as they feed, sometimes to several times their original size. The skin around the bite will form a lump surrounded by redness. Once the tick is removed, the lump usually goes away, although sometimes it stays around. Certain tick bites, although rare, can cause encephalitis (see Common Neurological System Conditions in chapter 12), Rocky Mountain spotted fever and other major problems.

Bites from certain spiders can be poisonous and will cause extreme pain and other serious symptoms. Snake bites also can be life-threatening. As for animal and human bites, the problem can be more than just a superficial wound. The possibilities of infection, tetanus and rabies are very real.

BEST RESPONSE: For the majority of the population, the usual bee, wasp or hornet sting requires only minimal treatment. If the sting is from a honeybee, the stinger may protrude from the skin, and you should carefully and quickly scrape it away with a fingernail. Grasping or squeezing could accidentally trigger the venom sac, causing more venom to enter the skin.

"For all stings, the affected area should be washed well with mild soap and water," says Kenneth S. Gray, M.D., F.A.C.E.P., diplomate, American Boards of Emergency Medicine and Family Practice, and co-owner and medical director of Doctors Care Medical Centers in San Diego. "Swelling can be controlled with an ice pack and elevation." However, Dr. Gray cautions, if symptoms from stings go beyond the local skin reaction to progressive swelling, uncontrollable itching or pain, or if such symptoms as difficult breathing, sweating, nausea and vomiting or fever indicate an allergic reaction or illness, medical help should be sought.

If you know you are allergic to stings, he notes, you should discuss with your physician the necessity of carrying an emergency kit containing an antihistamine and a hypodermic of adrenaline.

Chigger and flea bites will usually go away by themselves in a matter of a few days. If they are really troublesome, however, a physician may prescribe an antihistamine for the itching, a steroid cream for the irritating bite and antibiotics if an infection occurs.

If a mosquito has done you in, you should wash the affected area with mild soap and water to prevent infection. Application of calamine lotion will help relieve the itching. A baking soda paste also may be a soothing treatment. If there is significant swelling, ice packs can be applied.

Ticks like to nestle in the hair, the genital area and around the ankles. Check your body for these nasty little critters after you've been in the woods or fields. If you can find a tick before it embeds itself in your skin, it's a simple matter to throw it off in one whole piece. To remove a tick that's nestled into your skin, doctors commonly recommend rubbing the affected area with petroleum jelly (Vaseline) or gasoline to loosen the head. This cuts off the tick's oxygen supply, forcing it to drop off. If necessary, a physician can remove the head by making a small incision.

For spider bites, apply cold compresses and seek medical care if you become ill. Always see a physician after a snake bite, even if you know *for certain* the snake is nonpoisonous, says Dr. Gray. This is because any puncture wound has the potential to become infected or lead to tetanus. Also, get a good look at the snake so you can describe it accurately or pick it out from a photograph. Knowing what kind of snake bit you may help determine treatment. If it's dead, put it in a sack and take it to the emergency room with you. The general rule of snake identification is this: A snake with a triangular-shaped head is poisonous; one with a round head is not—the coral snake is an exception to this rule.

All bites from humans or animals in which the skin is broken should be seen immediately by a doctor. Tetanus shots—and, if the animal's a potential rabies carrier, a series of rabies injections—may be required.

Short of a portable plastic bubble, there's no way to insulate yourself from bites and stings. But for the determined, here are a few tips. Stay away from such insect hangouts as flower beds, orchards, vineyards, clover fields and garbage dumps. Sweet fruit, soft drinks, jellies and honey particularly attract insects. Wear shoes and socks (not sandals) and protective clothing when outside. Wear light-colored clothing made from smooth-finished fabrics. White is said to be the least insect-attracting color.

Be forewarned, however, that a mosquito can bite through many materials, so repellents should be applied to exposed areas of the skin and even to clothing. Repellents that contain deet (diethyltoluamide) are the most effective, but Dr. Gray cautions that you should follow the directions on the can carefully, and you shouldn't overapply repellents on infants and young children. "Remember, too, that repellents are not effective against stinging insects," says Dr. Gray.

ACCOMPANYING SYMPTOMS: If, after a tick bite, you develop flat red spots on the palms of the hands and soles of the feet, which then spread to the wrists, ankles, legs and arms and finally the trunk, and you have a fever and severe head and muscle aches, you could be getting Rocky Mountain spotted fever. You should seek immediate medical treatment. The disease occurs most frequently in the Southeast, from Maryland to Georgia, and is most prevalent in the spring and summer.

If, a few days after you are bitten by a flea, the bite becomes swollen and tender, you feel ill and feverish and you have swollen glands, you may have plague. You should see your doctor immediately. Plague is a serious illness, but it is curable if diagnosed and treated early.

SYMPTOM: **Blackheads and Whiteheads**

COMMON CAUSES: Blackheads and whiteheads are the scourge of acne (see Common Skin Conditions). They're not quite full-fledged pimples, but they're unsightly and bothersome just the same.

What causes these blemishes is a foul-up in the production process that takes place in your pores. The process itself is complex, but the flare-ups are basically triggered by dihydrotestosterone (DHT), a souped-up form of testosterone, which is a hormone secreted by both men and women (although men secrete about ten times the amount that women do).

DHT stimulates your sebaceous glands to produce oil. As a result, acne-prone skin produces hard skin cells at a faster-than-normal rate. At the same time, anaerobes, a certain kind of bacteria that thrive in the pores, irritate surrounding tissue. Dead skin cells, bacteria and other debris commingle with oil, forming thick plugs.

When these plugs form bumps under the skin, they appear as whiteheads. When they break through the skin, they appear as blackheads. This unsightly black color is the result of exposure to oxygen.

The role of diet in causing these blemishes is not clear, but most dermatologists believe it's genes that make your pores behave the way they do.

BEST RESPONSE: A real five-alarm case of blackheads and whiteheads should be seen by a dermatologist, who can prescribe special medicated creams to help control and alleviate the problem.

For normal cases and for those that pop up every now and then, you can control the problem yourself simply by avoiding anything that blocks the pores, advises Lyon Rowe, M.D., chief of dermatology at Kaiser Permanente Medical Center in Los Angeles, and associate clinical professor of dermatology at the University of California at Los Angeles. "This includes the creams, greases or oils you put on your skin. If you must wear makeup, switch to a water-based product."

You should also avoid sun exposure, he says. "Sun causes reddening and mild swelling of the skin, which might block the pores more. Rubbing the skin may do the same thing. You should wash and dry the skin gently. Skin products containing benzoyl peroxide are best for opening pores."

Finally, Dr. Rowe cautions against squeezing and poking at blackheads or whiteheads, because this can irritate the blemish and cause it to get worse or even become infected. And if you don't take corrective action, the popped blemishes will simply reappear in a short time.

SYMPTOM: **Bleeding**

COMMON CAUSES: It's happened to everyone—you prick your finger with a needle, fall on a piece of glass or run a kitchen knife across your hand. You cut your skin and damage the blood vessels underneath. As a result, you bleed. But unless you have a disease that causes uncontrollable bleeding, such as aplastic anemia, hemophilia or thrombocytopenia, cuts and scrapes are usually easy to fix.

BEST RESPONSE: There are three possible dangers from cuts—loss of blood, damage to the skin and infection.

First the blood. If a cut bleeds extensively or is "pumping blood," consider it a medical emergency that requires prompt first aid, and seek immediate treatment by a doctor.

For the usual cut, however, you should be able to control bleeding on your own by exerting firm pressure against the wound using a cloth compress (a clean handkerchief or towel works well). Press the cloth against the bleeding site for five to ten minutes or until the bleeding stops.

If, after the bleeding stops, you notice that the edges of the wound can't be brought together, or if damaged tissue extends out of the wound, sutures (stitches) will probably be necessary.

"Stitching should be done within four to six hours of the time of injury," says Kenneth S. Gray, M.D. "If there are serious lacerations of the face or a hand injury that involves nerves or tendons, your physician may refer you to a plastic surgeon or a hand surgeon."

Once the skin is broken, there is a danger that germs, always lingering on the skin, will rush in, make a meal of blood and damaged tissues and, in the process, contaminate the wound. Boils and carbuncles and impetigo (see Common Skin Conditions) may result. And no one wants those things if they can be avoided.

"I recommend washing the wound with a mild soap and lukewarm water," Dr. Gray says. "Over-the-counter antibiotic cream is fine for superficial wounds. Peroxide is generally not necessary, and Merthiolate is definitely out of style. Cuts should be bandaged until healing occurs. If the bandage gets wet or dirty, it should be changed. You should check the wound daily. If there is increasing pain, tenderness, swelling, heat, redness (including streaks) or pus in the wound, an infection has probably developed and you should see a physician.

"If it's been five years since your last tetanus booster, and your wound is dirty or requires stitches, you should get another tetanus shot," says Dr. Gray. A tetanus booster is recommended every ten years as a routine immunization, whether you are injured or not (see tetanus under Common Facial, Jaw and Mouth Conditions in chapter 8).

SYMPTOM: **Blisters**

COMMON CAUSES: The causes of blisters range from the common friction blister, caused when a shoe rubs your foot the wrong way, to the more chronic painful blisters of shingles (see Common Skin Conditions).

Blisters come in two sizes: small, called vesicles, and large, called bullae.

Small blisters are less than the size of a tackhead. If you've been bitten by an insect (see Symptom: Bites and Stings), the cause of your blister is not hard to figure out.

If one blister or a crop of them appears around the mouth, it could be a cold sore, or fever blister (see Symptom: Sores in chapter 8), which is caused by herpes simplex virus I. If the blisters appear on the vagina or penis, the cause could be herpes simplex virus II, a sexually transmitted disease (see Common Reproductive System Conditions in chapter 14). If the vesicles are on the toes, it could be athlete's foot (see Common Foot Conditions in chapter 9). If the blisters appear on the scalp or body in a ringed fashion and get larger and scaly around the edges, it's probably ringworm (see Common Skin Conditions).

Small blisters, which can appear anywhere on the body, can be a reaction to certain drugs. Also, the following substances are frequently associated with blister eruptions: iodides, sometimes included in vitamin pills and occurring naturally in shellfish and kelp; bromides; mercury; and phenolphthalein, an ingredient in laxatives.

Large blisters—bigger than a tackhead—are frequently the result of friction. You rake leaves and a blister appears on your palm; you wear new shoes and a blister pops up on your heel. This is the skin's way of protecting itself.

Large blisters are also characteristic of burns—those caused by bumping into a hot stove, spilling boiling water or a corrosive chemical on yourself or getting too much of the sun's rays (see Symptom: Burns).

Pemphigus is an uncommon but potentially fatal skin disease of middle-aged and elderly people that is characterized by large water blisters all over the body. The large blisters often first appear in the mouth, then spread to the skin, and leave a raw, crusted area when they break.

BEST RESPONSE: Because there are so many different causes for blisters, the course of action you take to get rid of them will vary according to the cause.

The garden-variety blister caused by friction from shoes or other equipment can be left as is and protected with adhesive tape and cushioned with foam rubber or moleskin, say doctors. Or, if the blister is very painful or infected, you can break it. This should be done by cleansing the area and puncturing the blister at its edge with a needle that has been sterilized with alcohol. Then press the blister so the fluid can escape. Trim away any ragged edges, since they may irritate the wound.

A person suffering from pemphigus needs immediate treatment. Hospitalization may be needed, and antibiotics or steroids are the suggested course of action.

ACCOMPANYING SYMPTOMS: If red patches on the face, scalp or arms turn into large, watery blisters that grow, then break and ooze a straw-colored fluid that forms a yellowish, itching crust, this is a sign of a skin infection called impetigo (see Common Skin Conditions). Treatment is general with antibiotics or antibacterial ointment.

If an infant or young child has blisters filled with fluid, and the top layer of skin detaches from the body, this is a sign of staphylococcal scalded skin syndrome. Medical treatment and a course of antibiotic therapy are necessary.

If blisters are accompanied by intense itching and jagged gray lines, this is a sign of infection by mites called scabies (see Common Skin Conditions). Call your physician.

SYMPTOM: **Blue Tinge**

COMMON CAUSES: Unless you've been dyeing blue Easter eggs or batiking a denim dress, blue skin—or cyanosis—usually indicates a lack of oxygen somewhere in the body.

A blue face, hands and feet, for example can indicate that the heart's not pumping enough oxygenated blood (see heart failure under Common Circulatory, Heart and Lung Conditions in chapter 5).

A blue arm or leg can indicate that an embolism—a blood clot or other solid particle that's cruising the bloodstream—has blocked the flow of blood into a limb. A blue tinge around the mouth can indicate that an embolism is cutting off the blood supply to the lungs.

If your fingers, toes, wrists or ankles sometimes turn blue in cold weather, however, the color could be caused by harmless contractions of the tiny arteries that feed these areas (see Raynaud's disease under Common Circulatory, Heart and Lung Conditions in chapter 5).

BEST RESPONSE: Check with your doctor immediately. If you have an embolism or blood clot, doctors say, you will probably be hospitalized and given medication to prevent new clots from forming. In severe cases, surgery may be necessary to actually remove the embolus. An untreated embolism, doctors caution, can cause the part of the body it affects to die. Heart failure also requires medical supervision.

If, however, your doctor determines that your blue fingers, toes, wrists or ankles are caused by overenthusiastic arteries that turn your blood supply off and on like a spigot, you probably need do nothing more than keep your hands and feet warm, wear roomy gloves and shoes, avoid cigarette smoke and leave downhill skiing and other icy sports to someone else. A glass of wine or a bottle of beer, doctors say, may also help chase away your "blues."

ACCOMPANYING SYMPTOM: If you have a child with a hacking cough who starts to turn blue around the mouth, this is a sign of croup (see Common Circulatory, Heart and Lung Conditions in chapter 5). You need to see a doctor immediately.

SYMPTOM: **Brown Patches**

COMMON CAUSES: Leopards are not the only ones who develop spots—humans do, too. Years of overexposure to the sun cause the skin to overproduce pigment in patches. These brownish patches are properly called lentigines but are most commonly referred to as age spots or liver spots, although they have nothing to do with the liver.

Some consider liver spots a sign that you're getting old, but they are really a sign that you've been getting too much sun. They're common in aging people with fair skin.

Similar spots and patches can appear across the nose, cheeks and forehead when you're pregnant—it's called "the mask of pregnancy"—or if you're taking birth control pills. This is due to a biochemical action of the sun on an increased supply of progesterone. A similar erratic pigmentation has been known to appear on areas of skin that have been exposed to perfumes containing oil of bergamot.

BEST RESPONSE: If you have age spots, you can cover them up with a masking makeup, but there is no cream—no matter what the advertisements may say—that will make them disappear.

If they really bother you, however, you can have the spots surgically removed by a dermatologist, who might use any one of a number of different methods.

To minimize further darkening and to prevent additional spots from forming, always use a sunscreen when outdoors. Bleaching creams should be used only under medical supervision, because they can cause irritation. And see your physician if the age spots change texture, color or size.

The brown spots or mask of pregnancy should disappear after delivery, although it may take several months or years. Similarly, brown patches caused by the Pill might vanish, but that could take a few years.

SYMPTOM: **Bruises**

COMMON CAUSES: You bump your hip against the side of a table or stub your toe. The result is a bruise, and what has happened is that fragile capillaries—tiny blood vessels under the skin's surface—have ruptured, spilling blood into the surrounding area. The fluid then seeped into deeper layers of skin, lodging there and creating a painful black-and-blue patch.

For the child trying out a new pair of skates or a new bicycle, a bruise is a purple badge of courage. There are other causes for bruises, however. Easy bruising can result as a side effect or adverse reaction to certain drugs such as anticoagulants, aspirin, sulfa drugs, quinine, quinidine, antihistamines, phenothiazines, antidepressants, local anesthetics, penicillin, mercury, bismuth, cortisone or anticonvulsants.

For a very few people, a bruise is a sign of trouble somewhere else in the body. Abnormal platelet function is a problem in kidney and liver disorders, and this can cause unexplained bruising or blood spots under the skin. Other causes of bruising are aplastic anemia (see anemia in Common Whole Body Conditions in chapter 19); thrombocytopenic purpura, a blood disorder; allergies and infections. Acquired immune deficiency syndrome, or AIDS (see Common Whole Body Conditions in chapter 19), is still another cause of purplish bumps under the skin that look like bruises but don't go away.

BEST RESPONSE: The basic first aid treatment for a bruise is application of ice as soon as possible after the injury, says Kenneth S. Gray, M.D.

That constricts the capillaries and slows the bleeding and swelling. You should also elevate the injured area.

If you feel you bruise too easily, or you find bruises on your skin for an unexplained reason, it may indicate an underlying illness that needs evaluation by your physician. If your doctor finds your bruising is related to a medicine you are taking, he or she may, among other things, recommend discontinuing or changing medication.

ACCOMPANYING SYMPTOM: If your bruising is accompanied by swollen gums that occasionally bleed, it could be a result of poor nutrition or deficiency of such nutrients as vitamin C, riboflavin or folic acid. It's best to see your doctor for diagnosis and treatment.

SYMPTOM: **Burns**

COMMON CAUSES: Spending too much time in the sun, getting too close to heat or fire and being exposed to chemicals can all cause painful burns to the body. What happens when the body is exposed to these conditions is not much different from what happens when you throw a steak on a fire. It cooks.

Burns of the skin are categorized by degree. First-degree burns are the least serious. They cause the skin to get red but cause little damage. Second-degree burns do cause damage. The outer skin blisters as a result of injury to the deeper skin layers, but there is no damage to the structures beneath. A third-degree burn is the most severe, causing severe damage to the outer skin and the layers beneath.

Sunburns can be categorized as first- and second-degree heat burns (third-degree burns do not occur from sun exposure). In a case of mild sunburn, the skin will feel hot and tight. It will also look pink to scarlet in color. In a severe sunburn, the color will be deeper, a reddish-purple hue. Swelling and blistering may develop.

Heat rash can develop soon after a sunburn (see Symptom: Rash). As the burn heals, the skin will darken and peel. Mottled discoloration may appear and last for months or years.

BEST RESPONSE: For a first-degree heat or chemical burn, all you need to do is rinse the wound in cool water or apply cool, moist compresses, says Kenneth S. Gray, M.D.

Never apply butter or grease, despite popular belief. This could facilitate infection. Also avoid putting antiseptics, ointments or sprays on chemical burns immediately after the injury. You could actually rub the chemical into your skin instead and increase the severity of the burn. Later on, after you're sure the chemical is completely gone, antibiotic ointments may be used.

"For all-over relief from a mild sunburn, try a soothing bath," says Carl S. Korn, M.D., Pharm.D., assistant clinical professor of dermatology at the University of Southern California in Los Angeles. "Pour a cup of white vinegar into a tub of cool—not hot—water, and hop in. That will reduce the redness and swelling. And drink plenty of water to replace lost fluids."

You can repeat with cold soaks for 10 to 20 minutes at a time, two to four times a day. In between soaks, you should soothe particularly sore and red areas. If your skin feels dry and flaky, Dr. Korn recommends using a light film of solid vegetable shortening. If you use too much, you can clog your pores, which can lead to prickly heat. A sprinkling of baby powder can also be soothing and will help ease you into your clothes.

The itching caused by sunburn can be relieved by taking aspirin (see Symptom: Itching). If your sunburn is severe—meaning the skin blisters and swells—see a physician. In the meantime, treat it as you would mild sunburn.

No one needs to experience more than one sunburn to realize that prevention is the way to go. Controlling sun exposure not only prevents burns but also prevents premature wrinkles and unwanted skin growths, both benign and malignant. Skin damage from the sun is cumulative, and those who are fair-skinned need to be particularly careful. Some suggestions: Stay out of the noonday (10 A.M. to 2 P.M.) sun. Don't be fooled by an overcast day—clouds and fog filter only a small amount of the sun's burning rays.

When you're going to be exposed to the sun, think of sunscreen as your second skin. The higher the number, the better the block, with 15 being practically a total eclipse. For best results, apply these preparations at least one hour before going out in the sun and reapply after swimming or profuse sweating. Be aware that certain drugs, such as tetracycline, diuretics ("water pills"), some antihistamines, tranquilizers and hormone pills, can cause a person to burn more easily because of photosensitivity.

ACCOMPANYING SYMPTOMS: If your sunburn is accompanied by fever, chills, nausea or vomiting, you have what is popularly known as sun poisoning. Medically, however, there is no such malady—it just means your reaction to the sun is so severe that your whole body rebels and you feel sick all over.

SYMPTOM: **Calluses.** *See* Symptom: Thickening

SYMPTOM: **Chafing**

COMMON CAUSES: Rub two wood surfaces together, and you get a campfire. Rub two skin surfaces together, and you get a chafing fire.

Chafing is a skin irritation that gets red and burns. If left untreated, it can even cause an odorous discharge over the affected area.

Chafing occurs mainly in the armpits, groin, buttocks and, for women, underneath the breasts. Athletes and those who are overweight are more prone to chafing. Heat, humidity and perspiration can also contribute to the problem.

Although chafing is usually a skin-against-skin problem, it is often caused by clothing, such as a soiled athletic uniform, rubbing against the skin.

BEST RESPONSE: You can prevent chafing by practicing good personal hygiene and wearing clean clothes—including clean athletic uniforms, says William Dvorine, M.D., in *A Dermatologist's Guide to Home Skin Treatment.* Applying antifungal powders to friction-prone areas prior to activity should help keep chafing from developing.

If chafing does develop, do *not* scrub with soap. This may irritate already damaged skin. Nor should you use any greasy ointments or ointments containing local anesthetics such as benzocaine. Instead, soak the chafed area with Burow's solution, an antiseptic solution, twice a day for five to ten minutes at a time, recommends Marvin H. Klapman, M.D., a dermatologist at the Kaiser Permanente Medical Center in Los Angeles.

SYMPTOM: **Chapping.** *See* Symptom: Dryness

SYMPTOM: **Clamminess**

COMMON CAUSES: Clamminess is described as a cold, dry sweat. There are a number of reasons why this happens—from the harmless clammy palms you get before making a speech to the more serious whole-body clamminess you can experience with a serious head injury or concussion (See Common Neurological System Conditions in chapter 12).

Other causes of cold and clammy skin are collapse of the circulatory system, shock and excessive sweating. Clammy skin also is one of the symptoms of heat exhaustion (see Common Whole Body Conditions in chapter 19).

BEST RESPONSE: Shock and head injuries are medical emergencies and require prompt attention by a physician. Heat exhaustion usually disappears after lying down in a cool place with the head lower than the body. Sip small amounts of cool fluids every few minutes to replenish lost water and salts.

SYMPTOM: **Coldness**

COMMON CAUSES: Those with cold hands may have a warm heart, but they're also likely to have cold feet. Some folks suffer from cold extremities because of a condition known as acrocyanosis.

The tiny arteries that supply blood to the hands and feet suddenly contract, and the affected extremities get less blood than they need. Waste products build up in the veins and give the skin a bluish color. The affected parts nearly always feel cold and may even be sweaty.

Acrocyanosis is fairly common, especially among women, and is not a sign of a major disorder. The condition is intensified by cold but the cause is not known.

Cold fingers can also be a sign of Raynaud's disease (see Common Circulatory, Heart and Lung Conditions in chapter 5). It's more common in women than men. Sometimes the hands and feet will feel cold as well. Attacks are usually brought on by cold or emotional upset, although the real reason for the malady is not known. As the disease progresses, ulcers can form on the fingers, causing pain and even disability.

BEST RESPONSE: Acrocyanosis does not need or respond to treatment. The best you can do is protect your hands and feet from extreme cold by wearing gloves and socks or by finding a warm body to snuggle up with at night.

Raynaud's disease, however, does require some attention. Mild cases can be controlled by avoiding cold and injury to the fingers and eliminating smoking. Attacks can often be ended simply by applying warmth. In severe cases, vasodilating drugs are sometimes successful in warding off attacks, if you take them before venturing out into the cold.

ACCOMPANYING SYMPTOMS: Coldness and pain in the legs can be a symptom of Buerger's disease, a condition affecting the blood vessels in the legs. Left untreated, it can lead to gangrene (see Common Skin Conditions). The same symptoms can also signal an embolism or blockage of the arteries in one of the extremities. You should seek immediate medical care.

If the skin on your hands, feet, nose and ears becomes cold, hard and pale and has no feeling, and you've been exposed to below-freezing temperatures, you may be a victim of frostbite (see Common Skin Conditions).

You should never rub a frostbitten area with snow! Rapid rewarming is what's necessary. This can be accomplished, doctors say, by immersing the affected skin in water that is around 100°F (this is water that is not uncomfortably hot for a normal forearm). Lower temperatures will do no good; higher temperatures might do harm. Rewarming will take ½ to 1½ hours and will be complete when the skin becomes pink. If, after warming, there is not full recovery of the affected part, see a physician as soon as possible.

SYMPTOM: **Cracking**

COMMON CAUSES: Cracked skin is almost always found on the backs of the hands, around the knuckles and on the fingers. If you've got it, you already know it's very painful. Sometimes it's a severe case of chapping that causes the problem. But cracking that occurs on the hands may also mean a bad case of dermatitis (see Common Skin Conditions) and is found in persons with sensitive, allergic or abused skin.

Cracking on the feet can mean athlete's foot (see Common Foot Conditions in chapter 9), a form of dermatitis or dry skin.

BEST RESPONSE: Cracked skin is an open invitation for germs to come in, set up housekeeping and cause an infection. For this reason, your cracked skin should not be ignored.

To treat cracked skin caused by chapping, you can soak your hands in cool water, dry gently and apply petroleum jelly (Vaseline) or moisturizing cream frequently, says Lyon Rowe, M.D. "Don't rub the cream in too vigorously. In fact, be gentle in washing and caring for your hands until the cracking clears."

If this doesn't work, you could have a case of dermatitis, and you should consult a physician.

SYMPTOM: **Crusting**

COMMON CAUSES: Crusting of the skin is the grand finale of many different skin ailments. It means blisters or other irritating lesions are drying up and going away.

The hallmark of the childhood disease impetigo (see Common Skin Conditions) is a sticky, yellowish crust on the face—particularly around the lips and nose.

Probably the most frustrating crusting malady is dermatitis (see Common Skin Conditions), because it is so difficult to keep under control. Even infants can suffer from dermatitis—the medical term is infantile eczema. This condition may result in large, weeping, encrusted areas all over an infant's body (see Symptom: Oozing).

BEST RESPONSE: If only a small area is affected, the usual treatment for impetigo is washing the crusty areas with an antibacterial skin cleanser and applying an over-the-counter antibacterial ointment.

If this doesn't do the trick right away or a large area is affected, an oral antibiotic, prescribed by a physician, is probably necessary.

There are many types of dermatitis and almost as many treatments. Also, successful treatment depends on finding the cause. For these reasons, your best course of action is to see a dermatologist.

SYMPTOM: **Dimpling**

COMMON CAUSES: This is not the Shirley Temple variety of dimples but the waffle-thigh kind known as cellulite that can lead women to try anything to regain that smooth girlish look. Simply put, cellulite is deposits of fat that almost always nestle in the thighs and buttocks.

Women have it more than men because of the difference in their anatomy. The fat in women's thighs is held in pouches of connective tissue that resemble a honeycomb. In men, the connective tissue is in a criss-cross pattern that supports the skin better. As women get older, the tissue shrinks and loses elasticity. The skin over the tissue contracts. If the fat cells don't shrink at the same rate, dimpling will appear on the thighs and buttocks. Another case of sexual discrimination!

If you notice dimpling in the skin of your breast, however, this is *not* a sign of cellulite. It can be a sign of breast cancer (see Common Breast Conditions in chapter 4).

BEST RESPONSE: Since some women are genetically predisposed to fat hips and thighs, cellulite may be something they can't escape. Eating a balanced diet, keeping body weight within normal range and participating in a regular exercise program (walking is probably best in the long haul) are the most sensible recommendations for keeping the dimpling problem to a minimum.

Sorry, but spot reducing does not work, nor do injections, body wraps, massage, creams or special diets. Ridding women of their cellulite (and their money) is big business for charlatans.

If you notice dimpling on any other part of the body, especially the breast, you should see a physician as soon as possible.

SYMPTOM: **Dryness**

COMMON CAUSES: Dry skin, or "winter itch," is a complaint of every healthy person at some time in life.

The problem gets worse the older you get, and for those who live in overheated homes in cold, dry climates and take too many long, hot baths, the skin on the lower arms and legs can get so dry that it resembles an alligator's hide or the bottom of a dry lake.

Dryness results from a lack of water—not oil—in the thin top layer of skin. The parts of the skin that contain lots of oil glands—namely, the scalp, face, back, chest and upper arms—don't have this problem because one of the functions of skin oil is to form a water-retaining layer on the surface of the top layer of skin. If your skin doesn't hold water or if you have underactive sweat glands, you're a sitting duck for dry skin.

BEST RESPONSE: Bathe or shower only as often as necessary, using a mild or superfatted soap or no soap at all in areas where you are dry, recommends Bernard Kirshbaum, M.D., clinical professor of dermatology at the Medical College of Pennsylvania in Philadelphia. Deodorant soaps are not really beneficial to your skin.

After bathing, pat yourself dry gently (try not to rub) and immediately apply a moisturizer. This will trap the water that was absorbed into the skin during bathing. Apply moisturizers or creams several other times during the day, too, but make the application after bathing a must.

If you have dry skin, you don't need expensive products to rid yourself of the problem, says Dr. Kirshbaum. You can use vegetable oils such as sunflower oil and the hydrogenated oils used for cooking, such as solid Crisco or Spry. These oils, according to Dr. Kirshbaum, are cheap, effective, safe and pure skin lubricants. If you want something more glamorous, cold cream is an acceptable alternative.

If you want to have hands that love to be touched, stop repeated exposures to detergents, cleansers and solvents. Avoid washing dishes if you can (doctor's orders), but protect your hands with rubber gloves if you can't. To achieve the best protection, you should wear white cotton gloves under rubber gloves. Apply lotion to your hands whenever they have been in water.

Finally, you should raise the humidity in your home by attaching a humidifier to the furnace or adding moisture to each room by resting pans of water on radiators or attaching a trough of water to room hot-air vents. Moisture from houseplants will also evaporate into the air and help humidify your home.

ACCOMPANYING SYMPTOM: If you have dry skin on your hands, legs or feet that forms into pink or red scaly patches, you probably are suffering from a type of irritant eczema (see dermatitis/eczema under Common Skin Conditions) that flourishes in the dry winter months.

One type is due to irritation from soap damage. Avoid washing these spots, and help them to heal by applying over-the-counter hydrocortisone cream. Another type results from stress and skin irritants as well as cold and dryness. Sunlight helps this condition. Any persistent patchy skin condition requires medical attention.

SYMPTOM: **Flaking**

COMMON CAUSES: The usual cause of flaking skin is one of the many forms of dermatitis or eczema (see Common Skin Conditions).

If you have flaking skin along the creases from your nose to the corners of your mouth, or in other skin creases, like the groin and armpits, it's probably seborrheic dermatitis. Irritant eczema and discoid eczema usually occur on the arms and legs, while housewife's eczema results from constant exposure of the hands and forearms to detergents, cleansers or chemicals.

What's causing the disease can be almost anything you're exposed to in your environment.

BEST RESPONSE: If your flaking skin looks like a form of eczema or dermatitis, you should see a physician for evaluation and treatment. The disease is almost impossible to clear up on your own.

Your doctor will begin treatment by trying to get to the root of the problem. If your doctor feels that your eczema is due to contact with some substance, patch tests may be used to identify the specific cause.

In treating eczema, your physician may recommend a steroid cream in a strength that is not available over the counter, or he or she may prescribe an antihistamine for severe itching. If your eczema has been complicated by a bacterial infection, antibiotics may be prescribed.

ACCOMPANYING SYMPTOMS: If you have flakiness between your toes and the area is red and itchy, with an unpleasant smell, it's probably athlete's foot (see Common Foot Conditions in chapter 9).

   If you have a sore on your inner ankle and the skin around it is red, flaky and itchy, you might have a varicose ulcer (see Symptom: Sores).

SYMPTOM: **Flushing.** *See* Symptom: Flushing in chapter 8

SYMPTOM: **Freckles**

COMMON CAUSE: Dorothy Parker lamented it best: "Four be the things I'd been better without: Love, curiosity, freckles and doubt."

   You can consider your freckles a sign that you've spent—or are spending—too much time in the sun. "Freckles are nests of pigment-producing cells that get darker when exposed to sunlight," says Madhu Pathak, M.D., Ph.D., of the Massachusetts General Hospital Dermatology Department.

   Babies aren't born with freckles, but they develop them early on, usually in the first three years of life. Blonds and especially redheads with blue eyes who spend too much time in the sun are usually those you see with freckles galore.

   Freckles don't fade. Only your tan does. The lightness or darkness of the spots only *appears* to change because a summer tan makes your freckles look paler in comparison. However, exposing freckles to the sun in order to "hide" them just won't work. It'll only work up the pigment-producing cells, the result being more freckles.

BEST RESPONSE: There is no "cure" for freckles. Once you have them, they're yours forever. But you can avoid expanding the freckle family by wearing a sunscreen when going out in the sun.

   And forget what you read about home remedies. Existing freckles cannot be removed. Applying lemon juice to freckles and sitting out in the sun will not fade the spots, but it will cause sunburn, which can create even bigger troubles for you.

If freckles are really bugging you, you can apply a cover-up makeup in a shade that blends with your natural color. In the long run, though, it may be best to enjoy what nature gave you and join the ranks of fearless freckle fanciers.

SYMPTOM: **Hives**

COMMON CAUSES: Hives or wheals are a very common disorder, in which red, itchy bumps develop on the skin. These bumps sometimes have a white center of variable size, and they frequently join together to form large, irregular patches.

Individual wheals almost always clear within one day, and frequently disappear within an hour or two. New wheals may continually arise, however.

In most cases, hives are irritating but harmless. They are often caused by allergies. The allergic trigger can be foods such as shellfish, strawberries, nuts or food additives, and a reaction can occur within 30 minutes to two hours after the food is eaten. Such drugs as penicillin, aspirin, codeine, nonsteroidal anti-inflammatory drugs and others can bring on hives, as can handling certain plants or being in contact with animal hair or dander. Only rarely are pollens, dusts and molds the problem.

Some people are sensitive to certain bug bites or stings. Chigger bites are a common cause of hives. The allergic reaction that follows insect stings can be extremely serious (see Symptom: Bites and Stings).

In some cases, physical factors, such as light, vibration, cold or pressure can cause hives. One form of pressure-induced hives is called dermatographism—literally, "skin writing." Wheals appear at the site of a scratch or scrape within 5 to 10 minutes and usually fade in 10 to 15 minutes. About 4 percent of young adults get this reaction even after such minor traumas as pressure from clothing, chair seats, hand clapping or enthusiastic kissing.

In spite of this list of possible causes for hives, in about nine out of ten sufferers it is impossible to discover what triggers their hives. Whatever the cause, though, tension and stress of any kind usually make hives worse.

Hives can occur anywhere on the body. When the face is affected, the lips and skin around the eyes can swell markedly. Although rare, hives can develop in the mucous membranes of the mouth and throat. This is potentially life-threatening because the victim can suffocate from choking.

Rarely, hives are part of a more serious disease, like lupus erythematosus (see Common Whole Body Conditions in chapter 19) or viral infections such as hepatitis (see Common Abdominal and Digestive System Conditions in chapter 1), infectious mononucleosis (see Common Whole Body Conditions in chapter 19) or upper respiratory diseases.

BEST RESPONSE: For most cases of hives, cool compresses and cool baths will soothe the itch. Heat, hot showers or baths should be avoided; they only make the itching worse. You can apply calamine lotion or cooled witch hazel to the skin.

If you have severe hives and chronic hives you should be treated by your physician, who may prescribe antihistamines. In acute or severe cases, the doctor may inject or prescribe steroids to reduce swelling and eliminate risk of suffocation. In most cases of chronic hives, however, corticosteroids are not recommended, since the side effects may be worse than the disease.

If hives develop in your mouth, call your local emergency number at once.

ACCOMPANYING SYMPTOMS: If your hives are accompanied by breathing difficulties, swelling over the entire body and a rapid pulse, you could be suffering from anaphylactic shock brought on by a hypersensitivity to insect stings, penicillin, anesthesia or a foreign serum. Anaphylactic shock is a medical emergency and requires immediate injection of adrenaline.

SYMPTOM: **Irritation**

COMMON CAUSES: Irritated skin can be like gum on your shoes—it never seems to go away.

Irritation can occur anywhere on the body, and the causes are endless. Have you been bitten by a flea lately or have other things been bugging your skin? Some people are sensitive to certain laundry additives, especially fabric softeners. Or your irritation could be due to adhesive bandages or tight dressings you've been wearing.

In men, it's common for the face to become irritated due to constant shaving and, in women, the cause is often makeup. The underarms can also become irritated, and deodorants and antiperspirants are usually the culprits here.

BEST RESPONSE: The best way to cure irritated skin is to identify the irritant and get rid of it. This will take some detective work on your part.

If the irritation is on the arms, legs or trunk, you can consider your clothes and laundry detergents the chief suspects. Put them to the test by using only 100 percent cotton clothing, as well as cotton sheets and pillow cases. Wash-and-wear fabrics can irritate sensitive skin. Do not use any laundry additives, especially fabric softeners. Instead, use low-suds detergents without additives. These measures should help alleviate the irritation.

In the meantime, you can soothe irritated skin with cool or tepid baths. Hot baths will make an itchy irritation more itchy. Applying moisturizing lotions is also helpful.

If you're a man and shaving is your problem, learning the *proper* way to shave will alleviate irritation. John F. Romano, M.D., clinical instructor in dermatology at New York Hospital-Cornell Medical Center in New York City, offers tips for a burnless razor shave.

For maximum softening, take your shower or bath before you shave. Use mild soap and warm (not hot) water on your face. Apply the shaving preparation (aerosols and brushless creams are best suited to men with dry or soap-sensitive skin), then wait two to five minutes for the beard to further soften. Run a clean, sharp blade under hot water and shave gently in strokes that follow the pattern of your beard growth.

To allow the toughest areas of growth to soften the most, you might shave in this pattern: upper cheeks, lower right and left sides of the face, upper lip, chin and then neck. Follow your shave with a thorough rinsing and pat dry. You can finish off the ritual with a gentle aftershave cream and/or a moisturizer to soften and protect the skin.

Men who are troubled with ingrown hairs should use a sharp blade razor and should shave with the grain of the beard, advises Dr. Romano. If you suffer from a severe shaving rash, you could rub a small amount of a steroid cream over the affected area after shaving to soothe and protect the tender skin.

Women with sensitive facial skin should follow a few basic steps to make wearing makeup more comfortable.

Before applying makeup, make sure your skin is well moisturized—even apply a thin layer of plain petroleum jelly (Vaseline) under your lipstick. When applying eye makeup, leave a thin, makeup-free zone along the edge of each lid and never use eyeliner on the inner rim of your eyelid. Brush mascara only on the outer two-thirds of the lashes. Never go to bed without gently removing makeup. Best of all, give your skin a one-day rest from makeup once a week.

For men or women who develop underarm irritation, the first thing to do is stop the use of all deodorants and antiperspirants. Do not shave in the area, and avoid washing with soap. And there's no need to worry about offending others. To control odor, suggests Marvin H. Klapman, M.D., apply a compress or a washcloth soaked in Burow's solution, an antiseptic lotion, to the armpits twice a day for five or ten minutes each time.

If your underarm is inflamed, Burow's solution compresses and over-the-counter cortisone cream applied two to three times a day may be helpful.

After the irritation has subsided—it can take several days to a week—you can start wearing deodorants and antiperspirants again. But don't go back to your old kind. Instead, use a hypoallergenic roll-on cream that can be dabbed on. Sprays cover too large an area. Fifty percent of all sweat glands are in an area about the size of a quarter, located in the center of the deepest part of the armpit. This is the spot where you should apply your deodorant or antiperspirant.

SYMPTOM: **Itching**

COMMON CAUSES: Itching is like eating peanuts—you can't scratch just once and be satisfied. And whereas itching may drive you nuts, scratching can make it itch even more.

It's most likely that you're scratching some lump, bump or rash that has popped up on your body. Itchy bumps, for example, could be hives (see Symptom: Hives), which are often caused by a reaction to foods, drugs, physical agents or bites. Sunburns can also cause itching (see Symptom: Burns).

If you're scratching and notice a rash, it could be a reaction to poisonous plants, says William L. Epstein, M.D., professor of dermatology at the University of California at San Francisco and an expert on poison ivy. "The first thing you notice in poison ivy is the itch, then comes the redness, swelling and even sometimes blisters. But the itch comes first."

Poison sumac, which grows along the Eastern Seaboard and extends into Louisiana and Minnesota, and poison ivy or oak, which can be found in every state except Alaska and Hawaii, are the most common poisonous plants.

Although called a poison, the saps from these plants are actually allergens capable of causing an allergic skin reaction in about half the people who contact the plant. The plants usually must be damaged—cut leaves, broken stems—to expose the sap. But you can also get the rash by touching objects that have contacted the sap—clothes, tools, equipment, fingernails, even the skin itself. These carriers are called fomites. Smoke from burning the plant is also a fomite. If not washed off with soap and water, the plant sap loses its toxicity very slowly—shoes or boots contaminated with the oil can remain contaminated for months and even years—and cause the rash on contact.

If, however, you're scratching a rash that has a particular shape, mainly a butterfly design that goes across your cheeks and the bridge of your nose, you could have lupus erythematosus (see Common Whole Body Conditions in chapter 19).

If you're scratching lesions that look like flat and angular violet pimples, you could have lichen planus, an inflammatory skin disease that usually settles around the mouth, ankles and wrists. Whether the condition is due to a virus, a reaction to certain drugs or the result of an emotional upheaval is still up for grabs. Lichen planus can also make fingernails and toenails ridged.

Nearly all patients with dermatitis or eczema (see Common Skin Conditions) complain of severe itching, which may be worse at night. Fungus infections such as athlete's foot (see Common Foot Conditions in chapter 9) are also notorious itchers. The rash and blisters that come from chickenpox and shingles (see Common Skin Conditions) can also cause itching.

Bug bites are common reasons for scratching. Chigger bites,

particularly, can drive you crazy (see Symptom: Bites and Stings). Lice (see Common Skin Conditions), which attach to hair and clothing, can cause severe itching. The same is true of the crab louse, which likes to make its home in the pubic region.

Sometimes, however, your skin can be itching for no apparent reason at all. There are no bumps, no lesions, no rashes. The most common reason for such itching is dry skin (see Symptom: Dryness). Such itching can be psychological in origin, and stress plays a prominent role in flare-ups.

Occasionally, a disease is the cause for the itching. Diseases that sometimes cause itchy skin include diabetes mellitus and anemia (see Common Whole Body Conditions in chapter 19); hyperthyroidism (see thyroid disease under Common Whole Body Conditions in chapter 19); several types of hepatitis (see Common Abdominal and Digestive System Conditions in chapter 1); chronic pyelonephritis (see Common Urinary Tract Conditions in chapter 18); leukemia (see Common Whole Body Conditions in chapter 19) and diseases of the lymph glands, such as Hodgkin's disease. One of the symptoms of both phlebitis and varicose veins (see Common Circulatory, Heart and Lung Conditions in chapter 5) is itching around the site of the affected vein.

BEST RESPONSE: If there is an obvious cause for your itch, treatment can be relatively simple, say doctors. Any measure that you can use to relax, such as exercise, meditation or biofeedback, may provide some relief.

But what can you do to ease your itching *now?* Take an ice pack or a towel soaked in ice water and put it directly over the itching area, suggests Thomas Goodman, M.D., author of the *Skin Doctor's Skin Doctoring Book.* For all-over itching, get into a tub of cold water and stay in it until you feel better. After your cold-water soak, put on any moisturizer or medication you are using to treat your specific skin problem.

Antihistamines can help relieve itching. Plain aspirin (not aspirin substitutes) can also help, especially in the case of itching caused by sunburn, says Dr. Goodman. He suggests trying two 5-grain (325-milligram) aspirin tablets four times daily. If aspirin upsets your stomach, take it with food. Don't take aspirin, however, for the itching of hives or welts. "It may make you worse," Dr. Goodman says. Instead, antihistamines are a good choice to relieve the itch of hives.

If you have run into one of the poisonous plants, wash as soon as possible—one to three minutes after exposure is ideal—to prevent the rash. Don't use soap. Rubbing alcohol, according to Dr. Epstein, works best at extracting the toxin from the skin. Then wash off with ordinary water. Clothes and equipment exposed to the poison also need to be washed with soap and water.

To treat the symptoms of poison ivy, calamine lotion is still the favorite of many, especially when blisters have formed, because it relieves the itching and absorbs the blister fluid. Don't use calamine that contains benadryl or zirconium, says Dr. Epstein, because the benadryl may cause further irritation.

Because itching is the most troublesome symptom in lichen planus, mild tranquilizers or antihistamines are often prescribed. Steroid ointment usually reduces the rash.

The first step in dealing with lice is to get rid of them. Laundering or dry cleaning clothing and spraying other fomites with antiparasite spray should be sufficient. To treat the skin problems caused by lice, an over-the-counter cortisone cream may help. If the problems persist, see your doctor. Prescription topical steroids may be needed.

If you have a "mysterious" itch, however, and can rule out dry skin, see your doctor. It could be a sign of something more serious.

ACCOMPANYING SYMPTOMS: If you're pregnant and have broken out in itching wheals or a rash, you could have one of a number of skin ailments that affect mothers-to-be. For the itching of pregnancy, doctors often prescribe steroid creams, but it's best to check with *your* doctor if you have this problem. Regardless of treatment, the itching usually goes away after your baby is born.

If you have an itching rash caused by poison ivy or some other poison, and your body starts to swell, see your doctor immediately. Your case is no longer considered mild, and system steroids will be necessary for treatment.

SYMPTOM: **Jaundice**

COMMON CAUSES: Jaundice is a yellow or greenish yellow tint to the skin that almost always indicates a serious problem elsewhere and often clears up a few days after birth.

The list of troublesome diseases that cause jaundice is long. Infectious hepatitis, cirrhosis of the liver and diseases of the pancreas and gallbladder (see pancreatitis and gallbladder disease under Common Abdominal and Digestive System Conditions in chapter 1) can cause skin to yellow. So, too, can cancer.

In addition, pernicious anemia, hemolytic anemia and sickle cell anemia (see anemia under Common Whole Body Conditions in chapter 19) can cause the problem. Finally, allergic reaction to a drug; extreme morning sickness and toxemia of pregnancy; yellow fever and relapsing fever, an infectious disease caused by bites from ticks or lice, can cause jaundice.

One of the exceptions to the rule that jaundice in adults is always a serious symptom is Gilbert's disease, a benign hereditary blood disorder. Affecting mostly young adults, the condition disappears by itself without treatment.

BEST RESPONSE: All cases of jaundice should first be evaluated by a physician.

ACCOMPANYING SYMPTOMS: If your skin turns a yellow-orange color and you are extremely fond of carrots or other foods rich in beta-carotene (such as green and yellow vegetables), you could have a harmless condition known as carotenemia, an excess of carotene (provitamin A) in the system. It is not the same as jaundice. To return your skin to its normal color, you should abstain from the offending food for two to six weeks. Then you can continue eating it—but in moderation.

SYMPTOM: **Liver spots.** *See* Symptom: Brown Patches

SYMPTOM: **Lumps and Bumps**

COMMON CAUSES: We end up with lumps and bumps for a lot of obvious reasons. Bites from ticks and chiggers, for example, can cause bumps (see Symptoms: Bites and Stings). And, you can get a lump when you fall down and bang your head. But what about those lumps that appear for no obvious reason?

A tender lump that suddenly appears in front or behind the ear, under the chin, on the side of the neck, above the collarbone or, less commonly, in the armpit or groin is usually an enlarged lymph node. The swelling is the body's way of handling an infection in the lymph glands. Sometimes, though, swelling could be a sign of malignancy.

A painless lump that appears on the back of the hand or wrist is usually a ganglion, which is actually a cyst on the skin connected to a joint or tendon. Painless lumps on the knuckles, wrists, elbows or knees are one of the signs of rheumatic fever (see Common Whole Body Conditions in chapter 19).

A sebaceous cyst is a pale lump beneath the skin. It's firm, movable and tender, and is usually found on the face, scalp, ear, back or scrotum.

Skin tags, also known as "senile warts," tend to run in the family. They're little fleshy nipples that hang from the surface of the skin and can get caught in clothing. You can have a few of these or hundreds, and the size can range from barely visible to over an inch in length.

If you have raised and warty-looking brown to murky yellow lesions on the trunk of your body, you probably have what is called seborrheic keratosis. These lesions also can be seen on the face or scalp. They appear to be stuck on the skin's surface and can easily be scraped off with a fingernail. More common in older men and women, seborrheic keratosis is ugly but harmless.

Syringoma is a benign tumor of the sweat gland caused by enlargement of a sweat duct. This type of tumor usually appears in women, under the eyes or around the nose.

Histiocytoma is a tough, raised lesion that is usually solitary and well rounded. These lesions are located on the extremities—near the elbows, knees and hips—and are a bodily reaction to repeated trauma in the area. They are not cancerous.

Sebaceous hyperplasia is termed "aged acne" because the shiny, yellow, waxy-oily tumors are really an enlargement of an oil gland and appear on the face. These resemble skin cancer but are not cancerous.

Actinic keratosis is considered to be a precursor of skin cancer (see Common Skin Conditions). It is characterized by raised, red and scaly bumps, which usually, though not always, occur in groups on sun-exposed areas.

Of course, the big worry with a lump is that it's a sign of cancer, which it *can* be. But most of the causes of lumps and bumps are quite harmless.

BEST RESPONSE: The lump caused by a swollen gland usually goes away in a few days, although it can sometimes linger past the time when other symptoms of infection—such as fever or sore throat—have gone. If you're worried that your swollen gland is hanging around too long and you're afraid you may have some serious disease (such as cancer), you should see your physician.

A ganglion often disappears on its own, although a doctor may insert a needle and drain the ganglion or may even surgically remove it. A sebaceous cyst is usually treated in the same way. If it's infected, the cyst is opened and drained and antibiotics are prescribed. If the cyst is a cosmetic problem, it can be surgically removed.

It's not difficult to remove skin tags—a doctor can do many at one sitting. The usual method is cutting or burning them off. When scraped off, seborrheic keratosis seldom recurs. Syringomas can be removed by a physician, but because of their location around the eyes and the danger of scarring, many doctors suggest leaving them alone.

If you think you may have sebaceous hyperplasia or actinic keratosis, you should definitely see a dermatologist. Sebaceous hyperplasia can mimic the sign of cancer, and actinic keratosis is a precursor of the disease. Any suspicious lump should be seen by a doctor.

ACCOMPANYING SYMPTOMS: If you have a lump that is hard, red, swollen, tender and painful, you probably have a boil, an infection of a hair follicle. They most often appear on the neck, face, armpits, back and buttocks. A boil can be treated by applying a hot, wet compress every few hours. Hot compresses help ease the pain and accelerate bursting. If you have a boil, you should take showers instead of baths to reduce the chances of spreading the infection to other parts of the body. You should also wash your hands thoroughly before preparing food. This is because the germs that cause the boil can multiply in warm food and produce toxins that cause food poisoning.

If you have recurrent boils or your boil doesn't go away within two weeks, you should see your physician.

If a lump is accompanied by swelling under one or both earlobes, and this was preceded by complaints of pain around the ear—especially when swallowing—and illness, the problem could be mumps. It's best to have a doctor confirm the diagnosis, since mumps can be confused with a swollen lymph gland.

SYMPTOM: **Marks, Dark-colored.** *See also* Symptom: Bruises

COMMON CAUSES: Children have been known to poke each other with pens and pencils, and sometimes the ink or graphite gets under the skin. The experience can leave a permanent black or blue discoloration—a form of cheap tattooing.

You can get brown to blue discoloration where the needle from an iron injection entered the skin. And in the elderly, reddish brown or purplish areas, sometimes as large as two inches across, can appear anywhere on the body but are most noticeable on the legs, forearms or backs of the hands. These markings are called senile purpura and are caused by bleeding under the skin. Blood seeps slowly from tiny vessels, weakened by old age. Although the blood is gradually reabsorbed, the underlying defect is irreversible, so the markings are likely to linger.

BEST RESPONSE: The discoloration from a pen or pencil wound doesn't need treatment unless it's causing pain or other symptoms, says Lyon Rowe, M.D. If it is causing problems, you can have it removed surgically.

Dark patches from iron injections will heal on their own, although it will take considerable time.

Doctors consider senile purpura harmless and the markings permanent. You should, however, have any discolored markings diagnosed by a doctor to make certain that they aren't really something more serious.

SYMPTOM: **Marks, Spider**

COMMON CAUSES: David A. Paslin, M.D., author of *The Hide Guide*, probably describes them best. Bloody spider marks on the skin, he says, "resemble the shape and outline of an all-red deciduous tree in winter, when viewed from a thousand feet above the ground. In the center is the large trunk filled at high pressure with blood. The blood gushes up the trunk and streams out the branches to fade away at the farthest twigs."

Spider marks can occur in pregnant women and in those taking estrogen and are a minor symptom in people who suffer from cirrhosis of the liver (see Common Abdominal and Digestive System Conditions in chapter 1). But many people have spider marks without underlying problems. They always appear on the face, arms and upper trunk.

BEST RESPONSE: Spider marks usually fade after pregnancy or after estrogen is discontinued. If you can't wait for time to heal your spider marks, they can be burned off using an electrocoagulating device.

Those with cirrhosis need to be under the care of a physician.

SYMPTOM: **Mole, Change in**

COMMON CAUSES: Moles have characteristics much like the people they invade. They have a long life (the life cycle of a mole is about 50 years) and they come in a variety of shapes, sizes and colors. And, like people, you can expect their appearance to slowly change over the years.

When moles first appear, they are flat and dark in color, looking much like a freckle. As they age, they can become lighter in color, larger or raised, and they can even develop hairs. Ultimately, most moles will disappear by seeming to fade into the skin or by rising up on a "stalk" and falling off, either on their own or through the friction of rubbing. All this is considered normal.

Changes that are not normal, however, may be signaling a malignancy (see skin cancer under Common Skin Conditions), says David A. Paslin, M.D. "The danger signs are unusual color change, bleeding, ulceration, crusting and satellite growths adjacent to the suspect lesion," explains Dr. Paslin. "The color changes vary. If the molelike growth has little blue or black nodules, beaded bumps or areas of pink or white, there is danger. If there is bleeding, beware." The risk of malignancy is also high if the growth ulcerates or crusts, or if dark-colored spots or nodules form beyond the perimeter of the mole.

Sun exposure is believed to be a major cause of cancerous changes in moles.

BEST RESPONSE: If you notice a mole taking on any of these abnormal signs, you should see your physician. If the doctor suspects a malignancy, all or part of the mole will be removed so that sections of tissue can be examined under a microscope. This procedure is harmless and simple. If a malignancy is found and the entire mole wasn't removed, your doctor will use the best procedure possible to completely cut out the malignancy.

Remember that even if your mole shows abnormal signs, it does not mean it's cancerous. "There are many bumps and lumps in the skin that look like but are not cancerous moles, including benign blood vessels and fibrous tumors, funny-looking, harmless moles and not-so-harmless pigmented basal cell cancers," advises Dr. Paslin. But if in doubt, have it checked out.

SYMPTOM: **Odor.** *See also* Symptom: Sweating

COMMON CAUSES: Exercise, hard work, strong emotions and other forms of stress cause the apocrine glands, located primarily under the arms but also in the groin, to produce tiny droplets of milky sweat. But perspiration itself doesn't smell. Odor is caused when bacteria lounging on the skin surface interact with the apocrine secretions, giving off a scent that can vary in strength from person to person.

Women generally don't sweat or smell as much as men do because they have fewer and smaller sweat glands. And little children normally don't have a perspiration odor at all because these glands aren't developed until puberty. The fact that you may have an odor problem stronger than the next person may simply be a matter of your sex or personal chemistry.

Normally it's the supersensitive teenager, the athlete or the rising young executive who worries about offending odors. Luckily, there is an easy answer to the problem.

BEST RESPONSE: Unless you're a coal miner or a chimney sweep, you don't need a daily whole-body scrub to wash away your problems. The only bodily parts that need daily attention are the sweat-producing areas, namely the armpits and groin. And a normal soap-and-water wash will do. "I'm not impressed with deodorant soaps as a way of stopping body odor, because they don't work as well on the bacteria as using a deodorant or an antibacterial ointment would," says Lyon Rowe, M.D.

Antiperspirants and combination deodorant/antiperspirants contain aluminum salts, which shrink the openings of your sweat glands to reduce the flow of the apocrine glands, Dr. Rowe explains. And, they contain antibacterial agents that control odor.

If you perspire excessively, look for an antiperspirant with a high concentration of aluminum chloride. Also, roll-on and cream products are the best choices.

SYMPTOM: **Oiliness**

COMMON CAUSE: Oily skin is caused by overproduction of the sebaceous glands just below the skin. It affects the face, neck, shoulders, chest and back, although the problem doesn't always affect all these areas at once.

People with dark skin whose ancestors came from the areas surrounding the Mediterranean Sea are more likely to have oily skin than those whose ancestors came from northern Europe. But this doesn't mean that your oily skin problem is your parents' fault.

Hormones can increase oil production beneath the skin, meaning pregnant women and women taking certain birth control pills can be affected. Stress also plays a role by triggering the adrenal glands in such a way as to hormonally induce excess oil production. Certain cosmetics, including hair preparations, can add extra oil to the skin's surface.

Eating oily foods, however, has nothing to do with the oiliness of the skin.

BEST RESPONSE: If your skin is extremely oily, skin experts recommend that you wash with a strong degreaser, such as Ivory soap, or a nongreasy, milky cleanser that leaves no sticky film behind. If your skin is mildly oily, washing thoroughly twice a day should be adequate. If your skin becomes irritated, don't use that particular soap for a day or two.

SYMPTOM: **Oozing**

COMMON CAUSES: Oozing is a sign that a bad case of dermatitis (see Common Skin Conditions) is getting out of hand. It's most often seen in dermatitis of the hands that has become infected with bacteria.

In babies, oozing is a sign of infantile eczema (see dermatitis/eczema under Common Skin Conditions). The rash that covers a greater portion of the body develops little red pimples. When the baby scratches, the areas weep or ooze, then join together and become crusted.

BEST RESPONSE: If your dermatitis has reached the stage of oozing, you should see a doctor. While you are waiting for an appointment, however, Thomas Goodman, M.D., suggests the following measures.

Soak your hands for 15 minutes, four times daily, in cool tap water or cool Burow's solution, an antiseptic lotion. After each soaking, apply an antibiotic ointment.

For the baby who suffers from infantile eczema, do not use anything on the baby's skin until you consult a doctor. In the meantime, dress the baby in cotton clothing, but don't keep the youngster too hot by overdressing.

SYMPTOM: **Pain**

COMMON CAUSES: Pain is a symptom you can't ignore. The advantage to pain (if there is an advantage) is that it alerts you to the fact that there is something wrong somewhere. It usually signals some kind of injury or inflammation of the skin.

Take skin infections. Any skin wound, whether it's caused by injury or surgery, can be complicated by infection. There can be redness, heat, swelling and pain.

Painful and tender skin is also associated with phlebitis and varicose veins (see Common Circulatory, Heart and Lung Conditions in chapter 5), and it's the kind of pain that puts you to bed without even being told.

One of the most painful skin problems is shingles (see Common Skin Conditions), the adult localized version of chickenpox. Pain is more commonly felt during and after the appearance of a rash, which characterizes the disease. In older adults, however, the pain may go on for months or even years—a condition called postherpetic neuralgia.

BEST RESPONSE: Pain usually requires "doing something." Any complication from a wound or injury should be evaluated by a physician.

Phlebitis and varicose veins are serious conditions that also need the attention of a doctor.

For the pain from shingles, doctors sometimes recommend acupuncture or nerve-blocking injections for severe cases. In the early stages of the disease, antiviral drugs can be given.

ACCOMPANYING SYMPTOMS: If your pain has been preceded by tingling sensations in the hands and feet, spreads slowly along both arms and legs to the trunk and is followed by numbness, this could be a sign of damage, called peripheral neuropathy, to the peripheral nerves. See your doctor immediately.

SYMPTOM: **Pallor**

COMMON CAUSES: Pale skin can be a sign of something worse to come, like a fainting spell, motion sickness or vomiting. It also goes hand-in-hand with nausea and can be a telling sign that an emotional upset ("Why so pale and wan, fond lover?") is taking its toll. But pale skin can also be a sign that something serious is wrong somewhere in the body.

Pallor is also associated with anemia (see Common Whole Body Conditions in chapter 19) and a whole raft of heart-related diseases, including angina pectoris (see Symptom: Pain in chapter 5); atrial or ventricular fibrillation and rapid heartbeat (see Symptom: Palpitations in chapter 5); rheumatic fever (see Whole Body Conditions in chapter 19) and endocarditis, an inflammation involving the lining of the heart.

A perforated ulcer (see Common Abdominal and Digestive System Conditions in chapter 1) and hyperthyroidism (see thyroid disease under Common Whole Body Conditions in chapter 19) are other common conditions that can cause the skin to turn pale.

BEST RESPONSE: If you're having emotional problems or feeling stressed but otherwise feel fine, you can ignore your pale looks. The pallor will go away along with your stress and problems. But if you're looking pale for an unexplained reason, especially if you're not feeling up to snuff, it's time to seek medical advice. Only your doctor can tell if there's something wrong somewhere else in your body.

SYMPTOM: **Peeling.** *See also* Symptom: Flaking

COMMON CAUSES: Peeling skin is nothing more than dead skin that dries up and falls off. Its most common cause is a bad sunburn. But there are a few disease-related reasons why skin peels.

Peeling, especially on the palms or the palm side of the fingers, is known to occur in diseases associated with fever. It's also associated with dermatitis (see Common Skin Conditions) and fungus infections such as athlete's foot (see Common Foot Conditions in chapter 9). Allergies to medicines and chronic sweaty palms can also cause peeling skin. And, say doctors, your skin can peel for no reason at all.

Infants and young children with staphylococcal scalded skin syndrome will experience peeling or detachment of the outer layer of skin from the body. Peeling of the skin (and the tongue) is also an aftereffect of scarlet fever.

BEST RESPONSE: Treating the peeling skin of sunburn is like bolting the barn door after the horse has left. There is nothing you can do about dead peeling skin except let it take its course. Slathering the body with moisturizer, however, will help minimize the problem.

If your peeling is minor, however, it's best to leave it alone. If the area feels dry, use a little moisturizer; if it feels itchy, use a ½ percent hydrocortisone cream. Fungus infections, however, should be treated by a doctor, because they're difficult to clear up on your own.

Children with staphylococcal scalded skin syndrome should be under the care of a physician.

SYMPTOM: **Pimples**

COMMON CAUSES: Most eruptions of pimples are acne (see Common Skin Conditions), which is common in teenagers undergoing hormonal changes and in adults who are under stress.

Parents often blame teenage acne on eating the wrong foods (like greasy french fries or chocolate). You should forget the food excuse, however. Except for the occasional person who reacts poorly to a certain food, food is not the major cause of acne. Poor hygiene is.

But teenagers aren't the only ones who break out in pimples. Adults get pimples, too.

Pimples can be caused by medications or other substances containing iodine or bromine. Dilantin, a drug used to treat epilepsy, may produce acnelike eruptions, as can other medications. Then there's an acne common to painters, which is caused by the chlorinated hydrocarbons found in paints, varnish and lacquers, as well as in various oils.

People suffering from Cushing's disease, a pituitary gland disorder, often have acnelike eruptions on the skin. Pimples are also associated with acne rosacea (see Symptom: Redness in chapter 13), although the most annoying symptom of this condition is a bulbous, red nose.

Injury of the skin from shaving (see Symptom: Irritation) sometimes causes small pimples to erupt, but these are different from teenage acne. The condition is called folliculitis, and the pimples are small versions of boils, often caused by staphylococcus bacteria. Folliculitis can actually erupt around hair follicles anywhere on the body—it's just more bothersome on the face.

BEST RESPONSE: Acne is one of those conditions in which time is the healing factor. If properly treated, however, acne can easily be controlled.

The best way to treat a mild case of acne (or any pimples) is to keep the skin as free of oil as possible, suggests Marvin H. Klapman, M.D. Washing your face thoroughly two or three times a day with a mild bar soap, and shampooing frequently, is a good start. Overly vigorous scrubbing probably will not help—it can lead to further irritation.

If cleaning alone does not do the trick, over-the-counter drying agents such as benzoyl peroxide can help. Avoid wearing makeup except the non-oily type, and wash your face thoroughly afterward.

Finally, don't pick! You could end up with worse and more permanent problems—scars and pits—than you started with.

For severe acne, characterized by a large number of festering pimples, or pimples covering a large area of your body, you should see a physician. You may need antibiotics. Tetracycline and erythromycin are usually prescribed.

For cystic acne, the most severe form, the prescription drug Accutane (technically known as 13-cis-retinoic acid or isotretinoin) has been found effective. There are some side effects to this drug, however, so it's best to have a frank discussion with your dermatologist before trying it. All women of childbearing age, however, should be cautious about using Accutane, since there is a very great risk of causing congenital abnormalities in the baby if expectant mothers take the drug.

ACCOMPANYING SYMPTOMS: If your pimples are accompanied by intense itching and contain short gray lines, you could be suffering from scabies (see Common Skin Conditions) and should see your doctor.

SYMPTOM: **Pitting**

COMMON CAUSES: Pits or scars are tiny craters in the skin that result from acne (see Common Skin Conditions), especially from cystic acne. Picking and squeezing pimples, even in mild cases, can lead to pitting and scarring.

What happens in cystic acne is that common, everyday teenage pimples develop into more serious abscesses and cystic masses that can last for a month or more. They eventually rupture and heal, leaving unflattering pits and scars.

BEST RESPONSE: Pitting doesn't have to be a lifetime wound. There are a few basic techniques that dermatologists can use to remove existing pits and scars. The most common are dermabrasion and collagen injections. In dermabrasion, a technique somewhat similar to sandpapering is used to plane the skin. It is not recommended for people with dark skin, since skin color may become mottled from the procedure.

Collagen injections pose no such risk and can be used by almost anyone, regardless of skin color. During this procedure, sterile liquid collagen is injected into the scar, "plumping" it up to the level of the surrounding skin.

If you or your teenager has pitting from acne, it would be best to check with a dermatologist to see if either of these methods could be used to give you back your smooth skin.

For this reason, the problem should be evaluated by a dermatologist.

SYMPTOM: **Rash**

COMMON CAUSES: Rash is a vague term used to describe a whole rash of ailments—possibly every skin malady known to man. That's because at some time in almost any skin problem, you'll notice some form of red, irritated skin. But a rash in and of itself is usually not a serious symptom.

Babies often can get diaper rash from a *Candida* (yeast) infection, caused by not changing soiled diapers often enough or not washing and rinsing cloth diapers thoroughly. Sometimes the rash is a reaction to a fabric softener or harsh soaps.

An elderly person or anyone who, for a number of reasons, has no bladder control, can develop a rash. If not checked, the rash can spread up the abdomen or the back and down the inner thighs.

Prickly heat or heat rash also can affect babies and those who are bedridden. The problem is due to heat and humidity. The body produces perspiration faster than skin pores can pump it out, forming bumplike blisters filled with trapped sweat. The red rash, which occurs mostly on the trunk and neck, is itchy and causes a prickly sensation.

Victims of pellagra, a niacin deficiency, can develop a rash that will show itself as red, symmetrical spots on areas of the skin exposed to sunlight or rubbed by clothing. The spots later turn brown and become larger and scaly.

Sometimes you can develop a red rash if you become sensitive to a medicine you have been taking for a long time. The rash may be accompanied by other symptoms, such as an overall sick feeling. Drugs that are known to cause these reactions are penicillin, tetracycline, aspirin, barbiturates, sulfa drugs, diuretics ("water pills") and other medicines.

In a mild case of lupus erythematosus (see Common Whole Body Conditions in chapter 19), a skin rash that takes on a butterfly appearance over the nose and cheeks may be the only symptom.

BEST RESPONSE: Years ago, Benjamin Spock, M.D., recommended exposing baby's sore bottom to the air, and that's still probably the best prescription around for diaper rash. Next best is changing diapers as soon as possible after they become wet or soiled. Disposable diapers or sterilized diapers distributed by diaper services are preferable.

If you use cloth diapers, you should soak them in an antiseptic solution to eliminate infectious agents, wash them in a mild soap and rinse them several times to remove all traces of soap or detergent. Bathe baby's bottom with warm water but not soap. Sprinkle lightly with cornstarch. For a mild rash, use a cream that contains zinc oxide and an oil.

Keep in mind, though, that diaper rash is sometimes hard to get rid of despite adequate care and hygiene.

For prickly heat, move yourself or your baby to a cool environment. In hot, humid weather, an air-conditioned room is best for sleeping. For immediate relief from prickly heat, take a cool (but not cold) bath and add a cup of cornstarch or baking soda to the bath water.

Pellagra, which needs to be diagnosed by a doctor, can be successfully treated with supplements and improved diet.

If you suspect that your rash is due to a drug reaction, you should see your physician, who may take you off or change your prescription. If you develop the telltale butterfly rash of lupus, you should see your physician.

ACCOMPANYING SYMPTOMS: There was a rash of them in the 1970s and early 1980s—now it looks like the cause of that rash has been found. We're speaking of the trendy disease known as hot tub folliculitis, caused by the pseudomonas organism. Three to four days after relaxing (or whatever) in hot tub splendor, you may notice a painful, itchy rash all over your body. As if that isn't enough, you may also have fever, chills, headache, earache, sore throat and general malaise. The condition is brought on by a less-than-clean and less-than-hot hot tub.

You can treat hot tub rash with white vinegar and water. If the affected area is small, dab on a solution of half water and half vinegar. If a large area is affected, add a bottle of vinegar to a cool or tepid bath and soak for a few minutes a day. Repeat if needed.

If you have a rash that is extremely itchy, it's probably a result of contact with some sort of poison—ivy, oak or sumac (see Symptom: Itching).

If your baby's diaper rash is persistent and begins to pimple and ooze, it's a sign that infection has set in and you should see your pediatrician.

SYMPTOM: **Rash, with Fever**

COMMON CAUSES: If you have a rash and a fever, it means there's a lot more wrong with you than just an irritation or an allergic reaction. Rash with fever almost always means an infection of some type in the body.

Rash and fever are common signs of many childhood diseases, such as chickenpox, measles, German measles and roseola (see Common Skin Conditions). It's also a sign of the adult version of chickenpox known as shingles (see Common Skin Conditions).

Other infectious diseases which cause rash and fever include meningitis (see Common Neurological System Conditions in chapter 12), occasionally characterized by a deep red or purplish skin rash; rheumatic fever (see Common Whole Body Conditions in chapter 19), commonly characterized by a red, ring-shaped rash on the torso; and infectious mononucleosis (see Common Whole Body Conditions in chapter 19), which sometimes causes a flat, red rash.

Erysipelas, or Saint Anthony's fire, is a rare strep infection caused by an open wound. The skin is painful and warm. The rash is raised and varies in color from dull red to scarlet. Tender spots appear beyond the margins of the rash.

BEST RESPONSE: All cases of rash with fever should be seen by a physician to make the proper diagnosis.

In most cases of chickenpox, however, the diagnosis can be made over the phone. Relief can be obtained by soaking in a lukewarm starch or baking soda bath for ten minutes two or three times a day, according to Benjamin Spock, M.D., and Michael B. Rothenberg, M.D., authors of *Baby and Child Care.*

"Use a starch that dissolves in water, or bicarbonate of soda (one cupful for a small tub, two for a large one)," they recommend. Do not rub the scabs off, and keep the child's hands clean and fingernails short to help prevent infecting the scabs that will eventually form as a result of the rash. To relieve the itching of chickenpox, calamine lotion and antihistamines are often prescribed.

Bed rest is necessary for measles, and a doctor should monitor the progress of the disease. An effective measles vaccine is available and should be given to every child. Gamma globulin can be given to the unvaccinated exposed child.

In children, German measles is a mild disease, but if contracted by a pregnant woman, the illness can seriously affect the unborn baby. For this reason, it's best for everyone to be vaccinated against German measles.

The rash of roseola is not a problem, but the fever is. Sponging with cool water or alcohol is helpful in getting the fever down.

Scarlet fever can be a serious disease and should be treated with antibiotics by a physician.

ACCOMPANYING SYMPTOMS: If you know you've been bitten by a tick, and begin to experience rash, fever and muscle pain, you could have Rocky Mountain spotted fever. The disease responds to antibiotic treatment, but if left untreated, it can be fatal.

SYMPTOM: **Rings, Red**

COMMON CAUSES: If you have a ring formation of tiny red blisters that grows outward, and the lesion is scaly and itchy, you probably have ringworm (see Common Skin Conditions), an extremely contagious fungus infection (it has nothing to do with worms).

But there are other skin problems that form rings that have nothing to do with ringworm. A condition called pityriasis rosea is characterized by scaling, pink oval spots on the skin. Psoriasis (see Common Skin Conditions) is characterized by bright red rings or patches of silvery scales.

BEST RESPONSE: If you are not sure what is causing the rings, see a dermatologist for diagnosis. If it is ringworm, your doctor will treat it with antifungal drugs.

Prevention is a matter of cleanliness. All parts of the body should be washed with soap and water, especially hairy areas and folds where perspiration collects. Make sure you dry thoroughly, since fungi thrive in warm dampness.

There is no known cure for psoriasis. But it's known that ultraviolet light, the kind that comes naturally from the sun, is effective in treating the disease. A side effect, of course, is that ultraviolet light can burn the skin, leading to even more serious problems, says Jim Storer, M.D., of the Psoriasis Treatment Center of Tulane University in New Orleans. He recommends that victims of psoriasis work up to spending 30 minutes in the sun in the middle of the day. But, he cautions, "You can bake yourself too much and the psoriasis will flare. Never do it to the point of burning."

Additional treatments for psoriasis include the use of shampoos and other products containing tar. There are many new treatments. If you suspect you have psoriasis, see a physician. If you're diagnosed as having the disease, make routine checkups a part of your life.

SYMPTOM: **Roughness.** *See* Symptom: Dryness

SYMPTOM: **Scar, Change in**

COMMON CAUSES: The scar that forms following a skin injury usually becomes less noticeable as time goes by. Sometimes, however, scars grow out of proportion to the size of the injury that caused them, due to excessive collagen formation during the healing process. This is called keloid formation, and it most often occurs after acne, an operation, burns, vaccination or severe injury. It also sometimes occurs for no apparent reason. Keloids are generally considered harmless and noncancerous.

BEST RESPONSE: The usual treatment for keloid formation is steroid injections or cryotherapy, but it is not always successful. If you have a tendency toward keloid formation, you might want to keep this in mind, since removal of a mole could lead to a keloid much worse in appearance than the mole itself.

Some success has been reported in treating keloid formation by applying ordinary zinc tape to the scars. In a study supported by the Swedish Medical Research Council, the size of the scar was reduced to the level of the surrounding skin in half the patients, redness was decreased in all the patients and itching decreased in all of those who suffered from it. Unfortunately, this tape is not yet available in the United States.

SYMPTOM: **Scarring.** *See* Symptom: Pitting

SYMPTOM: **Sores**

COMMON CAUSES: Sores are skin tissue that has been ruptured or abraded as a result of friction or injury. An ulcer is a sore that's getting worse—a festering sore.

A common type of body sore is bedsores, or pressure sores, caused by spending too much time in the same position in the same place. Bedridden persons are almost always the victims. At first the skin on the buttocks, heels, elbows or other bony prominences is red, shiny and painful. If untreated or neglected, bedsores can develop large ulcerations that can become infected and even gangrenous. If the ulcer develops a black crust, don't be fooled into thinking that this is a scab and a sign of healing. Actually, it may be a sign that the ulcer is getting deeper and needs to be treated by a doctor.

Have you been cultivating roses or doing other gardening? Your ulcer could be a result of a rare skin disease called sporotrichosis. That's when you puncture your skin with a thorn or splinter that is contaminated with the offending fungus. The spores enter your wound and within two weeks you have a crusty but painless ulcer that doesn't want to heal. The result is an infection that can spread to the lymph nodes directly above it.

Another lymph-related problem that can show up as sore skin is lymphadenitis. This results when an infected toe or finger causes the skin over nearby lymph glands to become red, tender and abscessed.

BEST RESPONSE: "There is a common mistake caregivers make in attempting to treat bedsores, and that's applying medication to the sore without first ridding it of infection and debris," says Melba Connors, R.N., the skin and wound care nurse at the University of California at San Diego Medical Center. "Debridement is best done by a physician with special instruments," she says. "If infection is present, the doctor will prescribe antibiotics.

"Treatment cannot begin until the sore is cleared up to a nice, pink, stable wound," says Connors. The doctor will then "pack" the wounds, using such treatments as wet-to-wet dressings or opaque dressings to promote healing. Healing time is slow, she says, and can take up to several months.

"That's why the *best* way to treat bedsores is prevention," she says. "Excellent care of the patient is essential. The skin should be kept clean and supple, and moisturizing cream should be used after each cleansing.

"Most important, pressure on the sensitive areas must be relieved," says Connors. Bedridden patients should have their position changed at least every two hours. A wheelchair patient must be able to shift position every 10 to 15 minutes, even if the patient is using a pressure-relieving pillow. Also, there are special mattresses on the market designed to relieve pressure for those who are healing from bedsores.

Lymphadenitis and sporotrichosis should be treated by a physician. For lymphadenitis, your doctor probably will incise and drain the wound and apply moist compresses to relieve pain. Antibiotic treatment may also be prescribed.

If sporotrichosis is suspected, your physician probably will take a sample of pus from the ulcers before making a diagnosis. If the diagnosis is positive, medication can then be prescribed to clear up the disease. Sporotrichosis can be cleared up in a few weeks with antifungal medications.

ACCOMPANYING SYMPTOMS: A shallow, oozing ulcer located on the inside of the leg just above the ankle could be the result of poor circulation, a condition common in the elderly and in pregnant women. It is called a varicose ulcer. Once formed, the ulcer can remain unchanged or it can heal, then return again.

If you have a varicose ulcer, your physician may recommend wearing elastic stockings or an elastic bandage during the day. You should also avoid standing for long periods, but should exercise regularly by taking short walks. When sitting or sleeping, the affected ankle should be higher than the chest. All these measures will aid circulation. The ulcer itself also may require treatment by a physician—this will vary depending on the severity of the ulcer.

The most common form of skin cancer (see Common Skin Conditions), basal cell carcinoma, starts as a lumpy sore that grows and becomes ulcerated. The lesion has a hard border and a raw moist center that may bleed. A common site is the face, although sometimes basal cell carcinoma can appear as a flat, slow-growing sore on the back or chest.

Unlike other malignant growths, basal cell carcinoma almost never spreads to other parts of the body, but it must be treated by a dermatologist to prevent further destruction of tissue.

SYMPTOM: **Stretch Marks**

COMMON CAUSES: Stretch marks are red, slightly depressed streaks that show up most often on the abdomen and occasionally on the breasts in approximately half of all pregnant women during the last three months of pregnancy. But it is not an exclusive problem of mothers-to-be.

People who have gained or lost a considerable amount of weight can also get stretch marks, as can youths who develop muscles too rapidly. Any sudden change in skin volume generally can cause stretch marks.

BEST RESPONSE: There is no known treatment for stretch marks, says Lyon Rowe, M.D. Creams or ointments, no matter what their claims, are not effective. After pregnancy, the marks will become silvery in color, but they won't disappear entirely. Generally, says Dr. Rowe, "some of the streaks will stay, some will go away. It depends on the type of skin you've inherited."

SYMPTOM: **Sunburn.** *See* Symptom: Burns

SYMPTOM: **Sweating**

COMMON CAUSES: One wag once defined nervous tension as being wet in all the dry places and dry in all the wet places. We all know what that's like!

In fact, excess sweating is common. Heavy exercise causes it. So, too, does hot and humid weather, being overweight, fever, menstruation and menopause. Those with an overactive thyroid (see thyroid disease under Common Whole Body Conditions in chapter 19) are also known to sweat more than the next guy.

But for some people, just the least bit of exertion—even tinkering with the kitchen sink—can cause the pores to flood. In fact, some people sweat so much—on their palms, in their armpits, even on the soles of their feet—that they must change their clothes several times a day. The problem even has a name—hyperhidrosis.

Is your sweating problem happening only at night? If you frequently break out in a cold sweat at night and you can exclude heavy drinking, fever or a too-hot bedroom as the cause, it could be a sign of a number of diseases. Night sweats, for example, are a sign of leukemia (see Common Whole Body Conditions in chapter 19).

BEST RESPONSE: Unfortunately, there isn't much you can do about overactive sweat glands, says Lyon Rowe, M.D. Diligent use of antiperspirants and deodorants and frequent changing of clothes will help keep the problem to a minimum.

For those with hyperhidrosis, there is a solution—surgery. "We're talking real problem sweating here," says Dr. Rowe. Which is why the condition first requires evaluation by a physician. The surgery requires removal of some of the skin in the armpits. For excessive sweating of the hands and feet, an electrical treatment called iontophoresis is used.

If you break out in night sweats for no explainable reason—lowering the room temperature, for example, does not help—see your doctor for an examination.

ACCOMPANYING SYMPTOMS: If your excess sweating is accompanied by chest pain, you could be suffering from angina or a heart attack (see myocardial infarction under Common Circulatory, Heart and Lung Conditions in chapter 5). Excess sweating accompanied by faintness, nausea, panting, rapid pulse rate and pale, cold, moist skin, are signs of shock. You should seek medical attention immediately for both of these conditions.

SYMPTOM: **Thickening**

COMMON CAUSES: Most cases of hard, thickened skin occur on the feet or hands as corns and calluses.

Corns are smaller than a pea and develop on the toes. They hurt. Calluses are larger (about one inch in diameter) and develop on the bottom of your foot or over a bunion. They're caused by putting more weight on one part of your foot than another when you walk. And they can hurt, too.

You may also get calluses on the palms of your hands, especially if you do heavy manual work or you've raked leaves, swung a tennis racket, rowed a boat or worked out on the parallel bars.

Some forms of dermatitis (see Common Skin Conditions) also can cause hardening of the skin. Scleroderma, or hidebound skin, is the extreme of hardened, thickened skin, where the face becomes masklike and the hands often clawlike. Scleroderma is a progressive disease of the skin and connective tissues and involves some of the internal organs as well. It usually affects middle-aged women, and the cause is unknown. The progress of this disease is usually fairly slow, and spontaneous recovery may occur.

BEST RESPONSE: What's good for a callus is also good for a corn. And unless you suffer from diabetes or a circulatory disorder (in which case you should be under a doctor's care), you often can handle the problem yourself. Thomas Goodman, M.D., suggests you use the following method.

Soak the affected area in warm water for 30 minutes. Then rub and scrub at the area with a pumice stone or corn and callus file. If you have very thick calluses, apply 40 percent salicylic acid plasters. Tape one in place for one to three days, then remove the tape, soak the corn or callus in hot water and rub it away with a pumice stone or a corn and callus file. Then apply some petroleum jelly (Vaseline) to the area.

Remember that the acid should only be applied to thickened areas, because it is caustic and the surrounding normal skin could become irritated. If this happens, discontinue treatment.

To minimize friction and pressure while healing, apply moleskin or foam rubber pads around corns and calluses. Diabetics and people with circulatory problems should not use commercial corn and callus removers, since they could cause serious complications.

If the problem is in your feet, wider-toed shoes and a custom-designed shoe insert from your podiatrist or orthopedist can redistribute your weight and help keep corns and calluses from recurring. Should they become a chronic problem, however, a new technique developed by Lowell Scott Weil, D.P.M., a Chicago podiatrist, may do the trick.

The technique involves injecting—almost painlessly—liquid collagen under the corn or callus. "The collagen is like a sponge," explains Dr. Weil, "and the body reacts to it by filling in the holes with its own collagen." The injected collagen is gradually eaten up by the body until what's left is natural, body-made collagen. The process literally causes the body to regenerate itself and form a small cushion under the corn or callus, relieving the pain. It's similar, Dr. Weil says, to "an internal Dr. Scholl's."

About 6,000 corns and calluses have been treated with injected collagen so far, and the technique, reports Dr. Weil, has been successful approximately 70 percent of the time. It works best in people over 50 and worst in those with deeply embedded calluses on the bottoms of their feet. The collagen will eventually wear down under normal foot stress, but wearing an arch support prescribed by your doctor should prolong its effectiveness. Nevertheless, says Dr. Weil, a "booster shot" every one or two years may be necessary.

Scleroderma needs to be diagnosed by a doctor, but there is no specific medication for the disease.

ACCOMPANYING SYMPTOM: If you notice your skin is hardened and you also have trouble seeing at night, you could be suffering from vitamin A deficiency. Treatment should be supervised by a physician.

SYMPTOM: **Warts**

COMMON CAUSE: Warts are gray, firm and irregularly shaped lumps that can show up anywhere on the body, although the hands and fingers are the most common spots. They are caused by a virus and can spread easily.

Warts are usually painless. However, a wart on the bottom of your foot (see Symptom: Warts, Plantar in chapter 9) can feel like a boulder in your sock, and warts on the face can be particularly troublesome for men who shave.

BEST RESPONSE: Because warts can spread easily, they should be treated either by applying chemicals such as salicylic acid, available over-the-counter, or by electrosurgery or freezing with dry ice or liquid nitrogen. This procedure needs to be done by your doctor.

Less orthodox home remedies for removing warts have been tried with some success. Success has been reported with topical application of prescription vitamin A acid. Applying tape snugly over a wart for three weeks has been found by some to work wonderfully well, as has applying a drop of castor oil or vitamin E oil and then covering the area with tape.

There is also another, though somewhat unusual treatment. According to a report in *Plastic and Reconstructive Surgery,* taping the inner side of a banana skin to a plantar wart can be successful.

SYMPTOM: **White Patches**

COMMON CAUSES: White patches—small areas of skin that look pale or bleached—are usually the result of one or two problems: vitiligo or tinea versicolor.

Vitiligo is the result of inactive melanocytes, the skin cells that normally give you color or pigment. White patches may appear on the face, neck, fingers and backs of hands, nipples, navel and genitals, though not necessarily on all these areas, and may spread to the entire body.

These patches are more noticeable on people with darker skin. The exact cause is not known, but one theory suggests that it is linked to a history of diabetes, thyroid disease or a special type of anemia. Up to 20 percent of vitiligo patients report that other family members have this condition.

Tinea versicolor, on the other hand, is a yeastlike fungus infection that causes white patches on the oilier parts of the body—back, chest, arms, neck and sometimes the face. Certain conditions make a person more susceptible, says Denise Buntin, M.D., assistant professor of dermatology at Tulane University Medical School in New Orleans. Those living in warm climates and/or those who perspire excessively are more likely to develop tinea versicolor.

BEST RESPONSE: Vitiligo can be a difficult disease to treat. Usually chronic, it requires treatment by a physician. A topical steroid may be prescribed by your doctor to stimulate the return of pigment.

If there is no relief, you could need a medication called psoralen, which is either painted on or taken orally in pill form. The drug must be paired with ultraviolet light. The treatment is called PUVA (psoralen artificial ultraviolet light) therapy and is lengthy, lasting from several months to a year or more. "There are potential side effects," cautions Dr. Buntin, and for this reason the process is supervised carefully.

The treatment of tinea versicolor is much simpler and can be carried out at home, says Dr. Buntin. Wash the affected areas every night for two weeks with an over-the-counter selenium sulfide shampoo, such as Selsun Blue. The lather must be left on for 10 to 30 minutes before washing it off. Sulfur soap can be used in a similar manner. You can also use an over-the-counter antifungal cream, like Micatin, twice daily.

You should notice an improvement in 7 to 14 days. If you notice that the spots don't scale when you scratch the edges with your fingernail, take it as a sign that the treatment is working.

If you're not sure whether you have vitiligo or tinea versicolor, Dr. Buntin feels it's safe to try the home treatment with selenium sulfide shampoo first. If it doesn't work, then see a dermatologist to determine whether your problem is vitiligo, a particularly stubborn tinea versicolor or something else.

Remember that even when your tinea versicolor is clearing, it can take months for the skin color to even out. And tinea versicolor often reappears. While you're waiting for your patchy skin to return to normal, you can cover the troublesome areas with a special cosmetic cream.

SYMPTOM: **Wrinkles**

COMMON CAUSES: The experts tell us that middle age is the prime of life—a time when self-acceptance, wisdom and experience help us to realize our full potential.

The mirror tells us that middle age is the time when little wrinkles appear at the corners of the eyes and mouth, the skin beneath the chin starts to hang loose and the area under the eyes takes on extra baggage.

But age alone isn't what causes the skin to wrinkle. The abuse you've been putting it through over the years is what's really to blame. It's the environmental insults that make some skins age sooner than others, according to Albert Kligman, M.D., Ph.D., professor of dermatology at the University of Pennsylvania School of Medicine in Philadelphia. Specifically, excess sunlight, heat, wind and cold are the biggest abusers.

Sunlight and heat damage the skin's collagen and elastin fibers. These fibers give skin its strength, its elasticity and its resiliency. Collagen is what keeps the skin from overextending. Wrinkles are the result of repeated damage to collagen and elastin fibers and, once present, can't be reversed.

Frequently used facial expressions (such as squinting or puckering from puffing on a cigarette), the use of harsh soaps and heredity also contribute to the aging process.

And, says Dr. Kligman, females with dry skin tend to wrinkle earlier than males who have tougher, oilier skin. Black-skinned men wrinkle the least of all.

BEST RESPONSE: Since overexposure to the sun is the main element in aging your skin beyond its years, it makes sense to cover up your hands and face when outside. Be smart—wear a protective sun hat and sunglasses and wear a sunscreen (the higher the SPF—sun protection factor—the better) if you plan to be outdoors for more than a few minutes.

Riding in a convertible with the top down may make you feel like a kid again, but it can make you look like your grandmother sooner than you'd like. The combined effects of sun and wind only increase your chances of premature aging. If you're a smoker, you shouldn't be—if you want to look younger longer. The lines created as you pucker to take a drag will eventually pucker even when you aren't smoking.

To prevent wrinkles, you should moisturize the skin. For maximum moisturizing, apply petroleum jelly (Vaseline) to your face, hands and neck and leave it on overnight. Don't slather it on, and rub it in well. Do this twice a week just before you go to bed. Next morning, wipe it off with a nondrying lotion, and proceed with your regular routine of makeup and moisturizing.

Make sure that the air inside your home is moist. When the relative humidity is below 30 percent, the skin gives up water to the air and becomes dehydrated. This accentuates existing lines and wrinkles.

Finally, what about facial exercises and cosmetic surgery? Most doctors agree that facial exercises do the same thing to your face as smiling or frowning—they make wrinkles worse.

Cosmetic surgery shores up the sagging skin and provides a firmer appearance. How long the results last, however, varies from one patient to another. One Hollywood star is said to have had her face lifted so many times, there was nothing left in her shoes!

SYMPTOM: **Yellowing.** *See* Symptom: Jaundice

Common Skin Conditions

Acne. Acne affects more than 80 percent of all teenagers in varying degrees of severity. Girls get it earlier but more mildly than boys, and it's worse in those with oily skin.

The disease is characterized by blackheads, whiteheads and pimples, which appear on the face, neck, shoulders, upper chest and back. Some lesions develop into abscesses and cystic masses, which hang on for a month or more until they finally rupture and heal, leaving scars and pitting.

The reason that teenagers are plagued with this malady is that production of hormones increases at their time of life. The hormones stimulate the sebaceous glands, which produce an oversupply of sebum, an oily substance. This, plus other biochemical changes taking place in the body, clogs up the pores, resulting in acne.

Many adults get acne, too, because of stress or, in women, because of hormonal changes connected to the menstrual cycle. Acne should be treated in a total program of skin care and medication.

Chickenpox. Chickenpox is a highly contagious childhood disease that starts as a reddish, flat rash usually on the trunk of the body, although in severe cases the pox seem to be everywhere, including the inside of the mouth.

This initial rash rapidly evolves into small, clear blisters, producing the characteristic "dewdrop on a rose petal." Within a few hours, the blisters break and dry into crusts. New pox continue to appear for three or four days, and they usually itch. The disease is no longer contagious when the rash is dried and crusted. Before the pox appear, some children feel sick and run a fever, but some don't feel sick at all.

Since most cases of chickenpox are mild, the normal course of treatment is bed rest and forcing fluids during the fever stage. Petroleum jelly (Vaseline), calamine lotion and emollient baths can help reduce the itching. Also, children should be kept from scratching the rash, because it can result in scarring and opens the way for other infections.

Dermatitis/eczema. Dermatitis and eczema mean the same thing—inflammation of the skin. Whereas the condition is common, it isn't at all simple—dermatitis comes in many varieties, each with its own name and characteristics.

Atopic dermatitis, also called general neurodermatitis, is a chronic, complex skin disorder that begins early in life and is associated with a tendency to such allergies as asthma and hay fever. Atopic dermatitis shows up in infants as infantile eczema, may reappear in childhood and often, except for the most severe cases, disappears by adulthood. The eruptions appear as dull red, scaly patches of thickened skin covered with bloody crusts from scratching. The disorder usually affects the elbows, knees, neck and face.

There is no known cure for atopic dermatitis. Many medications—including steroid ointments and moisturizers—are effective for awhile but soon lose their usefulness. Treatment is aimed at preventing scratching and avoiding infections, especially in the diaper area. Certain immunizations and childhood illnesses (such as chickenpox and measles) are made worse when a baby has infantile eczema.

Contact dermatitis is the skin's response to an irritant or allergen that has come in contact with it. The skin's response to poison ivy, for example, is a form of contact dermatitis, as are the skin eruptions that occur after using hair and face cosmetics or wearing clothes or shoes that contain certain chemicals that you may be allergic to.

Hairdressers are particularly prone to hand dermatitis caused by dyes, the rubber in gloves and the nickel in salon instruments. To cure contact dermatitis, the cause must be found. Dermatologists frequently use patch tests to aid in the search.

The cause of seborrheic dermatitis is not known. In adults, body creases become red, flaky and itchy. The areas from the sides of the nose to the corners of the mouth may be affected, as well as areas in the groin, armpits and under the breasts. Dandruff is common. Dermatologists often treat seborrheic dermatitis with antiseborrheic shampoos on the scalp and tar medications and cortisone creams on the affected areas. The condition comes and goes over several years.

Babies get a special form of seborrheic dermatitis called cradle cap. Initially, dry scales appear on the scalp, then eventually turn into yellow, greasy, scaly patches that sometimes extend over the eyebrows and behind the ears. If the dermatitis is on the face, there are small red blotches and pimples, which become redder when the baby cries. On other parts of the body, the dermatitis occurs as red, partially scaly patches.

Housewife's hand dermatitis is very common and is the skin's way of letting you know you're doing something with your hands that it can't tolerate. The skin will become dry, rough and reddened, especially over the knuckles. It may thicken, crack, flake and itch.

To treat this type of eczema, you must identify and then avoid the irritant that has caused the problem—is it dishwashing liquid, household cleaner, shampoo or, as is usually the case, water? Moisturizers and cortisone cream are frequently prescribed to clear up the lesions.

Irritant eczema is common in elderly people who bathe too frequently. There is mild redness, flaking and irritation, most commonly on the legs.

Dyshidrosis begins with small, fluid-filled blisters that form deep in the skin of the palms of the hands and sometimes the soles of the feet. The blisters break down to become red, itchy, scaly patches. An attack usually lasts two to four weeks and then clears up by itself. If it does not, soaking your hand or foot in Burow's solution, an antiseptic lotion, may be helpful, as might moisturizers or cortisone cream.

Discoid eczema is another type of eczema that usually clears up on its own after several months. The cause of the condition isn't known. It appears as disks of red, flaking, weeping, itchy skin—most commonly on the arms and legs.

Frostbite. This is freezing of the skin and deeper tissues caused by exposure to extremely cold temperatures. It most commonly occurs on the feet, hands, ears and nose. The likelihood of frostbite depends on temperature (the skin normally freezes at 31°F, and deeper tissues freeze at tissue temperatures between 14° and 29°F), wind velocity, duration of exposure and such factors as a person's age and physical condition.

Frostbitten skin is hard, pale and cold and has no feeling. When it's thawed out, it becomes red and painful. The worst cases of frostbite result in the death of the tissue, a condition known as gangrene. It almost always results in the loss of the affected part. It usually takes a month after the injury to determine how much of the body part will be lost. If frostbite is treated quickly, however, it may have no long-term ill effects.

Gangrene. Gangrene can occur in dead skin that can never be revived. There are two types, dry and wet.

Dry gangrene occurs when the flow of blood to certain areas is stopped or reduced. The cause can be frostbite, but more commonly it's the result of poor circulation due to diabetes, hardening of the arteries or an arterial embolism. If the gangrene is not caught in time, the area that is deprived of oxygen dies and turns black.

Wet gangrene results when either a wound or dry gangrene becomes infected. Pus, gas bubbles and an unpleasant smell emanate from the wound. This type of gangrene spreads rapidly and is extremely serious.

The last stop for both dry and wet gangrene is amputation. But before resorting to that, physicians can use a number of drugs—vasodilators and anticoagulants for dry gangrene, antiserum for wet gangrene and antibiotics for both types. To prevent further spread of wet gangrene, high-pressure oxygen treatment may be ordered.

German measles.   A rash is often the first sign of German measles, which more properly goes by the name rubella. It's a contagious disease that commonly occurs in children but can strike at any age.

The rash is flat and reddish, appearing first on the face and neck and quickly spreading to the arms, legs and body. It rarely itches and usually lasts about three to four days. Enlarged lymph nodes in the neck are very common.

In a child, German measles is generally a very mild disease, but in a pregnant woman, it can cause abnormalities in the unborn child. Because of this, it's best for everyone to receive the rubella vaccine.

Unless there are complications (such as pregnancy), the recommended treatment is nothing more than bed rest.

Impetigo.   This highly contagious bacterial skin infection is usually seen in children around the nose and mouth. If the skin is broken—from a scratch, an insect bite or an injury—the bacteria jump in and cause a reddish sore that quickly develops an oozing yellow crust.

To treat impetigo, a physician usually recommends washing the affected area with an antibacterial skin cleanser and applying an antibacterial ointment. Internal antibiotics also are frequently prescribed.

Researchers from the University of Alabama Internal Medicine Program in Montgomery found that applying an ointment containing bacitracin, neomycin and polymyxin to the injured skin of children at a day-care center helped prevent impetigo from developing. Any time your child suffers a cut or scratch, you should apply one of these antibiotic ointments, which are available over the counter.

Lice.   There are three types of lice—those that attack the scalp, the crab lice that go for the pubic and genital areas but like other hairy places, too, and those body lice that attach themselves to clothes or underwear or occasionally can be seen on the abdomen, chest and back.

Whereas different lice have a different preference for where they make their home, they're all alike in their eating habits—they bite the skin and suck blood. This causes severe itching.

You can get lice only by being in contact with another person who's harboring them—animals don't get lice.

Usually no treatment is needed for the skin problem caused by body lice. However, lice that attack the scalp or genitals do require treatment.

Measles.   Measles is a disease that can be picked up easily. Just handling a handkerchief used by an affected person can cause you to get it.

For the first three or four days, measles has no rash. Caused by a virus, it begins like a bad cold that's getting worse. When the rash does come out, it's usually around the hairline. The rash is reddish and flat and soon spreads to the body, arms and legs, becoming bigger and darker colored.

Measles can make you sick. The fever is usually high, and there's a dry cough, red, sore eyes and the potential for very serious complications. Although considered a childhood disease, it can strike at any age.

Bed rest, medications for cold and plenty of fluids if there is fever make up the usual course of treatment.

Psoriasis.   Psoriasis, unfortunately, is one of the mystery diseases. No one knows why you get it and no one knows how to cure it. Psoriasis appears as silver- to gray-scaled red patches on various parts of the body. The elbows, knees, trunk and scalp are the most common sites for flare-ups.

Fingernails are often affected, causing the nails to split, discolor, pit and separate from the bed. Psoriasis is not contagious, but the condition can be triggered by a slight skin injury or an infectious illness. Stress and anxiety often bring on the disease or make it worse.

It's best to have a physician diagnose and treat this problem. Although psoriasis can't be cured, it is controllable. One common treatment is exposure to sunlight. Application of coal tar derivatives may also be effective. The more resistant cases of psoriasis require more intensive measures and involve greater risks.

Ringworm.   Ringworm is not caused by a worm but by fungi—parasites that feed on the body's dead skin and perspiration. Highly contagious, it can be spread by an animal or by another person who has the disease.

Ringworm is easily identified by its ring formation of blisters or bumps, a red lesion that grows ever outward. Healing takes place in the center while the infection spreads to the periphery. Scaling and itching are severe. Ringworm can occur anywhere on the body.

Topical treatment of body ringworm with antifungal medications doesn't always work well; a systemic antibiotic for fungus infection is effective but needs a doctor's prescription. It's best to see a doctor under any circumstances; ringworm can be hard to diagnose, since there are a number of other skin diseases that can produce rings.

Roseola.   This contagious childhood disease starts suddenly, with a high fever (103° to 104°F) that lasts three to four days, after which time a reddish, flat, slightly raised rash appears on the chest and abdomen.

When the fever falls, the child feels and acts well. The rash may last only a few hours or for several days.

Although fever is high, the disease is considered mild. Treatment generally includes nonaspirin pain relievers such as acetaminophen (Tylenol) and tepid sponge baths to bring the child's temperature down.

Scabies.   This infection is caused by tiny mites that burrow under the top layer of the skin, lay their eggs and cause very itchy skin. There are scabies mites that infect humans and some that infect animals. Unfortunately, the animal type can be transmitted to humans.

Diagnosis of scabies is sometimes difficult, but intense itching that stays around and is worse at night should be investigated by a physician. This is especially true when people who are in close contact with each other have similar symptoms.

Most adults, and children under six years of age, should always have scabies treated by a physician. All members of the same household should be treated if any one member is treated. Clothing and bedclothes that may contain the mites or eggs should be laundered or dry cleaned. Items that cannot be cleaned can be put away in a closet for a week. Without contact with skin, scabies will die.

Shingles.   The official name for this adult disease is herpes zoster, and it's caused by the same virus that causes chickenpox in children. Shingles, in fact, is often a relapse of the childhood disease, but it's usually seen in those beyond age 50.

Shingles in adults acts quite differently, and is much more serious, than chickenpox in kids. It starts with four or five days of fever, chills, general discomfort and a painful rash that looks similar to the chickenpox rash but is confined to one area of the skin. The rash eventually crusts over but the pain may linger on.

What happens in shingles is that the virus lies dormant in nerve cells near the spinal cord and, once activated by some stress or trauma, the rash and pain follow the pattern of that particular group of nerves.

On the chest, for example, the pattern of rash and pain will run in a narrow strip from back to front, because that's how the nerve endings are arranged. Sometimes the ophthalmic nerves are involved, causing temporary blindness or permanent scarring of the cornea. If the facial nerves are affected, the result can be extreme pain and paralysis.

Shingles is one of those diseases with no known cure, and the pain can be so intense that it causes loss of sleep and work. Most therapy is aimed at reducing symptoms while the disease runs its course. Wet compresses can be applied to the affected areas, and aspirin can help relieve the discomfort.

Some sufferers have had success with acupuncture treatment or vitamin therapy. Vitamins B_{12}, E and C may be particularly helpful, but should be used only with your doctor's approval and supervision. Some physicians use nerve-blocking injections to relieve the pain, and there are several antiviral drugs that can be administered early in the disease.

Skin cancer.   Skin cancer comes in three forms—basal cell, squamous cell and malignant melanoma. Most basal cell and squamous cell cancers are not life-threatening and can be totally cleared up with proper treatment. Malignant melanoma, however, is cause for concern.

Basal cell is the most common type of skin cancer and appears as a small, pale patch that enlarges slowly, producing a central "dimple" and eventually an ulcer. Part of the ulcer may heal, but the main portion remains ulcerated. Some also show color changes.

Basal cell cancers can appear almost anywhere on the body, but are most likely to be seen on sun-exposed areas. They usually appear on the face and are most common among fair-skinned people.

Squamous cell cancer often looks like basal cell and most frequently appears on the lower lip, the ears and the hands.

Malignant melanoma is the most serious type of skin cancer and, if not treated promptly, it can be life-threatening. This type of cancer is characterized by blue-black or black discoloration of the skin. At times, small spots may be scattered around the major one.

If you have such a black or blue-black spot, especially if it changes size or shape, you should see a dermatologist as soon as possible. Melanoma spreads quickly and early diagnosis and treatment are essential. If it is removed early and completely, it is curable.

By visually examining an unusual growth, blemish, sore or discoloration, a dermatologist can usually determine if it's benign, precancerous or malignant. A biopsy, where a small portion of the tissue is removed and examined under a microscope, will confirm or deny the doctor's suspicions.

There are a number of ways to treat basal and squamous cell skin cancer, such as surgery, cryosurgery (freezing), radiation therapy or electro-desiccation technique, in which cancerous tissue is dried with a high-frequency current applied through a needle electrode. A malignant tumor is usually excised. If the skin tumor is large, a skin graft may be needed to cover the scar. Topical chemotherapy is often used for precancerous lesions.

Chapter 16
Teeth and Gums

SEE YOUR DENTIST OR DOCTOR IMMEDIATELY IF:

- *A tooth is knocked out or broken*
- *A tooth turns black or gray*
- *New spaces appear between your teeth*
- *Pus appears at the gum line when you floss or brush*
- *Your gums are red, swollen and tender*
- *You discover a lump on your gum*
- *Your gums have pulled away from your teeth*

Would you like to know how to make the trip to your dentist's office as benign as a trip to the hairdresser?

Most dentists agree that if everyone would practice *preventive* dentistry— that is, floss, brush the teeth, get regular professional cleanings and use a bacteria-killing mouthwash, most dentists would have to find a part-time job just to keep busy. Unfortunately, though, too many people don't take proper care of their teeth. They find the routine too bothersome.

But modern dentistry has found other preventive techniques that the cavity-prone might find more appealing—like eating certain cheeses or chewing a select kind of chewing gum, and quite possibly even buying a trendy chewy candy.

No one's really quite sure why, but researchers have found that five grams—less than an ounce—of aged cheddar, Swiss or Monterey Jack cheese before meals or snacks totally eliminates the acid production of plaque. Plaque is a soft film of bacteria, saliva and minute food particles that sticks to the teeth and puts you at higher risk for developing cavities.

Of course, what's good for your mouth is not necessarily good for your waistline. And three or four ounces of such high-fat cheese a day might increase your weight (not to mention what it's liable to do to your arteries!).

But no such caveat exists for chewing gum. Studies with a handful of volunteers at the University of Iowa's Dows Institute for Dental Research clearly indicate that chewing a sorbitol-containing gum for at least ten minutes after snacks or meals actually neutralizes acids that form on dental plaque and lead to cavities.

"If you don't have a problem with decay, keep doing what you're doing," cautions Mark E. Jensen, D.D.S., Ph.D., a researcher at the institute and director of the university's Center for Clinical Studies. "But if you do have a problem, brush regularly with a fluoride toothpaste, use a fluoride rinse and chew a sorbitol-containing gum after meals."

A *dentist* advocating gum? It may sound like heresy, but there really is a simple, scientific explanation for the gum's effect, says Dr. Jensen. It stimulates the flow of saliva and actually squirts it between the teeth into those little crevices where decay breeds. What's more, Dr. Jensen particularly recommends it for schoolchildren.

"We know they're not going to brush after lunch," the researcher ruefully says. "And the teachers are going to hate me for this, but if your kids have a decay problem, stick some gum in their lunchbox."

Gum in *school?* Right, says Dr. Jensen. And one day he may even say the same about candy. Preliminary research at the Dows Institute indicates that Gummi Bears, a gelatin candy that has inspired a television series and bounced its way into the mouths and hearts of millions of children, may possess a cavity-reducing ability similar to that of sorbitol gum. With its rubberlike form and citric acid, which apparently combine to produce the same effect as the chewing gum, the candy acts like an inexpensive Water Pik, stimulating saliva and squirting it between the teeth.

Of course, it needs the same ten-minute chewing action as the sorbitol chewing gum and a Gummi Bear, even a handful of Gummi Bears, doesn't normally last that long in the mouth. And Gummi Bears also contain sugar and corn syrup, two long-proven cavity producers.

Whether the positives found in Gummi Bears outweigh the negatives is a matter of dental debate. In the meantime, though, make sure you stick by the old standbys, no matter how boring the routine. Floss, brush, use a mouthwash and visit your dentist regularly.

SYMPTOM: **Bleeding**

COMMON CAUSES: Are your gums bleeding ever so slightly—just enough to stain your toothbrush or your dental floss? Do you see red when you push against your gums with your fingers? If so, you're probably in an early stage of periodontitis (see Common Tooth and Gum Conditions), an infection caused by a collection of food, bacteria and mucus in the spaces between the gum and the base of your teeth. Left unchecked, it can result in no teeth, little gum and a lifetime of ill health.

"If the gum doesn't always bleed when you push on it but does sometimes under the pressure of food or the toothbrush, you're in Stage One," explains Thomas McGuire, D.D.S., who practices preventive dentistry in Carmel Valley, California, and is the author of *The Tooth Trap*. And you're lucky. At this stage, which Dr. McGuire calls "the twilight zone between healthy gums and disease," the damage is reversible.

If your gums bleed frequently, though, or if your gums regularly bleed when you brush, bite or sleep, leaving traces of blood on your pillow, or if you have not only bleeding gums but also bad breath and occasional pain or tenderness, you've just arrived at Stage Two, says Dr. McGuire. Stage Two is trouble. It represents full-fledged disease, and it's more difficult to treat. If ignored, it leads to loss of bone in your jaw and, eventually, to the loss of all your teeth.

But frequent bleeding can also mean a disruption elsewhere in the body. Leukemia (see Common Whole Body Conditions in chapter 19) makes otherwise healthy gums painful and bloody. And pregnancy, though a joyous occasion for the expectant parents, is troublesome for the soon-to-be mother's mouth. In fact, it's so common for pregnant women to show signs of tender and bleeding gums that it has its own name—pregnancy gingivitis. This disorder is related to the natural hormonal changes that occur with pregnancy.

Sudden bleeding can result from a recent tooth extraction or dental surgery. This can happen several hours after the original bleeding has subsided, as a result of some sort of disruption of the blood clot. Generally, however, it is nothing to be alarmed about, and you can usually stop the bleeding by using some home first-aid measures.

BEST RESPONSE: Bleeding gums should never be ignored, even if they only bleed a bit, caution dentists. Consider them a sign of disease and make an appointment to see your dentist.

Your dentist will give you a thorough examination, including cleaning your teeth, to check for signs of periodontal disease. If the disease is in an early stage, say dentists, further deterioration can be reduced by a program of meticulous care, including frequent brushing, flossing, use of an antibacterial mouthwash and professional checkups.

If the symptoms are severe, antibiotics may be necessary. Also, a series of dental cleanings in which the teeth are scraped of their infected buildup may be required. In advanced cases, gum surgery may be needed or affected teeth may have to be extracted.

If you're pregnant, however, and merely suffering from a case of pregnancy gingivitis, such drastic measures do not apply. A good program of good home dental hygiene will help reduce the bleeding. However, you should have the condition confirmed by your dentist.

If your bleeding is not being caused by a dental problem, your dentist will refer you to a physician, who will examine you and probably order blood tests to check for some other disease.

If you've recently had a tooth pulled or your wisdom teeth removed and the socket is now bleeding, don't rinse your mouth, advises Howard B. Marshall, D.D.S., a periodontist in New York City. Instead, cut some gauze or clean washcloths into two-inch by two-inch squares. Roll the gauze pad into a ball and place it over the bleeding area. Then watch TV, go for a walk, read a book—do anything but talk or anything else that keeps you from biting down on the gauze for at least 30 minutes.

If the bleeding hasn't stopped by then, try biting on a wet tea bag, says Dr. Marshall. And if the bleeding continues after 30 minutes of gritting teeth on tea, you've become a dental emergency. Call your doctor or dentist and arrange to see him or her immediately. "Keep the area under continued pressure from the gauze ball or tea bag while traveling to the office," Dr. Marshall adds.

SYMPTOM: **Chipped Tooth**

COMMON CAUSES: One common cause of a chipped tooth is an accident, like smacking the teeth against something hard such as pavement or a dashboard. But you can also wind up with a cracked tooth from biting on something hard, like a piece of small bone in a hamburger or even a large filling. Tooth grinders also can end up with chipped teeth.

BEST RESPONSE: A tooth that's been chipped should be checked by a dentist. If just a small piece of enamel is chipped, and the tooth is not sensitive or loose, you can call the dentist, explain what happened and get a regular appointment, dentists agree.

If a large piece of a tooth is broken or you see pink tissue at the center of the tooth, however, you should get prompt professional attention. Just call your dentist and let him or her know that you're on your way. Then go. If it's after hours or your dentist isn't in, go to the nearest emergency room, where you usually will be given pain medication, or you may be treated by a dentist.

SYMPTOM: **Crooked Teeth**

COMMON CAUSES: The most common cause of crooked teeth is heredity—you may have inherited your father's large teeth and your mother's small jaw. However, crooked teeth can also be a sign of advancing periodontitis (see Common Tooth and Gum Conditions). As bone deteriorates in the jaw, the teeth lose their firm anchoring and change the way they sit in the mouth.

People with a bad bite are notorious for gum disease and early loss of teeth, says David Hamilton, D.D.S., an orthodontist in New Castle, Pennsylvania. "Food can't be chewed properly, and the crooked and crowded teeth are much more difficult to keep clean and therefore decay free."

BEST RESPONSE: If your crooked teeth are an unappreciated present from your parents, don't despair. It's possible to correct these problems anytime during your life, doctors agree, and decrease your chances of having dental problems later on. Braces or spacers are not just for children. And don't be shy about putting some metal where your mouth is. Roughly 20 percent of those who wear "railroad tracks" are adults. In fact, because some adults feel about as comfortable wearing braces as they would their kids' parachute pants, braces are now available in an almost invisible plastic.

You might also want to ask your dentist whether or not you could benefit from bonding, a procedure in which nontoxic, tooth-colored materials are fused onto crooked front teeth. Bonding often works wonders against gap-toothed grins, but it requires replacement every four to seven years.

If you're interested in the procedure and would like to find out which dentists in your area practice bonding, write to the American Academy of Esthetic Dentistry, Suite 948, 211 East Chicago Avenue, Chicago, IL 60611.

If your crooked teeth are not a cosmetic problem but a disease problem, you should see your dentist as soon as possible for treatment. Teeth that have become so loose that they're shifting around and becoming crowded and crooked are a sign of advanced disease. Once gum disease has reached such an advanced stage, treatment becomes more costly, less satisfactory (from a cosmetic standpoint) and more essential with each passing day.

SYMPTOM: **Discharge**

COMMON CAUSES: Pyorrhea is an outdated but very descriptive name for gum disease, and it is almost always the cause of oozing or discharge of pus along your gum line. The very word means "flowing pus": *pyo* is pus and *rhea* is flow. And together they mean trouble.

If a milky, green or yellowish discharge has spontaneously appeared at the base of your teeth, your gums are probably in bad shape; you probably have some bone loss.

Your gums can also produce pus well before they reach this terminal stage (see periodontitis under Common Tooth and Gum Conditions). In fact, the best way to test the health of your gums is with a little judicious prodding, explains Howard B. Marshall, D.D.S.

"Take the index finger of one hand and use it to help hold back the upper lip. Now, with the index finger of the other hand, press firmly on the upper gum with the tip of your other finger and slowly move the pressing finger down toward the tooth over the gum triangle. See if it bleeds or if you get a thin, milky, whitish yellow fluid from the gum space."

If you do, you're in trouble. Your condition may be reversible, however, with periodontal treatment by a dentist.

BEST RESPONSE: If the pus appears only when you floss or press at your gums—that is, if the pus doesn't appear all by itself or in the company of blood—then you can probably repair any gum damage at home, dentists say.

Careful, conscientious plaque control with regular brushing, flossing and rinsing with a solution of equal parts of 3 percent hydrogen peroxide and water should get rid of the fluid within a few weeks.

You'll still need to see your dentist, though, because your gums should be checked with a dental probe to make sure there isn't a pocket of infection around a tooth. Also, for pus to form, there must be tartar under the gum line, which must be removed by a dentist or hygienist.

SYMPTOM: **Grinding Teeth**

COMMON CAUSES: Most tooth grinding, or bruxism, as doctors call it, occurs at night. Most bruxism is either the result of misaligned teeth or an unconscious means of relieving tension (though inducing it in your dentist), or both.

But grinding your teeth because you have an ax to grind is counterproductive at best. The action of gnashing, gnawing or grinding is very hard on the teeth. It erodes them quickly and can eventually cause more unevenness in the bite, which, in a vicious cycle, causes yet more tooth grinding.

Misaligned teeth are a major cause of tooth grinding. If your teeth don't fit together comfortably, you'll struggle to reposition them. You may not be aware you're doing it, but you'll continually move your lower jaw from side to side.

BEST RESPONSE: Treatment of tooth grinding usually requires cooperation from you and expertise from your dentist. Ask your dentist to check the relationship of your top teeth to your bottom teeth to identify any irregularities that may be causing the problem. And ask whether you could benefit from an oral splint—a small clear plastic disk that is worn at night. It separates your top and bottom teeth from each other so you chew on the disk instead of your teeth.

But the splint, though it can give a temporary reprieve to your embattled enamel, is not a permanent cure. Often the top of the tooth or teeth must be reshaped to eliminate the tooth or teeth that are interfering with a proper bite. Managing stress and tension is also important.

The cure for tension, doctors agree, is to find and eliminate the sources of it in your life. Biofeedback, stress management and professional counseling arc all helpful. Your teeth will relax when *you* do.

SYMPTOM: **Loss of Filling or Cap**

COMMON CAUSES: Most people lose a filling or cap (also known as a crown or jacket) because new decay has set in, a part of the tooth or filling has been broken or the tooth under the filling or cap was not properly prepared to receive it.

BEST RESPONSE: You must see your dentist as soon as possible.

For a cap that's fallen out, some dentists suggest that you rinse it off, glop it full of petroleum jelly (Vaseline) or denture cream and stick it back on its stump until you can get to the dentist.

For a filling, just stick a small piece of cotton directly over the hole that your filling left behind. Do not, dentists warn, put an aspirin against the tooth or gum. This is a remedy that is far more likely to burn your gum than reduce your pain.

SYMPTOM: **Loss of Tooth or Teeth**

COMMON CAUSES: Other than the natural course of human development, baseballs, football helmets and the backyard fence are just a few of the tooth-knocker-outers of childhood.

Of course, you needn't be young to lose a tooth. You can be hit by a baseball at any age. But if you're over the age of 20, it's more likely that you'd lose teeth to advanced gum disease (see periodontitis under Common Teeth and Gum Conditions).

BEST RESPONSE: If your child's tooth—or even your own—has been knocked out, the only good response is to get to a dentist *at once*. If you remain calm, follow some simple advice and get to a dentist within 20 to 30 minutes, the tooth can be replanted, say dentists.

To save the suddenly homeless tooth—even if it's "just" a baby tooth—and to ensure its successful reimplantation, you must first find the tooth. If it's still in your mouth, gently push it back into its socket. If it's on the ground, pick it up by the crown, *not* the root, dentists warn. Above all, treat it gently. And don't wash it.

"The tooth will need all the tiny little nerve fibers clinging to it, if it's to survive," says Cherilyn Sheets, D.D.S., a spokesperson for the Academy of General Dentistry, practicing in Inglewood and Newport, California. "You can easily destroy them in washing the tooth." Instead, gently wipe off any dirt that's collected on the tooth, then set it back in its socket or hold it in your mouth between your cheek and gum.

"The tooth should remain constantly bathed in saliva," explains Dr. Sheets. If the victim is a very young child and will not keep the tooth in his or her mouth, a parent or other adult can hold the tooth in his or her own mouth. The most important thing is to keep the tooth moist during the period before treatment.

If for some reason you can't keep the tooth in its natural habitat—if the child whose tooth it was is too young to hold it and you can't or won't—you can put the tooth in milk. This is the best readily available substitute for replacing the tooth in the socket, according to Frank Courts, D.D.S., Ph.D., associate professor of pediatric dentistry at the University of Florida Health Center in Gainesville.

Most people, unfortunately, wrap the tooth in a piece of tissue or hold it in their hand, he says. This is the worst possible response. It can kill the tooth's nerves, as well as its chance for implantation.

If you've lost your tooth to gum disease, however, none of these measures will help. A tooth that falls out because of disease cannot be saved. But don't throw the tooth away. Your dentist may be able to use it as part of a temporary bridge.

You can possibly prevent losing more of your teeth by seeing your doctor immediately and going through a course of treatments to get rid of the infection of periodontitis.

SYMPTOM: **Lump**

COMMON CAUSES: A lump in the gum can be small and firm, like a pea. Or it can be large and squashy, like an underinflated beach ball. But in either case, the lump probably indicates an abscess.

An abscess usually develops from one of two processes. It may result from an infection within the tooth itself, which means the nerve is dying or has died, or it can be caused by food or bacteria trapped in a pocket between the tooth and gum.

In neither case is the outcome pleasant. The infected area—either at the base of one of the teeth or along the gum, depending on the cause of the abscess—will fill with pus and other by-products of the infection. As the abscess grows, it will bloom and swell like a pimple. You may feel intense pain, although the pain is frequently gradual and aching.

How can you tell if one of your teeth is abscessed? "Tapping or biting on the tooth will really make it hurt," says Norman Wood, D.D.S., Ph.D., chairman of the Department of Oral Diagnosis at Loyola University School of Dentistry and author of *The Complete Book of Dental Care.* Therefore, you probably won't want to repeat this test too often. You might instead check whether your sore tooth feels "high" to bite on. Does it, in other words, seem to touch before your other teeth when you bite gently?

"An abscessed tooth actually does touch first," Dr. Wood explains, "because the quantity of pus and/or inflammation at the root end forces the tooth slightly out of the socket."

You can sometimes identify an abscess that's settled in your gum— and not just in a tooth—by its location, according to Cherilyn Sheets, D.D.S. A tooth abscess will normally appear as a lump located high up on the gum, away from the pinkish white part of the gum, called the gingiva, that holds a tooth in place. A gum abscess will often be closer to the edge of the gum line.

Sometimes, though, just to confuse the issue, you can have a tooth abscess and a gum abscess at the same time. These are the hardest to treat and may mean tooth extraction.

BEST RESPONSE: Call your dentist and set up an appointment as soon as you can. An abscess is a dental emergency and it needs to be medically treated.

In the meantime, you can help yourself and your sore mouth in several ways. If you are in considerable pain, some dentists suggest you take an over-the-counter pain reliever, such as acetaminophen (Tylenol). You can also soak a wad of cotton in oil of clove and put it on the tooth. Or, Dr. Sheets suggests, you can try holding lukewarm water in your mouth for a few minutes.

If you still have pain, you can try using cold water or ice. But, cautions Dr. Sheets, unless you have a specific kind of abscess, the cold will cause excruciating pain. So if you use ice, make sure you tell your dentist if applications of cold relieved the pain. "If your dentist knows that ice relieved your pain, he or she should also know instantly that your problem is a particular type of abscess, and can treat it accordingly," explains Dr. Sheets.

If you can't reach your dentist, look in the Yellow Pages for an endodontist who will see you as soon as possible. Or just go to a hospital emergency room.

If for some reason you're out of touch with civilization (the third day out on a seven-day safari) and you can't get to your dentist right away—and *only* if you can't—you can temporarily relieve the major discomfort of an abscess by lancing it, suggests Howard B. Marshall, D.D.S. But it shouldn't be attempted on any abscess that isn't soft and coming to a head like a pimple.

"Sterilize a needle in the blue part of a flame, holding the needle with tweezers so as not to burn your fingers," suggests Dr. Marshall. Let the needle cool. Next, under good light and looking at the swollen abscess in a mirror, pierce the head of the abscess to a depth of about one-eighth inch. Gently squeeze the surrounding tissues and try to milk out any pus or blood mixed with pus. If you are not successful the first few times you try, do *not* continue.

And turn around and head for a doctor. Dr. Sheets cautions that you must still see your dentist as soon as possible. Although the pain may be relieved by the lancing, the underlying infection still exists and must be treated.

Once you've gotten to your dentist, he or she should try to save the tooth with a procedure called a root canal. If the dentist doesn't, ask why. If you're not satisfied with the answer, you'll still have time to seek a second opinion. Most teeth can be saved if treated properly, as long as there is enough bone remaining around the root of the tooth to give it good support.

SYMPTOM: **Pain**

COMMON CAUSES: A toothache is your tooth's way of telling you it's in serious trouble. If the pain is continuous and really acts up when you bite or chew, you may have an abscess—a pus-filled sac—around the bottom of the tooth, inside the gum (see Symptom: Lump). If the pain occurs *only* when you bite down on a hard object, you may have a cracked tooth.

Frequently, however, a toothache is caused by an infected sinus (see sinusitis under Common Nasal Conditions in chapter 13) or wisdom tooth, temporomandibular joint disorder (see Common Facial, Jaw and Mouth Conditions in chapter 8) or simply by decay.

But don't ignore the pain even if you think it's just decay. By the time a decayed tooth starts to hurt, it has already disintegrated to the point that bacteria have attacked the nerve buried deep inside the tooth. Keep ignoring the tooth's cry for help and the pain *will* disappear: As your tooth dies it loses the ability to let you know what's going on.

BEST RESPONSE: You need to see your dentist. But if the pain hits in the middle of the night or while you're in flight from Philadelphia to San Diego, head for the bathroom and vigorously rinse your mouth with warm water, suggests the Academy of General Dentistry. Flossing can also help by removing any trapped food that may be affecting your tooth. If swelling is present, apply a cold compress on the outside of your cheek.

Some dentists also suggest soaking a wad of cotton in clove oil and placing it on the aching tooth, while others suggest that an over-the-counter painkiller such as acetaminophen (Tylenol) can also be helpful. Many dentists suggest you do *not* take aspirin, however, because aspirin encourages bleeding.

SYMPTOM: **Receding Gums**

COMMON CAUSES: Gums typically recede for many of the same reasons hairlines do—aging, genetic susceptibility and overbrushing. But unlike hair loss, gum loss is not untreatable, is not inevitable and, most important, is not benign.

Unfortunately, overbrushing "literally 'skins' the gum off the neck of the teeth," says Howard B. Marshall, D.D.S. Dubbed the "dental chain-saw massacre" by one tooth professional, this abrasion occurs when you use too firm a brush in too firm a horizontal, back-and-forth fashion.

But too little brushing can be as harmful to your health. Gingivitis or the more serious periodontitis (see Common Tooth and Gum Conditions) can both cause the gums to recede. You may first notice this when you or someone else remarks on what long teeth you've got. In fact, your teeth haven't lengthened; your gums have gotten shorter. And more of each tooth now shows.

BEST RESPONSE: See your dentist if you suspect your gums are receding. He or she can check the health of your gums and help you determine the cause of whatever gum loss has occurred.

But while you're waiting to see your dentist, begin practicing a little moderation in your brushstroke. Instead of scrubbing your teeth and gums with all your might, dentists suggest, brush gently in a circular motion at a 45-degree angle aimed at the gum rather than with a back-and-forth motion.

Whatever you do, though, don't stop brushing; inadequate dental hygiene will make any and all gum problems worse.

SYMPTOM: **Redness**

COMMON CAUSES: The causes of red gums seem to be loosely tied to age. If gums are red between the ages of 3 and 30 months, a good bet is that the redness is caused by teething. If they're red only at the very back of your mouth and you're between the ages of 17 and 21, you may have an impacted wisdom tooth that has become infected. And if you're old enough to wear dentures, the redness could very well be caused by denture pressure (see Symptom: Slipping Dentures).

Red gums can also be caused by advancing gum disease (see periodontitis under Common Tooth and Gum Conditions), the same herpes virus that causes cold sores and, less frequently, an allergy to your mouthwash or toothpaste.

BEST RESPONSE: Unless you're sure the redness is caused by teething, take your baby to the doctor. Teething, however, is such a normal part of human development that you can feel comfortable just handing your baby a cold, hard object on which to gnaw.

Wise mothers will keep a supply of solid plastic teething rings in the freezer or fluid-filled ones in the refrigerator. These are filled with a harmless substance—in some cases, treated drinking water—that can't harm your baby if one of his or her newly emerged little fangs just happens to puncture the material.

Massaging the gums with a loving finger can also help your baby, and some doctors suggest that you occasionally apply a solution of equal parts of 3 percent hydrogen peroxide and warm water. Old-fashioned treatments such as giving your baby a bit of whiskey in his or her bottle are not only ineffective but can be downright dangerous.

If you're an adult and can rule out denture trouble as the source of your symptom, you'd better get to your dentist. Any infection or disease must be treated by a dentist.

ACCOMPANYING SYMPTOMS: Parents and even some pediatricians frequently blame baby's crying, rashes, fevers, sneezing, spitting up, eating disturbances, sleeping disturbances and a million other accompanying symptoms on teething. There may or may not be a relationship. But be aware that such symptoms can be indicative of other problems and that attributing them to teething can be unwise.

In one hospital over a 12-month period, for example, 50 children ranging in age from 3 to 30 months were hospitalized with symptoms of diseases that were attributed by their parents to the teething process. All but two were found to have a significant infection. One had spinal meningitis.

SYMPTOM: **Scalloped Edges**

COMMON CAUSE: Teeth with ornamentally scalloped edges are not the newest teenage craze. They're nature's way of helping teeth cut through the gums more quickly and evenly.

BEST RESPONSE: Ignore them. They'll soon wear down as your hungry child puts them to use.

SYMPTOM: **Sensitivity**

COMMON CAUSES: Occasionally, a tooth that has just been filled by the dentist will be extremely sensitive to hot and cold. This in itself is not a sign of trouble. If you haven't been to the dentist, however, you'd better consider it.

Sensitivity to temperatures and sugar can be a sign of tooth decay or a sinus infection. It can also signal advancing gum disease (see periodontitis under Common Tooth and Gum Conditions). It can also be caused by the irritation of grinding your teeth or by a tooth that has been chipped or broken.

A few benign reasons exist for sensitivity. Sucking on a lemon can cause the sensation for a short time after. So, too, can brushing your teeth incorrectly.

BEST RESPONSE: If your sensitivity is a result of a recent bout in the dentist's chair, do nothing. The sensitivity will go away by itself, usually within hours, although it's occasionally been known to take longer.

Otherwise, you should make an appointment to see your dentist as soon as possible. But until you can actually get there, some dentists suggest you brush your teeth with one of the over-the-counter toothpastes designed for sensitive teeth. It should relieve any discomfort.

You might also want to modify the way you clean your teeth—especially if your sensitivity is caused by incorrect brushing. Teeth should never be brushed side to side, dentists say. Brushing from side to side rather than down-on-the-uppers and up-on-the-lowers in a circular motion will wear your tooth's enamel along the gum line. The gum will get pushed farther and farther down the tooth until its thinnest part is painfully exposed to the rough-and-tumble life of paste and brush. That's what makes it feel sensitive. Your gums will return to normal when your brush stops beating them up.

SYMPTOM: **Slipping Dentures**

COMMON CAUSES: If advertisements for denture creams were accurate, loose dentures would be one of life's greatest woes. In ads, wobbly dentures topple love, destroy hopes, block job promotions and stomp self-esteem. Worst of all, loose dentures separate you forever from the joys of corn on the cob—unless you rush out and buy the sponsor's denture cream.

These ads are silly. Loose dentures are correctable without cream. But in one way, the ads are correct: Loose dentures do signal trouble.

The trouble is that the gums and jawbone inevitably shrink because of the constant pressure that's exerted by dentures. This shrinkage normally occurs after a few years of regular denture wearing. The result? Your new jaw structure and your old dentures no longer match. Your dentures seem loose. You'll probably also notice that your cheeks seem sunken, your lower jaw is protruding and you have to close your mouth farther to bite properly.

These problems are more than embarrassing. They're also a potential health risk. The chronic inflammation and pressure could lead to infection or even to cancerous changes in the gums. Also, if your loose dentures remain uncorrected, your jaw and mouth movements and your entire facial appearance may change drastically to cope with the gradual shrinkage.

BEST RESPONSE: "Denture creams work reasonably well in an emergency," advises Thomas McGuire, D.D.S. "But if your dentures start feeling loose or uncomfortable, head immediately to a dentist who specializes in prosthodontics, the making of dentures. In most cases, small adjustments in the dentures' fit should make denture creams unnecessary."

Proper care of your dentures will also help to keep them—and consequently your jaw—in good shape for a longer period of time, experts say. Always remove your dentures at night to give your gums a rest. Many dentures must be kept in water when they're not in your mouth or they'll warp, so make sure you carefully follow your dentist's instructions about storing them.

Also follow your dentist's directions about upkeep, making sure you clean your dentures daily. And conscientiously clean your remaining natural teeth and gums, especially around the base of your teeth.

The potential life span of your dentures ranges from six months to five years or more, depending on the condition of your gums and jawbone, the denture material used and how well your dentures were originally fitted. If you have full dentures, you should have them checked by a dentist at least every two years. If you have only a partial bridge, you should visit your dentist even more often—every six months or so.

But there *is* an alternative to dentures. If you're not happy with your dentures, think about getting oral implants—permanent tooth replacements—suggests Daniel Y. Sullivan, D.D.S., founder of the Center for Osseointegration and Reconstructive Dentistry in Washington, D.C.

Oral implants are now made of titanium, a highly biocompatible material that is also used by surgeons in hip replacements and skull plates. The implants are inserted into the bone tissue and allowed to bond to bone. Permanent tooth replacements attach directly to the implant fixture and will then prevent the shrunken-cheeked look that occurs due to bone loss.

Using a technique called osseointegration, which was developed by a Swedish orthopedic surgeon, Professor P. I. Branemark, the implants can be inserted under local anesthesia in the dental office. This technique has experienced a very high success rate—over 90 percent—for the past 20 years, says Dr. Sullivan.

"The procedure usually takes two surgical visits," says Dr. Sullivan, "and there is little or no discomfort. The teeth are permanent and even feel real. And you can chomp on an apple the rest of your life."

And don't hesitate to ask your dentist about permanent tooth replacements if you already have dentures. People who wear dentures actually make the best candidates, says Dr. Sullivan. And this technique will firmly reinforce any of your own teeth that may be failing.

SYMPTOM: **Stains**

COMMON CAUSES: Have you ever owned a white porcelain coffee cup? Have you noticed the cup, under a barrage of steady use and less steady washings, becoming slowly bruised by a brown stain? Then you've just had a clear and sobering illustration of how teeth become discolored.

"Anything that can stain white porcelain is equally capable of staining your teeth over a period of time," explains Cherilyn Sheets, D.D.S. "Long-term use of coffee, tea, carrot juice or any other colored juice, or smoking can all cause your teeth to appear yellow or brown."

Such discoloration is, on the surface, a real problem. Certainly, it's not pretty. You wouldn't wish brown-splotched teeth on good friends. But because it *is* on the surface, it's actually the least worrisome cause of tooth discoloration.

"This type of staining is known as an extrinsic stain," says Robert Mallin, D.D.S., a dentist in Metuchen, New Jersey. Extrinsic stains work their way onto the tooth from outside. They don't indicate anything about the internal health of the tooth.

"Generally, stains are harmless, if stain is all you have," adds Thomas McGuire, D.D.S. "The point is to use stain as a guide to how well you are taking care of your mouth."

The color of your stain is a good clue to its original source and also to whether it's a serious problem or not. "Stains can be many colors—yellow, orange, black, brown, red and even green—nice, earthy colors," Dr. McGuire says. And each indicates something different, although brown may be the color your teeth are most likely to turn. Brown is the color of coffee, tea, cola and tobacco. Putting any of these in your mouth (whether you smoke tobacco or chew it) will stain your teeth brown.

Usually the stain is most severe in dirty mouths, says Dr. McGuire. That's because it stains the mineralized plaque called calculus or tartar that clings to the teeth in a dirty mouth much more and much faster than it stains clean teeth.

Yellowed teeth, on the other hand, can occur in the healthiest of mouths. "Nature didn't give everyone pure white teeth. There are different shades of tooth color, just as there are of skin color," says Dr. Sheets. "Some people's teeth are simply more yellow than others' are."

Progressive yellowing is usually a consequence of aging. "The white part of your teeth (enamel) gets worn with age," Dr. McGuire explains. "The more enamel that is worn off means the more yellow portion of the tooth (dentin, the hard, bonelike bulk of your tooth) can show through."

But yellowing is almost never anything to worry about. Infrequently, your enamel can be worn away too fast by one of several rare diseases or by an abrasive toothpaste and overly aggressive tooth-brushing style. "The dentist should be asked about this if you think yours is wearing off too fast," Dr. McGuire says.

You may also want to ask your dentist about any green stains you notice on your child's teeth. A green stain is often visible on new teeth, especially at the point where the teeth and gum meet.

"It is caused by a membrane that helps form the teeth and happens to stick around after they erupt," Dr. McGuire says. "This is not serious and can usually be removed by a simple dental cleaning."

Rarely, greenish spots on your teeth are the guise taken by calculus.

Calculus contributes to and is formed as a result of gum disease, says Dr. Marshall. It needs to be scraped off by your dentist, or it will serve as a breeding ground for more bacteria. Luckily, your dentist or hygienist can remove it easily.

More difficult to treat and more serious is a tooth that appears to be turning black or gray. This is usually a tooth that's languishing or is already dead. The discoloration you're seeing is "intrinsic" staining.

"Changes that occur within the tooth itself cause intrinsic staining," says Dr. Mallin. Fillings composed of mercury/silver (amalgam) are a common cause, as is the death of the tooth's pulp.

Another variety of intrinsic staining is caused by drugs or other substances that stain your teeth from the inside out. The antibiotic tetracycline, for example, interacts with the newly forming enamel of a youngster's teeth, turning it permanently yellow, gray or brown. However, physicians are now warned about giving tetracycline to children during tooth development.

An *over* supply of fluoride also remains a hazard for the whiteness of your child's teeth. Too much fluoride in a child's diet while his or her teeth are forming can turn these same teeth yellow. A certain amount of dietary flouride itself is, however, essential to the health of forming teeth, and if the water supply is low in flouride, doctors regularly recommend it be taken as a dietary supplement. Otherwise, simply using a flouride toothpaste or getting a dentist-applied flouride treatment is sufficient. Check with your dentist or pediatrician to see how much your child should be getting and in what form.

BEST RESPONSE: "First of all, you should always brush your teeth as soon as possible after eating or drinking anything that could stain them, such as coffee," Dr. Sheets stresses.

"To get rid of the discoloration you already have, try using polishing toothpastes or even baking soda and water for a few days. These can often remove minor staining. If the staining still remains after a few days," she adds, "don't continue. Polishing toothpastes are abrasive and can remove tooth enamel, making your teeth seem even *more* yellow."

And if the color of your teeth troubles you, talk to your dentist. Professional cleaning or bleaching can often remove whatever surface staining you couldn't, although deeper discoloration or intrinsic staining will probably require more heroic measures. Stained teeth might benefit from one of several dental procedures available today.

One is bonding. In this procedure, a plastic material is bonded onto the surface of the discolored tooth or teeth. Bonding materials can be matched to the natural color of your teeth and should last four to seven years.

Another method is laminated veneers, in which a thin plastic shell is fitted onto the tooth. The shell can chip or discolor, though, so its life span may be short.

Porcelain veneers are also available. In this procedure, a half-crown is fitted onto the front of the problem tooth. A small amount of enamel must be removed to make room for the porcelain, then the porcelain is bonded to the tooth. Porcelain veneers do not discolor and generally do not chip as easily as plastic. They also have a long life span.

In extreme cases, a porcelain crown is fitted over the stained tooth. This procedure is expensive, but if it's well fitted, "a crown may last a lifetime and be indistinguishable from a natural tooth," the *British Medical Journal* reports. Unfortunately, the journal adds, "Bad crowning looks unnatural, causes periodontal disease, kills the nerve of the tooth, interferes with the occlusion [the way the teeth in each jaw relate to each other] and often falls off or breaks."

Discuss all of these options carefully with your dentist, advises Dr. Sheets. "Ultimately, you should ask yourself if the aesthetics of white teeth are worth the price. And, of course, only you can decide."

SYMPTOM: **Swelling**

COMMON CAUSES: "Sudden, acute swelling, if it involves only a part of your gums closest to the gum line, may be caused by something as minor as a popcorn hull or other bit of food lodged around your tooth," explains Cherilyn Sheets, D.D.S. "But swelling that outwardly looks like food is impacted could easily be something else."

There are many reasons why gums can swell, says Dr. Sheets. "Certain allergies can cause swelling of the gums, though this is not really common," she says. More often, though, sudden swelling, if it involves the mucosa—the movable tissue that makes up the bulk of the mouth tissue—means you have an abscessed tooth and the infection has broken through the bone to the mouth tissue (see Symptom: Lump).

Of course, swelling of the gums is not always sudden. Sometimes the swelling is, instead, "insidiously slow," says Robert Mallin, D.D.S. And this swelling almost always indicates advancing gum disease. If it's severe enough, the swelling can also mean that the disease is eating away at the bone in the jaw, which is every bit as horrible as it sounds.

Even if the gums are only slightly swollen, even if they bleed only "a bit," they're probably still diseased. "Healthy gums don't swell. Healthy gums don't bleed," Dr. Mallin emphasizes.

You can test the health of your gums, he adds, with a quick, simple home exam. Carefully dry off and look at a small section of your gum. "A healthy gum will appear reddish orange and stippled, like the skin of an orange," explains Dr. Mallin. "Diseased gums, on the other hand, appear smooth, glossy and red, like the skin of an apple."

Swollen gums, however, can also signal something other than gum disease. Impacted or infected wisdom teeth, for example, can cause a localized swelling. Leukemia (see Common Whole Body Conditions in chapter 19) can also cause swelling, accompanied by spontaneous bleeding, and so can oral cancer, although far more rarely.

BEST RESPONSE: "If your gums are swollen, go to your dentist," urges Dr. Sheets. "Swollen gums are one of your mouth's clearest warning signals. They mean something is wrong and that it needs to be treated."

The only exception to this rule involves swelling that you know is caused by food. When bits of food get under your skin, irritating you and your gums, use a toothbrush and a firm brushstroke to dig them out.

"Tooth floss may work the best of all," adds Dr. Sheets. She suggests putting a small knot in the floss before you pull it through your teeth. But she advises against using toothpicks; they are as likely to punch a hole in the gum as to remove the offending food.

SYMPTOM: **Toothache.** *See* Symptom: Pain

SYMPTOM: **White Spots.** *See* Symptom: Sores in chapter 8.

Common Tooth and Gum Conditions

Decay.   Unfortunately, he who eats will also decay—especially in his teeth.

Even though teeth are covered by one of the hardest substances in the body—enamel—acids produced by the action of bacteria on the sugars and carbohydrates you eat will erode the enamel and produce tooth decay. If the decay process isn't stopped, it progresses into the very center of your tooth, where it begins to attack the soft pulpy tissue that contains the tooth's life-giving nerves and blood vessels. That's when the pain makes you wonder if you saw the dentist this year or last year or even the year before that.

Too much sugar in your food is the number one cause of decay, dentists say. And they don't just mean chocolate bars. Recent studies indicate that some foods that are good for you in every other way actually produce the acids that cause cavities. Implicated are granola bars, wheat crackers, soda crackers, snack crackers, raisins, dates and other dried fruits—all the foods that caring parents offer their children instead of candy. Even orange juice, apple cider and grape juice are as cavity provoking as a soft drink, the studies show.

But the way to avoid the decay-causing properties of these foods, researchers say, is to avoid serving them one-on-one as a snack between meals. Eat or drink them only at mealtimes, researchers suggest, preferably with other foods that block acid production, such as aged cheddar, Swiss or Monterey Jack cheese. The idea is to mix up the good and bad foods in your mouth so that the bad food is less likely to attach itself to a tooth.

Another strategy is to provide tooth-friendly foods such as carrots, popcorn, peanuts and celery. But the best defense against tooth decay also includes twice-a-year professional examinations and cleaning, fluoride as applied and recommended by the dentist and what dentists call preventive home care—proper brushing, regular flossing and every-day swishing of a bacteria-killing mouthwash containing fluoride, hydrogen peroxide or chlorhexidine.

But if all fails, especially during the cavity-prone years of 4 to 14, don't despair. Researchers at the University of Alabama at Birmingham report that the more cavities children have in their first set of teeth, the fewer they have in their second.

Besides, having a cavity filled is no longer the horrendous experience it once was. The head-shaking vibration of old-fashioned drills is, along with the high-speed whine of their modern-day cousins, almost a thing of the past. Dentists in Israel, France and other countries are already using lasers to painlessly vaporize decay, while dentists in the United States are beginning to work with a chemical that dissolves it. Soon, researchers report, even your neighborhood dentist should be able to pump a solution of sodium and acid onto a decaying tooth, then brush the decay away.

Gingivitis.   Gingivitis, the first stage in periodontal disease, affects 90 percent of Americans at some time in their lives. Even children are not exempt.

Results from the first National Health and Nutrition Examination Survey indicate that almost four out of every ten children age 12 to 17 have some form of periodontal disease. Other statistics indicate that, by age 13, a full 80 percent of all American children have some degree of gingivitis.

Given this outline of children's gum problems, it should come as no surprise to find that gum disease is the major reason adults lose their teeth. And lose them they do. More than 20 million Americans have lost *all* their teeth, while an additional 14 million have lost either the entire set of uppers or lowers. Almost half of all Americans between the ages of 65 and 74 are toothless.

But tooth loss from gum disease can be avoided, dentists say, if only people would improve their dental hygiene as soon as they notice the inflamed and swollen gums of gingivitis.

Gingivitis is most often caused by plaque, a sticky deposit of mucus, food particles and bacteria that forms at the base of the teeth, along the gum line. It is sometimes, though rarely, caused by a vitamin deficiency, glandular disorders, blood diseases, drugs, stress or even heredity.

Irritation from plaque creates microscopic ulcers at the edge of your gums, researchers explain. The gum becomes infected and swells, and a pocket forms between the gum and a tooth—literally a trap for food particles and bacteria, which then combine with mucus to form plaque.

That's why the key to avoiding the long-term consequences of gingivitis, dentists agree, is to remove the plaque through daily flossing, after-meal brushing and regular cleaning by a dental hygienist.

If the plaque is not removed, it continues to build up and deepen the pocket around the tooth. Bacteria in the pocket attack the bone that surrounds and supports the teeth, and then the teeth become loose and begin to fall out. At this point, you no longer have gingivitis, dentists say, but a disease called periodontitis.

Periodontitis.   Periodontitis is the end result of untreated gingivitis. It's what your dentist writes on the bill when you're about to become one of the 20 million people without teeth.

But periodontitis can be dangerous to more than your molars. People with periodontal disease squirt a shower of oral bacteria into their bloodstream every time they chew. They bite down on a piece of food and the tooth literally pushes the bacteria around it into the bloody gum.

If you have rheumatic heart disease, congenital heart defects, prosthetic heart valves, prosthetic hips or even kidney disease, there's a very real danger that oral bacteria will travel through your bloodstream to settle on diseased or weak tissues, grow into a large colony and kill you.

That's why it's so important to improve your dental hygiene before gingivitis progresses to periodontitis. With good dental hygiene, gingivitis is reversible. Periodontitis is not.

But even though it's not reversible, you can stop periodontitis right in its tracks. You begin a vigorous program of brushing and flossing, as well as rinsing your mouth with a bacteria-killing mouthwash containing fluoride, hydrogen peroxide or chlorhexidine. And you can see your dentist frequently so that he or she can spot problems that encourage the growth of plaque. Your dentist can also shore up loose teeth, trim diseased gums to reduce bacteria-laden pockets and even bond synthetic material to teeth where the outer coverings have worn away.

You may not be able to regain the sharp-pointed mashers and grinders of your childhood. But with vigilant hygiene and professional help, you *should* be able to keep your beautiful smile.

Chapter 17
Throat

SEE YOUR DOCTOR IMMEDIATELY IF:
- *You have a cough that just won't go away*
- *You have a lump in your neck that lasts longer than two weeks*
- *Your throat feels swollen or as though you have a lump in it*
- *You can't open your mouth or you have difficulty swallowing*
- *You have a sore throat and a high fever—105°F*

Your throat is more than a passageway for rude noises, mashed potatoes and air. It's also a finely tuned defense mechanism that traps hostile germs.

Packed with a ring of infection-fighting tissue above, below and on both sides, it shoots down germs and frequently prevents them from going on to bigger and better things, like the lungs. Its main defensive weapons are the tonsils and—in children—the adenoids, which are positioned almost as though they're guarding the throat's entrance.

But sometimes the body's defenses are overwhelmed. The result is usually a sore and infected throat that can spread upward, downward or even in both directions at once. But there are plenty of other problems that can get you by the throat—in which case you and your doctor are going to get to know one another very well.

SYMPTOM: **Choking**

COMMON CAUSES: Choking can be triggered by anything from thick mucus to a roast beef sandwich. Eighty percent of inhaled or swallowed foreign bodies occur in children under age 15—usually because they are careless or surprised or unconscious when holding something in their mouth.

In adults, choking is usually triggered by food or bones that become stuck in the throat from eating too quickly or eating with dentures that

424

don't fit properly. Nearly 3,000 people choke to death each year because of something stuck in the throat.

BEST RESPONSE: If you are sitting next to someone in a restaurant who cannot speak, cough or breathe because food is lodged somewhere in his or her throat, try the Heimlich maneuver, says Kenneth Grundfast, M.D., chairman of the Department of Otolaryngology at Children's Hospital National Medical Center in Washington, D.C.

Grab the person in a bear hug from behind, make a fist and place the thumb side of your fist against the person's abdomen, slightly above the navel and below the rib cage. Then cover your fist with your other hand and use it to *press your fist into the person's abdomen with a quick upward thrust.* Repeat if necessary. Dr. Grundfast says this maneuver, which was named for the doctor who invented it, must be performed within four minutes or the person who is choking may die.

If you're alone and you start choking, adds Dr. Grundfast, lean over the edge of a hard (but not pointed!) table or chair and use it to provide the quick upward thrust.

Either way, the Heimlich maneuver works by suddenly compressing the lungs and increasing air pressure all the way up to the obstruction. The pressure then pops the object out of the throat, the same way a cork pops out of a champagne bottle.

Children *more* than a year old who are choking can also be helped by the Heimlich maneuver, says American Red Cross safety instructor C. P. Dail. If the infant is *less* than a year old, place the child over your arm in a head-down position and strike sharply four times between the shoulder blades with the heel of your other hand. If that technique doesn't work, turn the child over, supporting the head, and press down on the sternum—the hard bone found in the middle of your baby's chest—with two fingers positioned a finger's width below the midline of the nipples. If this doesn't work, try the procedure over again. The Heimlich maneuver is not recommended for infants. It's too easy to hurt a vital organ.

SYMPTOM: **Coughing**

COMMON CAUSES: Coughing can be caused by a foreign object lodged somewhere in the throat or lungs, a postnasal drip triggered by an allergy, a chemical irritant such as cigarette smoke or a variety of infections ranging from influenza (see Common Whole Body Conditions in chapter 19) and sinusitis (see Common Nasal Conditions in chapter 13) to pneumonia (see Common Circulatory, Heart and Lung Conditions in chapter 5) and tuberculosis.

Less frequently, a cough may be caused by a blood clot or tumor in the lung or even—should you be responsible for cleaning the chicken coop—an infestation of mold from the little chickies' droppings.

BEST RESPONSE: Never ignore a cough. Coughs are the body's way of getting rid of anything in the airway that doesn't belong there, whether it be smoke or soup or soap.

A "productive" cough—one in which mucus or some other substance is brought up out of the throat or lungs—is actually helping you by clearing possible obstructions from your airway. A "smoker's cough" is a good example of a productive cough. Many doctors suggest that you leave productive coughs alone or even help loosen secretions further by drinking extra fluids.

But an "unproductive" cough—one that never brings anything up—rarely does anybody any good. It just keeps you up all night. So get rid of it. "There are so many cough preparations on the market," says Kenneth Grundfast, M.D., "that it is hard to choose the best cough medicine. But there are two pharmacologic agents that help suppress coughs: dextromethorphan is one, and codeine is the other."

You'll probably need a prescription for codeine, but dextromethorphan is available over the counter under 50 different brand names. Cough suppressants should not, of course, be taken by people with asthma or chronic bronchitis (see chronic obstructive lung disease under Common Circulatory, Heart and Lung Conditions in chapter 5). And any cough that lasts longer than a few days should be evaluated by a doctor.

ACCOMPANYING SYMPTOMS: If you experience shortness of breath with an unproductive cough, if you cough up blood or if you cough up blood and have chest pain, see your doctor. You may have an undetected heart or lung disorder that requires immediate attention.

If your child has a harsh, barking cough, possibly accompanied by hoarseness and difficulty breathing, he or she could have croup (see

Common Circulatory, Heart and Lung Conditions in chapter 5). Check with your doctor.

SYMPTOM: **Hoarseness**

COMMON CAUSES: Hoarseness is either trivial or serious. There's nothing in between. It can be caused by an inflammation of the voice box (see laryngitis under Common Throat Conditions), by yelling too loudly and for too long, or by a cyst, swelling or cancer. It can be caused by an underactive thyroid (see thyroid disease under Common Whole Body Conditions in chapter 19), a cold, tobacco smoke, infection or stress, or by leprosy, growths or a weak, swollen artery. Growths can be benign, malignant or precancerous and occur mostly in men. Cancer of the voice box is almost exclusively restricted to smokers.

For the clergy, schoolteachers and entertainers, hoarseness is an occupational hazard.

BEST RESPONSE: If you become hoarse, says Kenneth Grundfast, M.D., your best response is to relax. "Don't try to whisper; just speak with a relaxed type of voice," he advises. "And sometimes voice rest is helpful. If you're in a busy environment that requires the use of your voice, just take a few days off."

Hoarseness that does not go away within two weeks is your tip-off that it's caused by something more serious than drinking or yelling. The effects of a Saturday night rock concert or a Monday night football game should disappear by Wednesday morning. If they don't, see your doctor. Even serious throat diseases such as cancer can be treated if they're detected early enough.

ACCOMPANYING SYMPTOMS: If you're hoarse and are also experiencing difficulty in swallowing and/or chest pain, see your doctor immediately.

SYMPTOM: **Soreness**

COMMON CAUSES: Most sore throats are caused by viral or bacterial infections (see pharyngitis under Common Throat Conditions) that are triggered by everything from the infamous strep of childhood to the notorious sexually transmitted diseases that haunt adulthood. One study of 763 adults with sore throats, for example, revealed that nearly one-third were infected with the organisms that cause pneumonia and chlamydia, a venereal disease.

Sore throats are also caused by irritation from tobacco smoke, certain foods, allergies, cancer or an injury. Bones, corn chips, potato chips and tacos, for example, can literally make small tears in the throat.

BEST RESPONSE: For throat pain due to infections, allergies or tobacco, any of the throat lozenges or sprays available over the counter that contain a local anesthetic such as benzocaine will reduce the soreness and pain, says Kenneth Grundfast, M.D. Frequent swallowing often helps as well, so be sure to drink plenty of liquids. But avoid orange juice, Dr. Grundfast warns. It's too acidic and can actually make your sore throat worse.

Saltwater gargles—two teaspoons of salt to a quart of warm water—may also reduce the pain, and increasing the humidity of your environment is usually helpful. "Turn up your humidifier until you can see moisture collecting on your windows," says Dr. Grundfast. "Then turn it down just a bit." Otherwise you'll have moldy oldies on your walls that can make your throat even worse.

Acetaminophen (Tylenol) may also relieve the pain, but if the pain is severe or if your sore throat lasts more than three or four days, it may have become infected by bacteria—even if it started out as a viral infection. Or it may have started out as a bacterial infection and it's just getting worse. In either case, you probably need an antibiotic. That's why any sore throat that lasts more than a few days should be examined by a doctor, who will take either a throat culture or a blood count. These are the best ways to determine what kind of germ caused your sore throat and what kind of antibiotic will kill it.

And remember, an untreated bacterial sore throat that's caused by streptococcus bacteria can, in as little time as a week, lead to complications such as rheumatic fever (see Common Whole Body Conditions in chapter 19).

If your throat feels scratchy because you just swallowed a piece of chicken bone, don't panic. To help the offending object along, some doctors suggest you eat one or two mouthfuls from the center of a soft slice of bread and wash it down with a drink of water. If you still have the sensation that something's in your throat, have your doctor take a look.

ACCOMPANYING SYMPTOMS: If you notice white spots on your tonsils or the sides of your throat, see your doctor. It's a sign that your sore throat is getting worse. You should also see your doctor if your sore throat is accompanied by a fever of 105°F.

If you have a sore throat and lose part or all of your voice, you probably have laryngitis (see Common Throat Conditions).

SYMPTOM: **Throat Clearing**

COMMON CAUSES: Throat clearing is usually the result of an allergy (see Common Nasal Conditions in chapter 13) that turns the postnasal faucet on to drip. It's also caused by nervousness and anxiety, or even the remnants of laryngitis (see Common Throat Conditions).

BEST RESPONSE: The best way to clear your throat once and for all if an allergy is causing excessive mucus is to get rid of the allergen. And laryngitis will disappear when your laryngitis bug decides to walk.

But if you're one of those people who constantly clears the throat with little "umph-umphs" every third sentence, the treatment is a little more complicated. The problem is that what seems to be an innocuous little habit is actually a nervous tic—just like blinking your eyes, grimacing, shaking your head, swallowing, jerking your thigh or shrugging your shoulder. Sometimes these tics are carried out in a pattern, such as shaking the head and then shrugging the shoulder. Sometimes they exist by themselves. But in either case they're usually a sign that you're having difficulty coping with some part of your life.

So how can you stop a nervous tic? The answer, say many doctors, is to figure out what part of your life is driving you nuts and then change it. If you hate making speeches, for example, don't tell the women's auxiliary that you'll be happy to introduce the main speaker at its next banquet. Let someone else do the honors. Or if the crowded aisles and spiraling prices of your supermarket get you uptight, ask a neighbor or other family member to trade shopping tasks every once in a while.

And find time for yourself. Tranquilizers don't really get rid of nervous tics such as throat clearing, but learning to relax can reduce the level of anxiety that triggers them. One relaxation exercise, for example, developed by a professor at Yale, can relax your whole body in seconds. Just sit down and allow your head and shoulders to droop gently forward. Let your chin hang toward your chest and take a deep breath. Then smile. You may feel so relaxed that you'll find yourself chuckling at the absurdity of it all.

And learn to share your problems. A neighbor over the back fence, a coworker at the next desk—everyone has similar problems. Remember, nothing's certain except death and taxes. Everything else is negotiable.

SYMPTOM: **Tickle**

COMMON CAUSES: Allergies and viruses seem to tickle the tonsils, or sometimes the sensation is actually an irritation caused by swallowing something hard or sharp.

BEST RESPONSE: Eat. Some doctors suggest that eating bland foods such as cooked rice along with a few sips of water will kill your tickle.

SYMPTOM: **Voice Change**

COMMON CAUSES: Other than the one at puberty, most voice changes occur in response to excessive yelling (see Symptom: Hoarseness), infections, aging, antihistamines, excessively dry air, anxiety or cancer. But if you don't smoke or drink, don't worry about cancer.

"In adults who neither smoke nor drink, cancer of the mouth and throat are nearly nonexistent," says Jerome C. Goldstein, M.D., executive vice-president of the American Academy of Otolaryngology—Head and Neck Surgery.

BEST RESPONSE: Rest and relaxation plus a little humidity may well do the trick, advises Kenneth Grundfast, M.D. But if your voice doesn't return to normal within two or three weeks, check with your doctor. And if you *suddenly* lose your voice, check with your doctor right away.

"People don't wake up without a voice," says Dr. Grundfast. "They wake up and it's a little hoarse and it gets worse and worse until finally they can't talk. But when somebody just loses their voice, it's usually hysterical," meaning the reason for the voice loss is more likely to be psychological than physiological. A little professional guidance may be necessary.

Common Throat Conditions

Laryngitis.   Laryngitis is an inflammation of the voice box—the part of your throat just behind where you can feel a bump with your fingers. It's caused by various infections, such as colds, sinusitis, bronchitis, flu, pneumonia, whooping cough, syphilis and measles, as well as by inhaling irritating chemicals.

Chronic laryngitis is usually caused by constantly inhaling industrial dusts or chemicals, although it can also be caused by thickened vocal cords or smoking. Generally, doctors will advise you to rest your body and your voice, avoid smoking and alcohol and drink lots of liquids. You may also want to avoid places where you'll inhale lots of dust. A well-ventilated and well-humidified area will probably make you feel more comfortable.

Laryngitis usually disappears within a week. If it doesn't, see your doctor.

Pharyngitis.   Pharyngitis is the $25 word your doctor may put on your bill after commiserating with you over your sore throat, because pharyngitis is nothing more—or less—than an inflammation of the throat. It is usually caused by colds, tonsillitis, adenoiditis or sinusitis. When caused by a virus, it's usually gone within three to six days. When caused by bacteria, it's likely to hang around until shot down by a fusillade of antibiotics.

To determine whether your sore throat is triggered by a viral or bacterial agent—particularly the strep bacteria that can cause heart, kidney and nervous system problems—your doctor will probably do a throat culture, a test in which he or she rubs a swab against the back of your throat and your tonsils. The substance on the swab is then analyzed to determine what's growing in your throat and what will kill it.

Quinsy.   Quinsy, which is also called a peritonsillar abscess, is an abscess painfully snuggled in between a tonsil and the side of the throat. It is usually indicated by fever, a large swelling on the affected side, severe pain, difficulty in swallowing and the inability to open your jaw. The uvula—that elongated teardrop of tissue hanging down into your mouth—is usually swollen, as are the lymph nodes on either side of your neck.

Quinsy can prevent breathing and swallowing. If you suspect you have it, seek medical help at once.

Strep throat.   *See* Pharyngitis.

Tonsillitis.   If you look in the mirror and open your mouth, you can see what appear to be lumpy bulges on either side of your throat. Those are your tonsils. Tonsillitis is an inflammation of the tonsils, usually in response to a viral or bacterial invasion. Years ago, doctors surgically removed tonsils as a matter of course. Today, they don't.

Generally, tonsillitis strikes hardest during two peak periods of childhood: between ages 3 and 7 and between ages 12 and 13. But it also occurs in adulthood. The tonsils are generally removed only if tonsillitis occurs several times a year. Just how many times is a matter of controversy, but many doctors seem to feel that if tonsillitis strikes between four and seven times each year, you should think about having the tonsils removed.

If you suspect you have tonsillitis, check with your doctor, who will probably want to do a throat culture. In this test, the doctor runs a swab along the inside of the throat and tonsils. The substance on the swab is then analyzed to determine what's causing the infection. If it is caused by bacteria, your doctor will probably prescribe an antibiotic. If it's caused by a virus, your doctor will probably tell you to go home, go to bed and reach for the acetaminophen (Tylenol).

Chapter 18
Urinary Tract

SEE YOUR DOCTOR IMMEDIATELY IF:
- *You're unable to urinate*
- *You see blood in your urine*

There are some things in life we all take for granted, and going to the bathroom is surely one of them. But our own very personal experiences can remind us that starting and stopping the flow of urine is not always a well-controlled activity.

There's a good reason for it. There are 12 known reflexes associated with storing and excreting urine, and something can go wrong with any one of them at any time, anywhere.

So here's a rundown on what can impair your bathroom skills—and how you can get them fixed.

SYMPTOM: **Bed-wetting**

COMMON CAUSES: Bed-wetting is usually a subtle neurological problem related to sleep disorders such as sleepwalking or night terrors. It is rarely a urinary problem. And it is seldom behavioral or psychological. It is not under a child's active control, nor is there any way a child can decide to urinate when asleep—as one popular myth goes—to "punish" his or her parents.

"Bed-wetting seems to be caused by a neurological immaturity," says Bryan P. Shumaker, M.D., a urologist at Henry Ford Hospital in Detroit. "It occurs as children move from deeper to lighter levels of sleep, and it tends to run in families."

BEST RESPONSE: Maturity usually puts an end to bed-wetting, says Dr. Shumaker. "It's not necessary to put kids through fancy x-rays and bladder exams."

433

But check with your doctor to rule out any unlikely organic problems, such as a spinal injury. Then be patient and just wait for your child to grow up, advises Dr. Shumaker. Fifteen percent of all bed-wetters outgrow the condition with each passing year. By puberty—somewhere between ages 12 and 14—most have stopped wetting.

If your child (or you) isn't willing to wait until his or her body matures naturally, however, you can try what's generally called a "wetting pad," says Dr. Shumaker. The wetting pad is a small pad that fits inside your child's underwear. When the first drop of urine touches it, a buzzer goes off. But the buzzer is to wake *you*—not your child. Then you can get the child to the bathroom.

Eventually, the child will learn to wake up when the buzzer goes off, and maybe even *before* it goes off. But a child can slip back into wetness even after being trained, cautions Dr. Shumaker, and you should use the pad only if you're willing to be patient.

Another option is a drug called Tofranil that your doctor can prescribe. It works by causing lighter sleep for a longer period of time, says Dr. Shumaker, the same effect caused by sleeping in a strange bed. In fact, he says, "many times a parent will come in and tell me how a mother or mother-in-law always claimed that the child never wet at Grandma's house. And that's probably true. But it was true because the strange bed or couch kept the child in a lighter state of sleep," not because Grandma was a better guardian.

If you do decide to go the drug route, Dr. Shumaker cautions, periodically halt the medication to see if the bed-wetting has stopped on its own.

And if you do decide to interfere with your child's natural course of development with buzzers or drugs, think about the message you're sending to your child. As Gilbert Simon, M.D., reports in his book *The Parents' Pediatric Companion,* "even when these methods make the child dry, there's still the danger of fostering an impression that the child is somehow defective, sick or incompletely developed and in need of other people or things to make him normal."

Instead, Dr. Simon prefers actively involving the child in methods used to control his or her *own* problem: for example, setting an alarm clock for half an hour before the usual wetting time, marking a calendar on bed-wetting days or getting the child to wash his or her own sheets.

SYMPTOM: **Incontinence**

COMMON CAUSES: "Occasional incontinence, the inability to maintain bladder control, is normal in a woman," says Richard J. Macchia, M.D., acting chairman of the Department of Urology at the State University of New York Health Science Center at Brooklyn, "because the continence (urinating) mechanism is very inefficient.

"We did a study, for example, a long time ago. My predecessor told one of the residents that even young women who have never been pregnant sometimes lose their urine. The resident didn't believe it. So he went over to a nurses' hall with a questionnaire and found a whole bunch of student nurses who had never had children. He also found that over 50 percent of these young, healthy women experienced an occasional loss of urine."

Men have less of a problem, adds Dr. Macchia, partly because a man's urethra, the tube leading to the urinary opening, is so much longer than a woman's and partly because the prostate gland, which surrounds the urethra, can help pinch the urethra shut when it's needed.

But incontinence can and does happen to both sexes. "The most common kind is urge incontinence," says Dr. Macchia. "You get an urge to go to the bathroom and can't get to the bathroom in time—maybe because the urgency is produced by an infection or maybe because you have arthritis and your feet have a hard time moving as fast as your bladder.

"The second most common type is stress incontinence. As men and women get older, the pelvic muscles—the ones you use to start and stop your urine—tend to relax," says Dr. Macchia. This is especially true if you're a woman who has had children or a man or woman who has gained weight. When you put added stress on your bladder by picking up a package, laughing or sneezing, the muscles aren't strong enough to keep the opening of your urethra closed.

The bladder is a muscle controlled by nerves. That's why neurologic diseases such as multiple sclerosis and Parkinson's disease or diabetes mellitus can make you incontinent. So can hyperactive muscle contractions or an abnormal growth of tissue.

However, "one important cause of incontinence in men is a

prostatectomy," adds Dr. Macchia. "The prostate sits very close to the continence mechanism, and sometimes even in the most experienced hands the removal of the prostate damages the continence mechanism."

BEST RESPONSE: An active exercise program aimed at strengthening your pelvic muscles, doctors say, can often cure mild incontinence. Contract the muscles that start and stop urination 25 to 50 times, repeating the exercise twice a day. Work up to 100 repetitions, doctors suggest, and do more if possible.

And limit your fluid intake, particularly caffeine-containing liquids such as coffee, tea and colas, while you increase the frequency of urination to every two or three hours. Don't wait for your bladder to tell you it's time to go; just go.

But you also need to see your doctor for an accurate diagnosis. If you're an older woman, for example, sometimes a course of estrogen pills will increase your ability to contract the muscles involved in holding your urine. Or sometimes a pessary, a device that's inserted through the vagina and wedged against the uterus, will shore up a droopy bladder.

If the problem is caused by an infection, a change in medication—sedatives, muscle relaxants and high blood pressure drugs, for example, can trigger or exacerbate urinary incontinence—or even surgery, you may need antibiotics.

Surgery is still a common solution to stress incontinence—with success rates between 57 and 96 percent, depending on the procedure used—but new research may provide nonsurgical alternatives in highly selective cases.

In one study, researchers used biofeedback techniques to treat incontinence in 39 people between the ages of 60 and 86. Nineteen of the study participants had stress incontinence, 12 had a hyperactive bladder and 8 had urge incontinence. Each attended one to eight biofeedback sessions, in which their bladders were filled with fluid through a catheter and bladder pressure was measured by a polygraph tracing that the participant could see. Watching the tracing and associating it with what they felt inside, participants literally trained themselves to improve bladder control.

The researchers also taught these volunteers various skills designed to improve their control when biofeedback equipment was not available. For example, those with stress incontinence alternated ten-second periods of muscle contraction with ten-second periods of muscle relaxation to learn how to contract and hold bladder muscles during three or four coughs. Those with hyperactive bladders who experienced involuntary bladder contractions learned to strengthen the pelvic floor muscles with stopping and starting exercises, and those with urge incontinence learned not to rush to the toilet when they felt an urge to urinate. Rushing increased pressure on the bladder, researchers found, so participants were trained to pause, relax their abdomen and proceed at a normal pace to the toilet, using the pelvic floor muscles to prevent incontinence.

After an average of 3½ training sessions, participants with stress incontinence reduced the number of times they were incontinent by 82 percent. Participants with weak bladders showed an average 85 percent improvement and participants with urge incontinence reduced their problem by an average of 94 percent. Moreover, the researchers report, 13 of the study participants were no longer incontinent at all, and an additional 19 had fewer than one accident per week.

SYMPTOM: **Swelling**

COMMON CAUSES: In an uncircumcised male, says Richard J. Macchia, M.D., swelling of the urinary outlet usually indicates an infection involving the foreskin and the cavity underneath.

For anyone, it's frequently your first warning that diabetes mellitus (see Common Whole Body Conditions in chapter 19) may be developing.

BEST RESPONSE: See your physician as soon as possible, says Dr. Macchia. If it's an infection, antibiotics are necessary to clear it up. If your doctor suspects diabetes, he or she will probably want you to take a glucose tolerance test.

SYMPTOM: **Urination, Burning during**

COMMON CAUSES: People, particularly women, frequently complain about a burning pain during urination. It signals a urinary tract infection. But in many patients, no infection can be found, says Richard J. Macchia, M.D. In such cases, he says, it's quite common to find no cause at all.

Sometimes the urinary tract is affected by a neighboring problem. "What appears to be a bladder problem," says Dr. Macchia, "is actually the first indication of a bowel or a gynecological problem."

Crohn's disease (see Common Abdominal and Digestive System Conditions in chapter 1) is one example. Since the bowel is very near the bladder, says Dr. Macchia, the irritation that hallmarks the disease sometimes spreads from the bowel to the bladder. All three systems are located together in the pelvis, Dr. Macchia points out, so it's easy for them to affect one another. Sexually transmitted diseases (see Common Reproductive System Conditions in chapter 14) can cause a burning sensation for the same reason.

BEST RESPONSE: "If the burning sensation is from a urinary tract infection," says Dr. Macchia, "the infection might be very transient—especially in the case of women. Women frequently clear the urine infection themselves simply by voiding (urinating). They flush out the bladder."

That doesn't mean that drinking lots of water to frequently flush your bladder will kill an infection, adds Dr. Macchia. What might help, however, is to acidify your urine by taking two 500-milligram tablets of vitamin C each day. He says that should make most of the germs in your bladder pack their bags.

But, he adds, "if the burning lasts a day and you wake up the next morning with it, go see a doctor." You may have a sexually transmitted disease or a bladder or bowel problem that requires medication.

ACCOMPANYING SYMPTOMS: Burning accompanied by itching may also indicate infection or inflammation of the urethra, whereas burning and a fever may indicate that you have a urinary tract infection (see Common Urinary Tract Conditions) that also involves the kidney. Check with your doctor as soon as possible.

SYMPTOM: **Urination, Frequent**

COMMON CAUSES: A healthy adult will usually excrete around 50 ounces of urine in a 24-hour period, divided among four to six occasions, none of which are after bedtime.

The number of times you run to the bathroom and the amount you urinate varies according to how much fluid you drink and how much fluid you lose—either through sweat, vomit or diarrhea. It also depends on the amount of caffeinated beverages or alcohol you consume, since both make your kidneys work overtime. Even how cold the weather is or how excited you get about your life makes a difference.

But when you take all that into consideration and you still seem to urinate too frequently, the cause could be cystitis, a urinary tract infection, bladder stones, kidney failure or pyelonephritis (see Common Urinary Tract Conditions); a prolapsed uterus (see Symptom: Bulge, Vaginal in chapter 14); diabetes insipidus (see Common Whole Body Conditions in chapter 19); an enlarged prostate; a vaginal infection; or an inflammation of the urethra.

"Of the 50 or so causes of frequent urination, the most common is a urinary tract infection," says Richard J. Macchia, M.D. "Another common cause is anxiety and stress. One also has to be worried about cancer— prostate cancer or bladder cancer especially—as well as a blockage of the urinary tract."

And don't forget medications. "Some medications can irritate the bladder," adds Dr. Macchia. "They can do virtually anything from causing more urine to causing urination frequency to accelerating the urine flow."

BEST RESPONSE: Fortunately, most of the infections, inflammations and irritations can be cleared up by antibiotics, doctors say. So you need to see your physician.

And let the doctor know what medications you've been taking, advises Dr. Macchia. "One of the things that any doctor should do is review them," he says. Your whole problem might be triggered by the seemingly insignificant ingredient in a drug you're taking for a completely different problem.

SYMPTOM: **Urination, Nighttime**

COMMON CAUSES: Getting up to go to the bathroom in the middle of the night may be more than a royal pain. It can also indicate the presence of chronic glomerulonephritis or cystitis (see Common Urinary Tract Conditions); prostatitis (see Common Reproductive System

Conditions in chapter 14); diabetes insipidus or diabetes mellitus (see Common Whole Body Conditions in chapter 19); a kidney infection; an enlarged prostate; anxiety or urinary retention.

"There are many causes for going to the bathroom at night," says Richard J. Macchia, M.D., "but there is also a psychological cause that's very strong. The urinary tract can be an end organ for anxiety—even if you don't think you are anxious. At every age it seems as though you have to have an orifice to worry about!"

BEST RESPONSE: "The question is, are you getting up in order to urinate or are you simply urinating because you're up?" asks Dr. Macchia.

If you wake up and go to the bathroom out of habit or because you feel bored and have nothing else to do, that's one thing, says Dr. Macchia. "But if you get up because you've got to urinate, see your doctor so he or she can establish a diagnosis."

SYMPTOM: **Urine, Changes in Flow of**

COMMON CAUSES: "Voiding [urinating] is a very complicated, coordinated thing," says Richard J. Macchia, M.D. "The urine is made up in the kidneys, then passes down through two little ureters [tubes] and into the bladder. The bladder is supposed to store the urine. It's supposed to keep it sterile and prevent it from refluxing back into the kidneys. And it's supposed to give you a signal for when it's time to urinate.

"Then, when you go to urinate, a coordinated series of events is supposed to occur: The bladder contracts downward and the sphincter muscle at the bottom of the bladder, which controls the outflow like a guardian at the front door, is supposed to open."

But sometimes the door malfunctions. Sometimes it stays shut, says Dr. Macchia, and sometimes it opens only a little. That's when the urine slows, the stream becomes weak or thin and sometimes you even dribble.

"Sometimes we don't find the cause," says Dr. Macchia honestly. "We just know that the bladder—for whatever reason—is not functioning properly."

Sometimes in men, however, a change in urine flow is caused by an enlarged prostate gland, cancer, a narrowed urethra (the tube leading from the bladder through the penis) or even a weakened bladder.

In women, says Dr. Macchia, the cause is usually a weakened bladder or a prolapsed uterus (see Symptom: Bulge, Vaginal in chapter 14), although extreme constipation, a little outpouching or bulge in the urethra or a narrowed urethra also pop up every once in a while.

"There is also something called the 'infrequent voider syndrome,'" says Dr. Macchia, "and it starts with young girls. Some girls, for whatever reason, tend not to go to the bathroom very often. And everybody thinks, 'Gee, this is a nice little girl; she doesn't have to go to the bathroom.' What happens over the years is that the bladder distends and—just like any other muscle you overstretch—it decompresses and becomes inefficient in voiding."

Little boys (and their grown-up counterparts) also have a bathroom problem called "bashful bladder syndrome"—the inability to initiate urination in the company of others. It is exacerbated, doctors say, when the person is confronted by a wall of urinals.

BEST RESPONSE: "If you notice a significant change in urine flow, see your doctor," advises Dr. Macchia. The doctor will talk to you, give you a physical exam and ask for a urine specimen. Sometimes your urologist will also want to do a cystoscopy, which is an internal examination of your urethra and bladder with a telescopic type of device about the width of a pencil.

A cystoscopic examination is done in the office, says Dr. Macchia, and for most women it's not an uncomfortable procedure because the urethra is so short—not much longer than an inch. Men are a different story. "Half the men can take it comfortably, and half need either general or spinal anesthesia," Dr. Macchia says.

Not all changes in urine flow need treatment, says Dr. Macchia. Only in severe cases where the change in flow really annoys you or makes life difficult does a doctor need to step in. Of course, there are exceptions to every rule. If an enlarged prostate causes urine to back up into the kidneys and damage them, says Dr. Macchia, you might want to consider surgery.

But a "bashful bladder" has the easiest solution of all, according to two Georgetown University doctors. When you're in a situation that normally causes a problem, the doctors suggest that you mentally calculate the multiplication tables in serial order, and everything will come out all right.

ACCOMPANYING SYMPTOMS: If you find it both difficult and painful to urinate, see your doctor. You may have prostatitis (see Common Reproductive System Conditions in chapter 14) or a urinary tract infection (see Common Urinary Tract Conditions) that requires an antibiotic.

If you pass less urine than usual, then begin to lose your appetite, feel increasingly nauseated and begin to vomit, see your doctor immediately. You may have a kidney problem that requires hospital treatment. The same is true if you pass significantly less urine than usual or stop urinating completely.

If you see blood in your urine—visible as a red or brown color—see your doctor.

SYMPTOM: **Urine, Discolored**

COMMON CAUSES: Normal urine can look different every day, says Richard J. Macchia, M.D. "The usual color ranges from crystal clear to a deep yellow. The color depends on a number of things, including your state of hydration. If you drink a lot, your urine becomes colorless. If you don't drink a lot, it comes out a deeper yellow."

Unusual colors, however, can be triggered by certain foods, medications and diseases. Red or brown urine, for example, frequently indicates blood. It's caused by such diseases as pyelonephritis, glomerulonephritis or kidney stones (see Common Urinary Tract Conditions); hemolytic anemia (see anemia under Common Whole Body Conditions in chapter 19); hepatitis (see Common Abdominal and Digestive System Conditions in chapter 1) or even tumors.

It also can be caused by eating beets. Fortunately, there is a quick way to tell whether the redness is caused by beets or by blood. Sprinkle a little baking soda into the urine. If the red goes away, then returns when you add a few drops of vinegar, you can be certain that beets—and not disease—caused the red. Be aware, however, that most people who react to beets by getting red urine are usually iron deficient.

Sometimes it seems as though your urine can turn any color in the rainbow. Antibiotics, carrots and spinach can turn it bright orange, for example, while antidepressants and anti-inflammatory drugs can turn it green. Pus, which indicates infection, can make it look milky.

BEST RESPONSE: "If you notice anything abnormal, see a physician," says Dr. Macchia. "If your urine is red, go right away. Blood in the urine in an adult is a tumor until proven otherwise, even though only somewhere between 5 and 20 percent of those who have blood in their urine are going to have one."

SYMPTOM: **Urine, Odorous**

COMMON CAUSES: "Urine is supposed to be sterile in the bladder," says Richard J. Macchia, M.D., and essentially without any odor. So, foul-smelling urine, unless it's been stagnating in a diaper or a toilet bowl for a few hours, is probably caused by a urinary tract infection (see Common Urinary Tract Conditions).

Sweet-smelling urine is usually caused by diabetes mellitus (see Common Whole Body Conditions in chapter 19). In people who already know they're diabetic, it indicates that their diabetes is not being properly treated.

BEST RESPONSE: See your doctor, says Dr. Macchia, who will probably prescribe antibiotics, if your problem is infection. Drinking large quantities of water may relieve your symptoms until you do.

Common Urinary Tract Conditions

Bladder stones. *See* Urinary tract stones

Cystitis. Cystitis is an inflammation of the bladder that has been caused by a urinary tract infection. It is common in women and uncommon in men, and it is usually indicated by a frequent urge to urinate, a burning pain when you do and blood in the urine.

Fortunately, drinking large quantities of water, emptying your bladder immediately after sexual intercourse, wiping yourself from front to back after a bowel movement and taking antibiotics will usually solve the problem.

Glomerulonephritis.   The most common form of nephritis, glomeru-lonephritis is an inflammation of the kidney that can follow an upper respiratory tract strep infection. The infection itself doesn't seem to cause the inflammation, although doctors suspect that the inflammation is an allergic reaction to a substance thrown off by the strep bacteria.

Unfortunately, the inflammation can damage your kidneys' glomeruli, which are clusters of renal capillaries that filter chemicals and metabolic waste products out of your blood. And when the glomeruli can't do their job, red blood cells leak through them into your urine, along with small amounts of protein. If the glomeruli are severely damaged, you may also feel generally unwell, with drowsiness, nausea and vomiting. Your body may swell with accumulated fluids, particularly around your ankles, and you will probably produce only small amounts of urine as your kidneys begin to fail.

Fortunately, many forms of glomerulonephritis are so mild that your doctor won't do anything but identify them. Other forms respond to steroid and cytotoxic drugs, but the use of diuretics—drugs that increase the amount of fluid excreted by your body—to control swelling is somewhat controversial. Iron, vitamins, medication to reduce your blood pressure and antibiotics to quickly squelch any new strep infec-tions can also help your kidneys fight off further inflammation.

Kidney failure.   Kidney failure is sometimes the result of mild, repeated inflammations that have scarred your kidneys. The attacks may have been triggered by pyelonephritis, glomerulonephritis, kidney stones, chronic excessive use of painkillers such as phenacetin, or even high blood pressure. Drinking large quantities of beer has also been known to cause it. Since one function of your kidneys is to control blood pressure, chronic kidney failure can cause high blood pressure as well as be triggered by it.

Kidney failure is usually indicated by frequent urination and lethargy. That's because the kidneys, which are supposed to filter waste products and chemicals out of your blood and send them on to the bladder for excretion, can no longer do their job. They can't limit the amount of water you excrete, nor can they clean out your blood.

If you have kidney failure, your doctor may suggest you eat low-protein foods, take iron and vitamin supplements, drink several pints of fluid a day and avoid any over-the-counter medications. There is no cure for kidney failure, doctors say, but the disease can be more closely controlled with this kind of treatment and close medical monitoring.

Three out of every four people who develop kidney failure will eventually progress to end-stage kidney failure, a condition in which the kidneys can no longer sustain life. If this happens to you, your doctor may recommend dialysis, a procedure repeated two or three times a week in which blood is pumped out of a vein into a blood-cleaning machine, then back to another vein. Or your doctor may even suggest a kidney transplant.

Fortunately, dialysis and transplantation have enabled more than half of those with end-stage kidney failure to lead comparatively normal lives for many years after the condition begins. Occasionally, a problem called dialysis dementia—a condition in which those on dialysis become dizzy, lose some of their memory and think they're somewhere other than on terra firma—develops, but researchers have discovered that one cause may be a biotin deficiency, which is easily remedied by adding the deficient vitamin to the diet.

Kidney stones.   *See* Urinary tract stones

Pyelonephritis.   Pyelonephritis is an inflammation of the kidney and its pelvis. The infection can occasionally be carried by your blood from another part of your body to your kidneys, but it usually comes from bacteria that work their way up the urethra, through the bladder, up the ureters and into the kidneys. The bacteria usually cause a urinary tract infection along the way that may go unnoticed, but when it hits your kidneys, it may be hard to ignore.

If you have pain—only half of those with pyelonephritis do—it is generally in your back, just above the waist. It spreads around the side of your body and down into your groin. It may occur on both sides, but one side is usually worse, and your temperature rapidly rises, often to 104°F. You may also feel like urinating constantly, even when your bladder is empty, and the process itself is likely to be uncomfortable. Your urine is usually cloudy or light red.

Pyelonephritis is common, particularly in women, because women get more bladder infections than do men. In women, it's a short trip from the outside of the body to the inside, and careless wiping after a bowel movement or wiping toward the urethra instead of away from it often leads to the introduction of fecal bacteria into the urinary tract.

Generally, bed rest and a bland diet with extra fluids, along with antibiotics, will help your body overwhelm any infection. If the infection becomes chronic, however, you may have kidney stones, a weak bladder muscle that is allowing infected urine to back up from the bladder to the kidney or, more rarely, repeated attacks of urinary tract infections.

Urinary tract infection.   A urinary tract infection can occur anytime the army of bacteria existing in the moist area outside the urinary opening decides to march. Generally they march through the opening and up the urethra and—when you don't urinate often enough—they proliferate in the bladder urine. From there they escape up through the ureters to your kidneys, leaving a trail of inflammation and swelling. These infections occur mostly in women.

Most infections hit the road with a short course of antibiotics, but in women they pop up for a return engagement somewhere around 20 percent of the time. Left untreated, they can cause pyelonephritis or cystitis.

Fortunately, Stanford University Medical Center researchers are developing a vaccine that may block bacteria from traveling from the bladder to the kidneys. Until it's ready, however, you might try to prevent recurrence by urinating after intercourse, not keeping a contraceptive diaphragm in the vagina for more than six to eight hours, wiping the genitourinary area from front to back after a bowel movement, keeping anything that touches the anal area during lovemaking away from the vagina, avoiding petroleum jelly (Vaseline) as a lubricant during intercourse, using tampons instead of sanitary napkins (which act as a culture medium for fecal bacteria) and urinating whenever you have the urge rather than waiting for the opportune moment.

Urinary tract stones.   Urinary tract stones are the pearls of your renal oyster. A grain of some hard substance—maybe just a mineral—gets caught in the kidney, urine crystallizes around it and the stone grows until the pain tells you it's there.

Generally, the pain of a kidney stone starts in your back, but as the stone works its way through your urinary tract, the pain follows right along. Over-the-counter medications such as aspirin or ibuprofen (Advil or Nuprin) may reduce the pain, but it won't go away until you get rid of the stone—either by passing it in your urine, having it dissolved by medication, having it removed by one of several procedures involving ultrasound or electricity or having it shattered by electrically generated or laser-generated shock waves while you sit relaxed or anesthetized in a tub of water. Most of these approaches will pulverize between 70 and 99 percent of all stones—a statistic that makes most open kidney surgery a thing of the past.

Occasionally, a stone will start in your bladder rather than merely using it as a pit stop. Bladder stones, however, are rare. And when this occurs, doctors can pass an instrument up the urethra and into the bladder, where the stone can be crushed into tiny pieces that are easily washed out of your body.

If you want to prevent the recurrence of any stones (they recur in two-thirds of those who get them to begin with), drink lots of water (8 to 12 glasses a day) and see a doctor for a formal evaluation to detect risk factors. Fifty percent of patients have an identifiable risk factor that can be eliminated by medication and/or diet modification.

Chapter 19
Whole Body Symptoms

SEE YOUR DOCTOR IMMEDIATELY IF:
- *Your arms or legs suddenly feel weak or unsteady*
- *Your temperature reaches 106°F*
- *You are diabetic and you feel lightheaded and lethargic and have a headache, chills or tremors*

L ike a stone dropped in a pond, with the ripples making ever-widening circles, many symptoms have more far-reaching effects than just throwing one part of your body out of whack. A fever hits, and your whole body cooks. Fatigue sets in, and exhaustion washes over you from head to toe.

Symptoms that affect the whole body are some of the hardest to diagnose. They're also the ones you tend to put off doing something about the longest because their very vagueness leaves you with the feeling that they're not too serious. But are they?

Doctors will tell you that any symptom that stays put like an uninvited relative is best confronted. When it comes to whole body symptoms, the best advice is to pay attention. Here's a rundown of some of the most common whole body symptoms and what they might be telling you.

SYMPTOM: **Appetite, Insatiable**

COMMON CAUSES: Have you developed an appetite that just doesn't want to quit? Is your stomach barking orders of "Give me more, give me more"?

If you've genuinely developed an insatiable appetite, it could be a sign of disease, says William Norcross, M.D., associate clinical professor of Community and Family Medicine at the University of California at San Diego School of Medicine.

There are three common diseases that are characterized by an

448

insatiable appetite, he says—diabetes mellitus (see Common Whole Body Conditions), hyperthyroidism (see thyroid disease under Common Whole Body Conditions) and depression (see Common Neurological System Conditions in chapter 12). Although appetite isn't the only symptom of these diseases, he notes, it could be the only symptom you're aware of right now.

Are you also drinking more fluids and urinating more than usual? "An increase in appetite, thirst and urination are the classic symptoms in a person with undiagnosed diabetes mellitus," says Dr. Norcross. "If you have hyperthyroidism, you may be losing weight in spite of your very healthy appetite. You may also feel nervous and intolerant of heat."

Are you feeling uninterested in life? Do you find your friends boring? Your sex life, too? If so, you could be suffering from depression.

Of course, your increased appetite doesn't have to mean you have some kind of disease. Some people eat all the time out of habit, not out of hunger. So, says Dr. Norcross, examine your conscience. Are you eating because you're *really* hungry or are you eating just because you feel like it or because you have nothing better to do?

To many people, food satisfies emotional needs, says Dr. Norcross. At least temporarily. Sometimes people eat because they're angry, lonely or bored. Such eating habits could be a sign of or result in an eating disorder (see Common Whole Body Conditions).

BEST RESPONSE: If you're eating all the time because of an insatiable hunger, you should see your family doctor, who will probably order a series of laboratory tests to see if you're suffering from diabetes mellitus or hyperthyroidism, says Dr. Norcross. If disease is the diagnosis, your appetite will return to normal once treatment begins and the disease is under control.

Treatment of the most common form of diabetes includes diet and exercise. Sometimes insulin injections or an oral medication may be required. The diet of choice, says Julian Whitaker, M.D., director of the Whitaker Wellness Institute in Huntington Beach, California, is one that's high in complex carbohydrates and fiber and low in fat, especially saturated fat.

A high-fat diet interferes with insulin's action, preventing it from lowering blood sugar. So blood sugar starts to rise—and trouble begins. Carbohydrates, on the other hand, do not have this effect. Fiber helps control diabetes, possibly by slowing the absorption of nutrients and thereby reducing insulin requirements.

Many foods high in complex carbohydrates are also rich in fiber. These include whole grains, fresh fruits and vegetables, rice, beans, corn, legumes and lentils. The foods to avoid are fatty red meat, cheese, whole milk, mayonnaise, egg yolks, fatty salad dressings and fried foods.

Exercise is also important. Walking, slow jogging, biking and swimming are activities that are frequently prescribed for patients at Dr. Whitaker's clinic. Studies show that exercise can improve glucose tolerance and reduce the insulin requirement in diabetic patients by improving the utilization of insulin in the body.

Treatment for hyperthyroidism often involves drug therapy and sometimes surgical removal of most of the thyroid gland or destruction with radioactive iodine.

If you're eating because you're depressed or if you have an eating disorder, you should also see your doctor, says Dr. Norcross. Psychotherapy may be recommended, and it is very helpful in treating depression, he says. In some cases, antidepressant medications need to be prescribed. Eating disorders such as bulimia also must often be treated with psychotherapy.

One thing you shouldn't do to control a runaway appetite is resort to diet pills, Dr. Norcross warns. Diet pills, whether they're over the counter or prescribed by a doctor, carry their own set of unwanted side effects, with high blood pressure, central nervous system disorders and even psychotic behavior high on the list. One cause is the active ingredient in diet pills, a substance called phenylpropanolamine, or PPA for short. PPA works by depressing the hypothalamus, the portion of the brain that controls the appetite.

"The problem with constant insatiable hunger is that it leads to obesity, mostly because the wrong foods are chosen to satisfy the hunger," says Dr. Norcross. "Get the high-calorie stuff out of the house and eat fresh fruits and vegetables to help satisfy your appetite." He also recommends exercising to quell hunger pangs. "Exercise has been found to curb your appetite—for a short time anyway."

ACCOMPANYING SYMPTOMS: If you have an appetite that's out of control and you follow your binges by purging your food or taking laxatives, you are a victim of bulimia (see eating disorders under Common Whole Body Conditions) and should seek professional help. In severe cases, hospitalization may be necessary to break the binge/purge cycle.

If you have a child with a voracious appetite who fails to grow normally or gain weight, he or she could be a victim of a variety of disorders, one of which is cystic fibrosis, a hereditary disease that affects the pancreas. It is characterized by lung complications and digestive problems. Treatment includes a diet that is high in calories and protein but low in fat. Supplementation with pancreatic enzyme granule preparations is usually required at every meal.

SYMPTOM: **Appetite, Loss of**

COMMON CAUSES: Kids can lose their appetite when their growth normally begins to slow—or when liver is served for dinner. Adults can lose their appetite during emotional times such as shock, anxiety or anticipation—or (for some) when liver is served for dinner. And no one is apt to feel like eating if he or she is coming down with a stomachache or the flu.

In the absence of such telltale causes, however, a loss of appetite can be a sign of disease. It can even be a serious symptom. Anorexia nervosa (see eating disorders under Common Whole Body Conditions) is a life-threatening disease. Its victims lose their appetite and diet to the extreme. It's most common among teenage girls, although anyone can be affected. Muscle and tissue wasting are the serious complications.

Medications for colds, heart diseases, asthma, tumors and epilepsy can cause you to lose your appetite. So, too, can a number of diseases. These include Addison's disease (see Common Whole Body Conditions); pernicious anemia (see anemia under Common Whole Body Conditions); hepatitis (see Common Abdominal and Digestive System Conditions in chapter 1); celiac disease (see malabsorption syndrome under Common Abdominal and Digestive System Conditions in chapter 1); kidney failure (see Common Urinary Tract Diseases in chapter 18); acute nephritis, an inflammation of the kidneys; cancer and heart disease.

Although rarely seen today, loss of appetite is also a side effect of the vitamin-deficiency diseases pellagra (niacin), beriberi (thiamine) and scurvy (vitamin C). It can also be caused by excessive intake of vitamins A and D.

BEST RESPONSE: "If you're unable to identify an event or a stress in your life that could be causing you to lose your appetite, you should see your family physician," says William Norcross, M.D. You should also take note of any other symptoms you may be experiencing and report them all to your doctor.

"If your loss of appetite is being caused by a personal setback or stress, your appetite will eventually return on its own," Dr. Norcross says. Until this happens, however, he suggests that you *not* force yourself to eat. Instead, just make sure you drink plenty of fluids—at least two quarts of fluid a day.

"You can take a daily multivitamin and, in this way, weather the storm," he says. "But if appetite loss continues for more than a week, regardless of the cause, you should see your doctor."

If anorexia nervosa is suspected, you should also see your doctor. Treatment includes psychotherapy and antidepressant drugs. In severe cases, hospitalization may be necessary.

If you can pin your loss of appetite on over-the-counter medication, simply stop taking the drug, and the feeling should go away. If prescription medication is at fault, you should discuss the matter with your doctor.

ACCOMPANYING SYMPTOMS: Check with your doctor if your loss of appetite is combined with any of the following symptoms: lack of sex drive, disinterest in friendships, unexplained crying spells, fatigue, trouble sleeping and difficulty concentrating and making decisions. You could be suffering from depression (see Common Neurological System Conditions in chapter 12) and may require psychotherapy and/or medication.

SYMPTOM: **Chills**

COMMON CAUSES: Other than the natural response to a cold winter's day, the most common cause of sudden chills is an infection, says Ted Ganiats, M.D., acting director of family medicine at the University of California at San Diego Medical Center.

Or, if you're a woman going through menopause, you may experience chills along with tingling sensations before you have a hot flash (see Symptom: Flushing in chapter 8).

BEST RESPONSE: Bundle up, says Dr. Ganiats. That's true regardless of the cause of your chill. It's best to dress in layers, so you can add and subtract as the chills come and go.

If you have any reason to suspect an infection, see your doctor. Left untreated, even the smallest bacterial ambassadors can become the vanguard of an invading army.

SYMPTOM: **Cold Sensitivity**

COMMON CAUSES: "People often think that their sensitivity to cold is due to poor circulation, but by and large, that's unlikely to be the cause," says William Norcross, M.D. "Unless you also have swelling of the ankles and legs, get muscle cramps or feel pain when exercising, poor circulation is not your problem."

The same thing goes for cold feet, says Dr. Norcross. "Having cold feet with no other symptoms poses no health risk. Some people have them and some people don't."

People who complain of being cold all the time are usually thin people, says Dr. Norcross. This is related to their sparse amount of body fat. Since body fat is an insulant against cold weather, thin people are especially sensitive to cold.

"Heavy people who have a higher percentage of body fat experience the opposite problem," Dr. Norcross notes. "They are sensitive to heat."

BEST RESPONSE: "There's no drug or other treatment for the cold that thin people experience," says Dr. Norcross. "Wearing extra clothing and staying in a warm room is the best strategy. And take heart—skinny people live longer!"

ACCOMPANYING SYMPTOMS: If you are sensitive to cold and are losing weight despite a healthy appetite, your face appears puffy and you're feeling fatigued and sluggish, you could have hypothyroidism (see thyroid disease under Common Whole Body Conditions), and you should see your doctor. Hypothyroidism is treated with lifelong daily thyroid medication.

SYMPTOM: **Drowsiness**

COMMON CAUSES: Do you find yourself drifting off to sleep at the most unlikely times—like while you're watching the shower scene in *Psycho* or while you're stuck in a gridlock in midtown Manhattan?

The most common cause of such midday drowsiness is insomnia or lack of sleep the night before (see Symptom: Insomnia). Scientists call this "short-term drowsiness." So if you were counting sheep all last night, you can't expect to be able to frolic with the flock today.

Certain drugs, such as cold tablets, antihistamines and most motion sickness medications, can also cause drowsiness while you're taking them.

But if you're chronically drowsy—if you sleep comfortably at night but still have trouble resisting the urge to take a snooze during the day—you could be suffering from a sleep disorder.

"Many people who suffer chronic drowsiness have sleep apnea or narcolepsy," says Martin Reite, M.D., director of the University of Colorado Sleep Disorder Center in Denver.

Sleep apnea is a condition in which the victims—usually overweight, older men—involuntarily but frequently stop breathing while sleeping. The immediate reaction is for them to wake up. They don't know what's happened, they just know they've awakened. Frequently, persons with this condition are also heavy snorers (see Symptom: Snoring in chapter 13).

Narcolepsy is a condition in which you experience recurrent attacks of uncontrollable urges to sleep. Most commonly, it appears in late childhood or early adulthood. The attacks can occur anytime—even when you're talking or driving.

"Narcolepsy is a biological illness that may be genetically acquired," says Dr. Reite. "The dream sleep of the sleep cycle actually comes on when the person's awake."

Sometimes narcoleptics are also cataleptic, meaning they respond to a certain emotion—even something as innocuous as a funny joke—by unconsciously experiencing muscle weakness. They may even drop to the ground and appear to be asleep. Their regular sleep is often troubled by their waking up during the night and feeling paralyzed.

Other, less bizarre, causes of chronic drowsiness include endocrine gland disorders, depression (see Common Neurological System Conditions in chapter 12), and drug and alcohol abuse. Also, drowsiness is part of a recently discovered syndrome that's brought on by the Epstein-Barr virus, the same virus that causes infectious mononucleosis (see Common Whole Body Conditions) in children and young adults. In adults, the virus keeps growing, and this invasion can lull you to sleep.

BEST RESPONSE: If you are chronically drowsy and you can't blame it on insomnia or medication, you should see your doctor. If a physical cause cannot be found, you might have to check into a sleep laboratory.

"The diagnosis of sleep apnea or narcolepsy needs to be made in a sleep laboratory where sleep recordings and other tests can be done," says Dr. Reite.

You usually check into a sleep laboratory for a night or a night and a day. Before settling in for sleep, a complete physical examination is done and a thorough medical history is taken. Often the sleeping partner is interviewed. You'll then be hooked up to electrodes and other sophisticated machines that measure brain waves, heartbeat, eye movement, air flow, muscle activity, oxygen levels and more. After all the data are analyzed, individualized treatment of the sleep disorder can begin. (To find the sleep laboratory nearest you, contact your local medical center or write to the Association of Sleep Disorders Centers, 604 Second Street SW, Rochester, MN 55902.)

"If it's found that sleep apnea is your problem, the treatment will have to be tailored to your individual needs and the severity of your illness," says Dr. Reite. Losing weight, taking certain medications, and using oxygen or pressurized air at night are frequently helpful, he says, as is wearing a special device that keeps your tongue from falling back and restricting your breathing.

A few people do require corrective surgery, but don't let that scare you away from a sleep lab, says Dr. Reite. Left untreated, sleep apnea can get worse. And since the amount of oxygen in your blood drops when you don't breathe, ignoring sleep apnea can lead to serious neurological and heart problems.

If the diagnosis is narcolepsy, however, you can probably help control your sleep attacks with naps and medication. You should schedule your time so that a short nap—one hour long or less—can be taken in the middle of the day. Also, do your most boring tasks when your alertness is at its peak (for most people, this is usually in the morning) and save the more active tasks for afternoon slump periods, says Robert Clark, M.D., director of St. Anthony Medical Center Sleep Laboratory in Columbus, Ohio.

You should follow your doctor's recommendation for dosage and timing of drugs, and you should contact your physician for treatment of even a minor infection, such as a cold, flu, bronchitis or sinusitis, since this can worsen sleepiness.

Finally, Dr. Clark suggests that you eat three regular meals every day, avoid late lunches and take note if certain foods increase your drowsiness. "Sweets, dairy products, apples, peanuts and peanut butter often appear to make sleepiness worse," he says. "You can see what your sensitivity is by avoiding all these foods, then adding one food at a time to see what the effect is."

Doctors have found that supportive counseling and self-help groups are very helpful if you suffer from narcolepsy, since this is a difficult disease to cope with. For safety's sake, doctors suggest you wear an identification bracelet that says you suffer from a sleep disorder. They also suggest that you avoid driving long distances, since the monotony can lull you to sleep. Working around dangerous machinery also should be avoided.

There is a device on the market called a "sleeper beeper" that attaches to the ear and responds to head movement with a wakening beep. The American Narcolepsy Association, however, doesn't recommend depending on these devices, since they may not always be reliable.

If depression is causing your drowsiness, see your doctor. You may require medication and psychotherapy to relieve your symptoms. There's no specific treatment for Epstein-Barr virus, however. It must simply run its course.

SYMPTOM: **Fatigue**

COMMON CAUSES: Do you feel like you're dragging your anchor? Lagging behind the pack? Are you dog-tired and bone weary? Do you have a strong desire to stop, rest or sleep? Then what you're suffering from is fatigue, and it's one of the most common complaints around.

Sometimes fatigue is a matter of doing too much yard work or playing too hard. Or the problem may simply be lack of sleep (see

Symptom: Insomnia). But, doctors say, fatigue also can be caused by a physical or emotional illness, or even by some seemingly obscure problem related to life-style.

Almost every disease, including the common cold, flu and allergies, will cause fatigue. But the other symptoms of these diseases are usually so obvious and overwhelming that fatigue is only a minor complaint.

There are some more serious maladies, however, that can often go undetected because fatigue is the *only* symptom you notice, and you may figure it's just "not serious enough" to investigate. The most common of these illnesses is anemia (see Common Whole Body Conditions). But you can also feel all in if you're suffering from infectious mononucleosis (see Common Whole Body Conditions), hepatitis (see Common Abdominal and Digestive System Conditions in chapter 1), a low-grade urinary tract infection (see Common Urinary Tract Conditions in chapter 18) or an infection of the female reproductive system. You can also lose your pep if you have high blood sugar—diabetes mellitus—or low blood sugar—hypoglycemia (see Common Whole Body Conditions)—or if your thyroid's out of whack (see thyroid disease under Common Whole Body Conditions).

If you're a woman, you may have less vim and vigor just before you menstruate. It can also be a complaint during menopause. And one of the earliest symptoms of pregnancy—even before you miss a period—is overwhelming fatigue.

Certain drugs are also notorious energy-robbers. Some pain relievers, cough and cold medicines, asthma/allergy/hay fever remedies and motion sickness pills are common over-the-counter drugs that can cause fatigue. And prescription drugs that can drag you down include those that reduce high blood pressure, prevent convulsions or relieve the symptoms of serious mental illness. Sleeping pills can cause a hangover sort of fatigue the next day. In addition, antihistamines, tranquilizers, muscle relaxants, sedatives, narcotics, birth control pills and certain heart medications can also sap your energy.

Another significant cause of fatigue is the way you live your life. It's the way you balance the good habits—eating well, getting regular exercise and pacing yourself—with the bad—constant dieting or overeating, smoking, drinking, not exercising and burning the candle at both ends—that can make the biggest difference in pepping you up or dragging you down.

Being overweight can also cause fatigue. Carrying all that excess baggage around can slow you down just as if you were dragging around a ball and chain all day. But obesity also loads you with a weight of a different kind. It can also wear you out psychologically, says Charles Kuntzleman, Ed.D., author of *Maximum Personal Energy.* "It affects your perception of yourself, making you self-conscious, which is energy draining. You're always mentally defending yourself: 'Hey, I'm okay; my waistline's just a little big.' "

Doctors say that smoking causes fatigue because it affects the delivery of oxygen to the tissues. And, strange as it may seem, when you begin withdrawing from your cigarette habit, you can also experience fatigue, since nicotine acts as a stimulant. But don't let that stop you from quitting. This kind of fatigue will soon blow over.

Then there's the matter of circadian rhythms. This isn't a new rock group—it's the body's internal alarm clock that, at different phases of the day, raises and lowers blood pressure and body temperature, triggering thousands of chemicals in the body to turn on and off. This chemical swing can make you feel dexterous or clumsy, sharp or foggy. You also can alter your rhythms by traveling across time zones, working variable shifts or otherwise changing your normal sleep times. Even the twice yearly, one-hour changes between standard time and daylight saving time can throw you off stride and give you a groggy feeling.

Are you as tired in the morning as when you go to bed at night? Does your fatigue appear for only minutes or at the most a few hours, and does it diminish as the day wears on? Has your fatigue been around—like an uninvited relative—for quite awhile? Then the cause could be psychological. Depression and anxiety (see Common Neurological System Conditions in chapter 12) are frequent causes of energy drain.

If you're a Type A personality—a workaholic—or you've recently been through a great amount of stress, you may also find yourself exhausted much of the time. In the past, Type A personalities and overstressed lives were strictly male territory, but now women, because of careers both inside and outside the home, display the label equally. Many of these women are overworked, stressed and tired.

BEST RESPONSE: If you're tired *most* of the time rather than just occasionally, your first step to recovery, doctors say, is to see your family physician. You should tell your doctor when the fatigue began, if it's constant or if it comes and goes.

What makes it worse and what makes it better? Do you have any other physical symptoms or have there been any drastic changes in your life? In other words, for the doctor to help you, you should tell it like it is and tell it *all*.

If you think your fatigue may be due to a medication you're taking, tell the doctor that, too. He or she may be able to substitute another drug, change the dosage or reschedule it to a different time of the day. With many drugs, however, fatigue is often only a factor when you first start taking them, says William Norcross, M.D. Your body can adjust somewhat with time.

Your doctor may also want to do a physical examination and order blood tests to determine if anemia, thyroid disease, infectious mononucleosis, hepatitis or diabetes is your problem. If you're a woman of childbearing age, a pregnancy test may be in order. If a urinary tract infection is suspected, your doctor may suggest a urinalysis.

Treatment of the most common forms of anemia includes an iron-rich diet, iron tablets or injections of either iron or vitamin B_{12}. If you suffer from an underactive thyroid, thyroid hormones probably will be prescribed, but if an overactive thyroid is what's troubling you, drugs, surgical removal of most of the gland or destruction with radioactive iodine may be in order.

Treatment for both infectious mononucleosis and hepatitis involves bed rest, increased fluids and a nutritious diet. If you suffer from diabetes mellitus, treatment includes diet, exercise and sometimes insulin or an oral medication (for more on treatment of diabetes mellitus, see Best Response under Symptom: Appetite, Insatiable).

Medical treatment, however, is not the answer if you suspect or are told by your doctor that your engine is starting to run out of gas because you're strung out and stressed. Rather, tension relievers and life-style changes are in order.

Try some tension-relieving exercises like rolling your head and shrugging your shoulders, taking a short walk or doing a few jumping jacks. And never sit for more than an hour and a half, suggests Dr. Kuntzleman. Breaking up a day with bits and pieces of exercise can be just as important as getting a full-blown workout.

Exercise in itself is a great fatigue fighter. Doctors say a daily 30-minute workout—a brisk walk, swim, jog, bicycle ride or other aerobic activity—will actually pep you up instead of wear you out. After you exercise, your heart will be more efficient, your blood will contain more energizing oxygen and your muscles will have a greater ability to use this oxygen. The end result will be more energy—not just for exercise but for whatever you do.

Before starting on any exercise program, however, you should check with your doctor to make sure that the activity you've chosen is the best one for you. And if you feel dizzy, nauseated or breathless, stop exercising and do less the next day. If these symptoms continue, see your doctor. Your problem could be something more than just fatigue.

Some other exercises that people often don't consider are yoga and meditation. "Yoga doesn't magically give you energy," says Swami Saradananda, director of the Sivananda Yoga Vedanta Center in New York. "What it does is release the energy you have by releasing pent-up tension in the body. Tension is basically energy that's blocked. When you release it, you make the energy you have usable."

Meditation, too, can help you achieve the seemingly impossible: You can be perfectly relaxed and invigorated at the same time. Sitting quietly in a relaxed position, with your eyes closed, and repeating a simple word over and over again while shutting off distracting thoughts can reduce your body's response to stress.

And when you think of fatigue, do you think of how you eat? You should. This is the first of a number of life-style changes that you can make to give you more zip. For starters, you should begin each day with a good breakfast high in complex carbohydrates (danish and coffee won't get you past 10:30 A.M.), then lighten up for lunch, especially if afternoon fatigue is your biggest problem.

Doctors and nutritionists suggest that most diets should be 55 percent or more carbohydrates, approximately 15 percent protein and less than 30 percent fat. Diets that are too high in fats can drag you down.

You should try to steer clear of the traditional pick-me-uppers— sweet stuff and coffee—which can zip you up quick but have the potential to drop you like a rock. Better snacks are fruit, yogurt and crackers. And if you must drink coffee, says Charles Ehret, Ph.D., senior scientist at Argonne National Laboratory in Illinois, drink it at British teatime, between 3:30 and 5:00 P.M. At that time it doesn't interfere with your circadian rhythms—and you might benefit from a slight pick-me-up, he says. By the time it lets you down, you'll probably be ready for dinner anyway.

If you're watching your weight, you shouldn't cut out the complex carbohydrates—the breads, fruits and vegetables—but should cut back on the simple carbohydrates (the sugary stuff) and fats. Avoid fad diets, since they may rob your energy and aren't usually effective for the long haul anyway.

Some find they can pep up with a shower. Hot, cold, lukewarm—it doesn't matter. It's the falling water that gives you a kick because it produces negative ions, molecules with an extra electron that can literally alter brain chemistry in the 30 percent of us who are ion sensitive.

If your sleep is thrown off course by shift work, experts at the University of Pennsylvania in Philadelphia suggest you avoid the trap of drinking more coffee and smoking more cigarettes. That only makes things worse. Also, one study showed that workers are more efficient if their shifts aren't rotated too often—three- or four-week shifts are better than one-week shifts. And shift changes that move forward are best—morning shift followed by evening and night—since this conforms more easily to your biological clock.

If you've traveled to a different time zone, don't sleep until it's bedtime in your new environment, no matter how tired you are.

Finally, if you're trying to put zest back into your life, consider the age-old benefits of getting away from it all. There's nothing like a change of scenery to rejuvenate the soul and invigorate the body. And—whether you're at home or at work—try to seek out those people who are energetic and upbeat.

"People who love, have fun and care give you good feelings about yourself and your energy levels," says Dr. Kuntzleman. Find them and treasure them.

ACCOMPANYING SYMPTOMS: If your fatigue comes on after strenuous exercise, you may have what some call "the mineral blues," a deficiency of potassium and magnesium in muscle cells. Both minerals can be lost through sweat, and when stores drop below normal, even a mild deficiency can bring on fatigue. The condition should be confirmed by a doctor. Both potassium and magnesium are abundant in nuts and soybeans. You'll also find potassium plentiful in fruits and vegetables, and magnesium in grains.

If your fatigue is accompanied by fever, night sweats, swollen glands, weight loss or a loss of appetite, you could be suffering from a serious ailment such as acquired immune deficiency syndrome, or AIDS (see Common Whole Body Conditions) or Hodgkin's disease, a form of cancer that affects the lymph nodes. You should see your doctor.

SYMPTOM: **Fever**

COMMON CAUSES: Everybody has a temperature, but you're some-body special if you have a fever. Normal temperature is 98.6°F, but that's only if the temperature is taken with an oral thermometer. With a rectal thermometer, normal is 99.6°F. And if you measure your temperature in the armpit, normal is 97.6°F, although a cold room will lower the reading and a hot one will raise it.

To further complicate the matter, there is a wide variation in what is considered normal. Some people can have a normal temperature of 98°F or even lower, and everybody's temperature fluctuates as the day progresses: It's lowest during sleep and highest between 4:00 P.M. and 8:00 P.M.

So before you decide you have a fever—an abnormally high temperature—consider *where* you're taking your temperature, *what* your normal temperature is and *whether* it's morning, noon or night.

The most common cause of fever is infection, and that covers a wide range of illnesses, from the seldom serious influenza (see Common Whole Body Conditions) to life-threatening meningitis (see Common Neurological System Conditions in chapter 12). Infections of the urinary tract (see Common Urinary Tract Conditions in chapter 18) and ear (see middle ear infections under Common Ear Conditions in chapter 6) are common. Arthritis (see Common Bone, Joint and Muscle Conditions in chapter 3), lupus erythematosus (see Common Whole Body Conditions), tumors and head injuries can also cause fevers.

It's important to know that fevers in children generally run higher than those in adults. A child probably will run a higher temperature than an adult for the same disease, but it doesn't mean that the child is any sicker. Fevers up to 104°F are common in children.

When should you worry about a fever? "I would be concerned," says Ted Ganiats, M.D., "if you suddenly develop an oral temperature of 101°F or more. Or if you've had a temperature of 100°F or more for over a week. But the real concern should be the other symptoms that are associated with the fever.

"If you have a runny nose and a little cough and a temperature of 101°F," he explains, "I'd say you probably have a cold and it'll run its course. But if your temperature is 101°F and you have harder-to-explain symptoms, like a stiff neck or a brand new rash, I'd say you should see your doctor."

Very high fevers—106°F and over—are usually a result of a body thermostat that's gone out of control. They're serious and should be considered a medical emergency. An example of this is heatstroke (see Common Whole Body Conditions), in which the body is unable to cope with high temperatures.

BEST RESPONSE: "When it comes to fevers, you have to use some common sense," says Dr. Ganiats. "There's a lot of evidence that fever is therapeutic and that it should be allowed to run its course. But there are also many people who feel better and get better when fever is treated."

The main thing to remember, says Dr. Ganiats, is that you should treat fever only if it's making you miserable. But it's more often children, rather than adults, who are bothered by fever.

Adult fevers can be treated by taking aspirin or acetaminophen (Tylenol) every four hours. Children can be given acetaminophen but they should *not* be given aspirin, says Dr. Ganiats. Aspirin use during a viral attack in children is suspected of somehow triggering a life-threatening condition called Reye's syndrome, a sudden, severe disease that affects the liver and the brain. Children also can be given lukewarm sponge baths; alcohol sponge baths should be used cautiously, says Dr. Ganiats, since the fumes may disturb an already ill child.

And if the fever in either a child or an adult doesn't return to normal within 24 hours and, more important, if other symptoms are present, check with your doctor. You may need an antibiotic or other medication to treat one of the numerous conditions that can cause a fever.

Heatstroke is a serious disorder that requires immediate medical care. While waiting for an ambulance, move the person to the coolest possible place—a shady area or an air-conditioned room. Remove excess clothing. Cool the person by sponging with cold water or wrapping in a cool, wet sheet. Fan the person with your hand, an electric fan or a blow dryer on the cold setting. In the hospital, body temperature is regulated while fluids and body salts are replaced.

SYMPTOM: **Heat Intolerance**

COMMON CAUSES: Those most likely to be heat intolerant are people who are overweight or those who suffer from an overactive thyroid, a disease known as hyperthyroidism (see thyroid disease under Common Whole Body Conditions), says William Norcross, M.D.

"The problem in obesity is that excess fat acts like a layer of insulation, and the person isn't able to give off the heat," explains Dr. Norcross. "So, even in a 70°F room, the overweight person can feel very warm."

Those with hyperthyroidism are bothered by the heat because the thyroid gland is responsible for maintenance of body metabolism, which in turn is responsible for energy output. Heat intolerance is one of the condition's many side effects. (Nervousness, insomnia and weight loss are also part of the syndrome.)

If you take certain medications, you also can be particularly vulnerable to hot-weather problems, especially if you exercise vigorously. The problem medications are diuretics ("water pills"), phenothiazines (drugs, like chlorpromazine, that are taken for psychiatric problems), amphetamines and barbiturates. Drinking alcohol can also make you intolerant of the heat.

Being sensitive to the heat, however, doesn't necessarily mean there's anything wrong with you. There are simply those who can and those who can't take the heat. If you know you're one of those who enjoys the crisp autumn woods more than the sweltering beach, your heat intolerance is perfectly normal.

BEST RESPONSE: Unless you move to a cooler clime, your sensitivity to the heat cannot be eliminated. But it can be reduced. For starters, if you're overweight, you can help by losing your excess poundage. And anyone sensitive to the heat can help maintain their cool by limiting physical activity during the summer months between noon and 2:00 P.M., when the sun and the heat are the most fierce.

When going outdoors in the heat, wear light-colored, lightweight clothing to reflect the sun's rays and to permit evaporation. Also wear a hat or visor. Indoors, wear the layered look, so garments can easily be shed when the temperature starts to rise. Also, it would be good to invest in an air conditioner, since comfort is what's desired most.

If you have hyperthyroidism, you should discuss your discomfort with your doctor. A change in treatment might be in order. If you suspect a drug is causing your sensitivity, you should discuss your discomfort with the doctor. A change in medication may be in order.

SYMPTOM: **Insomnia**

COMMON CAUSES: You snuggle under the covers with great expectations of pleasant dreams, but end up tossing and turning. Or the sandman comes quickly enough, but you wake up around 3:00 A.M. and, hours later, wearily greet the dawn. And if you thought last night was bad, just wait for today. You'll drag through it as if the air—and your brains— are made of cotton.

"The real problem with insomnia is that, because of lack of sleep or poor quality of sleep, the insomniac is not able to function well the next day," says Martin Reite, M.D.

Fortunately, for most people, insomnia lasts for only a couple of nights. It's just a bad reaction to some stress in life—be it personal strife, anxiety, excitement, jet lag or a change in your work shift.

Chronic insomnia, however, has more serious implications. "It's a symptom for which you have to make a diagnosis," says Dr. Reite. Any disease with chronic pain—arthritis, for example—can keep you awake. Or the pain of an ulcer can wake you out of a sound sleep. And any endocrine gland disorder, including thyroid disease, has the potential for causing insomnia, as does depression.

Fibrositis is a disease in which deep sleep is unattainable. It afflicts tense, perfectionist-type people. For them, the norm is shallow sleep that results in muscle spasms and pain in various parts of the body, called tender body spots.

And, contrary to popular opinion, alcohol and even sleeping pills can cause you to lose a night's sleep. Although drinking alcohol may knock you out fast, it interferes with the deep sleep of the sleep cycle, resulting in restless sleep, or even waking you up and keeping you awake. Sleeping pills impose the same unnatural sleep, causing you to feel groggy and sluggish the next day. Plus, their addictive nature can result in a vicious cycle.

Also, a change in life-style can have an effect on your sleeping habits. "Often insomnia can be traced back to within one week of retirement," says Michael Stevenson, Ph.D., director of the insomnia clinic and sleep disorders center at Holy Cross Hospital in Mission Hills, California. "Isolation, boredom, loss of social contacts and preoccupation with self all hit at once. Sleep goes right out the window."

There are also specific sleep disorders that can interfere with your rest, but it usually requires a kind bed partner to tell you about them.

Nocturnal myoclonus is repetitive kicking movements of the legs during sleep. This isn't just an occasional twitch but constant motion that has disrupted many a marriage when the spouse is literally kicked out of bed. The cause of the problem is not clearly understood, although it's a problem that's known to get worse as you get older.

Sleep apnea, another sleep disorder, causes the victim to wake up as a result of suspended breathing. It's usually associated with snoring and most often occurs in overweight, older men. Although sleep apnea doesn't *always* wake you up, it always causes poor-quality sleep, making you feel drowsy the next day (see Symptom: Drowsiness in this chapter, and Symptom: Snoring in chapter 13).

BEST RESPONSE: If you suffer from chronic insomnia—if you go through sleeplessness for nights on end—your first step is to see a doctor, preferably one who has knowledge of sleep problems, says Dr. Reite. "What you don't want is to go see a doctor and immediately come out with a prescription for a sleep medicine. If this is the case, you should try another doctor."

Dr. Reite says that a doctor sensitive to your sleeplessness will do a complete medical workup to find if there is a physical problem causing your insomnia. If the right questions are asked, he says, most insomnia problems can be diagnosed in the doctor's office. About 10 to 20 percent of insomniacs, however, will be suffering from a sleep disorder and will need to go to a sleep laboratory for diagnosis (for more on sleep laboratories, see Best Response under Symptom: Drowsiness).

For garden-variety insomnia, however, there are several things you can do on your own to reintroduce a normal sleeping pattern into your life, says Dr. Reite. And they begin with keeping regular hours. This doesn't mean that you have to go to bed at the same time every night, but it does mean that you should get up at the same time every day. That means no sleeping in until noon on the weekends. This will help establish a routine for your body rhythms, he says.

Avoid caffeine late in the day—even a cup after dinner is enough to keep some people up for the late, late show. The same goes for exercise. Exercise revs up the body, and a workout too soon before bedtime can keep you awake longer than you want. Exercise early in the day, however, may help you feel pleasingly tired later on.

Also, don't use alcohol as a sedative, says Dr. Reite. Alcohol may help get you to sleep initially, but you'll have an abnormal sleep cycle the rest of the night.

Maintaining a proper sleep environment is also important, says Dr. Reite. Your bedroom should be dark, quiet and as comfortable as possible. The temperature of the room should be cool, around 65°F. And your bed should be comfortable—for you.

A light snack before bedtime may also be helpful for some people. Some doctors suggest a glass of warm milk or a banana because they contain tryptophan, an amino acid that is converted into a substance in the brain called serotonin, which helps induce sleep. Food only contains small amounts of tryptophan, which is why it doesn't have the same effect on all people.

"Tryptophan certainly is not a cure-all for all types of insomnia. But you can give it a try with your doctor's supervision," says Dr. Reite.

The major no-no in fighting insomnia is taking naps in the afternoon, no matter how tired you may feel. It will only prevent you, once again, from going to bed tired, says Dr. Reite.

He also suggests that you get your mind off yourself. "Become other-preoccupied instead of self-preoccupied," he says. You can do this by increasing your social contacts. Get involved in a project, or do volunteer work.

If, however, you still can't fall asleep after 20 to 30 minutes, don't lie in bed fighting it, says Dr. Reite. Get up. Go to another room and read or watch television until you feel sleepy. Then go back to bed.

The best way to fight the sleeplessness that comes with changing time zones or shift work is to immediately get on the new time schedule, even if it means eating dinner when it's time for your coffee break. Also, don't go to sleep until the rest of the world around you has lights out, even if your own eyes have been at half-mast for hours.

ACCOMPANYING SYMPTOMS: If you have a child who has sleepless nights, is restless during the day, has a supershort attention span and is prone to temper tantrums, he or she may have what was once called hyperactivity but is now known as an attention deficit disorder (see Common Neurological System Conditions in chapter 12). You should discuss these symptoms with your doctor. Treatment includes a well-structured environment with regular mealtimes, bedtimes and playtimes, lots of loving attention, planning sessions with teachers and parents and occasional use of medication.

SYMPTOM: **Pallor.** *See* Symptom: Pallor in chapter 15

SYMPTOM: **Sweating.** *See* Symptom: Sweating in chapter 15

SYMPTOM: **Swelling**

COMMON CAUSES: Swelling or bloating is a sign of water retention, and it is such a severe problem in some people that their entire body seems to blow up like a balloon. Often the swelling is most noticeable in the feet and legs because gravity moves the fluid downward.

In many cases, there is no known cause for water retention. Some people are just more prone to the problem than others. However, it's most often a problem if you're overweight, as a result of the general inefficiency that goes with an overtaxed body; if you eat a high-salt diet, because of the large amounts of water-retaining sodium in the body; or if you're a heavy drinker, because of alcohol's effect on the liver and kidneys.

Water retention is commonly a side effect of drugs, with steroids, oral contraceptives or nonsteroidal anti-inflammatory drugs among the top offenders. And sometimes it's caused by disease. Heart failure (see Common Circulatory, Heart and Lung Conditions in chapter 5), glomerulonephritis and kidney failure (see Common Urinary Tract Conditions in chapter 18) and cirrhosis of the liver and some forms of hepatitis (see Common Abdominal and Digestive System Conditions in chapter 1) can all cause an accumulation of body fluid.

And, in women, water retention is quite common a week to ten days before menstruation and during menopause and pregnancy.

If your swelling is so noticeable in the legs and feet that your finger leaves an indentation after you poke at a spot, you may have what doctors call pitting edema. In many cases you can have a mild degree of pitting edema because of obesity or vein problems. In most cases it is not a sign of serious disease.

BEST RESPONSE: Diuretics ("water pills"), a type of medication that forces the kidneys to excrete excess water, are a standard treatment for fluid retention. Because of the serious nature of their potential side effects, which include mineral losses and electrolyte imbalance, plus their potential for abuse, many doctors are now prescribing only small doses given intermittently, or discouraging their use altogether when not absolutely necessary.

Instead, doctors say, a safer and more natural way to help reduce water buildup in the body is to reduce sodium in your diet. Sodium has the ability to enhance retention of water in the body tissues, slowing down its passage through the body and out through the urine.

Reducing sodium means cutting out salt at the table and eliminating salty snack foods, ham, bacon, processed lunchmeats, soy sauce, canned soups, bouillon cubes and packaged convenience foods. Eating a lot of licorice candy can cause salt and fluid retention.

If you're overweight, you should cut down on calories and get regular exercise to help you lose weight. If you're a heavy drinker, you should cut down on your alcohol intake, or, preferably, abstain forever.

Resting during the day with your feet up will also help relieve the downward gravitational pull of the fluid. For those plagued with swollen limbs, wearing support stockings or custom-made elastic stockings can ease the discomfort.

If, in spite of these measures, you continue to feel bloated, you should see your doctor.

Although pitting edema is not usually a serious problem, you should see your doctor as a precaution.

ACCOMPANYING SYMPTOMS: If you have swelling accompanied by heart palpitations and you have been taking diuretics for a long time, see your doctor. You could be suffering from mineral deficiencies.

Swelling in your feet and legs in the afternoon and evening is a common occurrence in late pregnancy. It is often caused by the pressure of the uterus on the vein that carries blood away from the legs. Swelling may also be a sign of toxemia, a serious complication of pregnancy. Getting early and frequent prenatal care is the best way to prevent this complication.

SYMPTOM: **Thirst, Excessive**

COMMON CAUSES: If you're vacationing in a hot, dry environment, you may be thirstier than usual, simply because you're losing water through perspiration. Exercising to the point of profuse sweating will also work up a thirst. This is quite normal and harmless, as long as you're replacing the lost fluid, says William Norcross, M.D.

But an excessive thirst for no explainable reason is the classic sign of diabetes insipidus or diabetes mellitus (see Common Whole Body Conditions).

Diuretic drugs ("water pills"), which force the kidneys to excrete excess water, sodium and potassium, can also cause excessive thirst.

BEST RESPONSE: "Excessive thirst is easily remedied by drinking fluids, and it's important that you replenish fluid levels to prevent dehydration," says Dr. Norcross.

Water is the best fluid for replacing diminishing supplies in the body, he says. You'll probably find that trying to quench your thirst with a sugary soft drink won't do the trick. That's because sugary drinks are delayed in the stomach and don't get to the bloodstream and out to the body's reservoirs—the tissues—efficiently enough.

Dr. Norcross also recommends avoiding coffee and other caffeine-containing beverages when in a hot environment, since the chemical acts somewhat as a natural diuretic, causing frequent urination. And don't even consider salt tablets, he cautions. They are potentially dangerous. There is sufficient sodium in the American diet to meet almost any need.

If you're taking diuretic medication, you should tell your doctor about the excessive thirst you're experiencing. It could mean you're excreting too much bodily fluid and a change in medication may be in order.

If, however, your excessive thirst has been unrelenting (and especially if it's combined with frequent trips to the bathroom), you should see your doctor, who will give you a test for diabetes mellitus or diabetes insipidus. Although the two terms sound similar, they are different in their causes and treatment.

Diabetes insipidus is caused by the lack of a certain hormone that regulates how much water is retained and excreted from the body. Treatment is with synthetic hormone, administered by nose drops, powder or injection. In some cases, surgery is necessary.

Diabetes mellitus, on the other hand, is a chronic disease characterized by high blood sugar and the body's inability to process the sugar efficiently. This type of diabetes is managed with diet, exercise and sometimes medication, such as injections of insulin or oral drugs that normalize blood sugar (for more on treatment for diabetes mellitus, see Best Response under Symptom: Appetite, Insatiable).

SYMPTOM: **Trembling**

COMMON CAUSES: Do you get the shakes when you have to give a speech or go for a job interview? Do you tremble when the weather gets nippy or after you've played handball for a couple of hours?

Nervousness, excitement, cold, heavy physical exertion and tension are all normal causes of trembling.

In fact, some people can inherit a tendency to tremble in response to fatigue, tension or anxiety. Usually, it's first noticed in puberty. It's not a sign of disease or anything serious.

Drinking too much coffee or tea, or taking caffeine-containing drugs, can give you the shakes. Prescription drugs, such as phenothiazine or other tranquilizers, can have a similar effect. Tremors can also be the sign of withdrawal from a bout with the bottle or from drug addiction.

Tremors also occur in cerebral palsy (see Common Neurological

System Conditions in chapter 12). And tremors that accompany old age are often due to arteriosclerosis (see Common Circulatory, Heart and Lung Conditions in chapter 5) and are caused by the hardening of the arteries going to the brain.

Occasionally, a person will be afflicted with intention tremors— tremors that come on when you try to do something. For some this can be due to a nerve disorder or nerve damage, but for most it is a relatively benign, inherited condition.

But tremors that usually come on when the body is at rest are a sign of the central nervous system disorder called Parkinson's disease (see Common Neurological System Conditions in chapter 12). If you rhythmically shake your hands or head, or both, when you're at rest, and the tremors get better or disappear when you use your hands, you could be suffering from Parkinson's disease. It's a common disorder of middle and old age.

BEST RESPONSE: If your trembling was triggered by a physical or emotional situation, you needn't do anything, say doctors. It will disappear once your body or the situation calms down.

If you're a coffee or tea drinker, or you're taking nonprescription drugs containing caffeine, you should avoid these stimulants and see if your tremors go away. If they're the cause of your problem, simply avoiding them is the cure.

Trembling that's here today, gone tomorrow is usually no cause for concern, say doctors. But if your tremors are recurring, you should see your doctor.

If the diagnosis is Parkinson's disease, long-term treatment, usually with drug therapy, psychotherapy and physical therapy, is in order. For more advanced cases, the drugs levodopa, amantadine or trihexyphenidyl can help control the tremors. Surgery is sometimes beneficial.

ACCOMPANYING SYMPTOMS: Hand tremors accompanied by nervousness, fatigue, excessive sweating, weight loss, rapid pulse and a pounding heartbeat are the signs of hyperthyroidism (see thyroid disease under Common Whole Body Conditions). You should see your doctor as soon as possible.

If you're a heavy drinker who's gone on the wagon, tremors accompanied by sweating, hallucinations and fever are a sign of delirium tremens, the d.t.'s. This is a sign of alcoholism (see Common Whole Body Conditions) and is best treated with increased fluids, vitamins and medications, in a hospital setting.

SYMPTOM: **Twitching**

COMMON CAUSES: Twitches, or tics, as they are often called, are brief, involuntary muscle spasms that can appear anywhere in the body. If you're overtired, for example, your eyelid can twitch. And as you're falling asleep, any part of your body may jerk involuntarily as if it's being possessed. Such twitches may be annoying or even scary, but they're harmless.

Between 12 and 24 percent of children suffer from fast, sudden and unexpected involuntary muscle jerks. These habit tics, known as transient tic disorders, begin before age 15 and can include nose twitches, blinking eyes, shoulder shrugging or jerking of the hand. They may last for two or three months, disappear and then reappear for one or two years. Then they may disappear altogether.

In less than 3 percent of the general population, however, the problem doesn't go away. It gets worse, and develops into multiple tics, a condition known as Tourette's syndrome. The tics can show themselves through vocal noises such as snorts, barks, grunts or even obscene language. The nervous habit of throat clearing is a form of tic.

BEST RESPONSE: If you twitch persistently, see your doctor for diagnosis. Transient tics in children are usually not treated because the symptoms are mild and the disorder ordinarily doesn't last longer than a year. If, however, the symptoms are persistent or are severe enough that they interfere with school or peer relations, doctors say, treatment is necessary. Psychotherapy can help in coping with the teasing and isolation that frequently occur. Specific medications can quiet twitches.

Tourette's is not a psychological or intellectual problem as was once thought, and treatment can be effective in overcoming the disability. Treatment is usually given in the form of closely supervised medication. Psychotherapy, biofeedback, hypnosis and sometimes surgery are also helpful.

The Tourette Syndrome Association is a national organization with regional groups that can provide information and support to affected persons and their families. Check your phone book, or with a local health agency, to find the group nearest you.

ACCOMPANYING SYMPTOMS: If you have painful twitching along the side of the face, this is a sign of tic douloureux (see Common Facial, Jaw and Mouth Conditions in chapter 8), and you should see your doctor. Treatment with pain medications or other drugs may relieve symptoms during an attack.

If your child has had a recent streptococcal infection, such as a strep throat, and now has uncontrollable tics and facial grimaces, this is a sign of Sydenham's chorea, also known as St. Vitus' dance. Closely related to rheumatic fever, it is a delayed complication of an inadequately treated strep infection. Treatment is with antibiotics, although recovery is slow, usually taking three to six months. Some doctors believe antibiotics are necessary until adulthood to prevent further infection. Medication may also be prescribed to control the twitching.

SYMPTOM: **Weakness.** *See* Symptom: Fatigue

SYMPTOM: **Weight Gain, Unexplained**

COMMON CAUSES: If you overindulge, you're likely to bulge. But what if your eating habits haven't changed and you're still tipping the scales?

In many cases, the problem is not that you're eating more but that your activity level has dropped off. It can also be a matter of age.

As age creeps up, so do the pounds. That's because metabolism naturally slows as you age. And if you don't compensate by eating less or exercising more, you're going to gain weight.

Some people start experiencing weight gain around the age of 30, says William Norcross, M.D., and an extra pound or two a year is common.

Unexplained weight gain, however, is often a telltale sign of an underactive thyroid, a disease called hypothyroidism (see thyroid disease under Common Whole Body Conditions). Other, though less obvious, symptoms are likely to be evident, including puffiness, a change in voice and brittle hair. Although a lot of people would like to blame their weight gain on their thyroid, doctors say that less than 2 percent of weight problems are caused by a sluggish gland.

But if you retain body fluid—something that is quite common in premenstrual women—it will show up as increased poundage on the scale. Water retention also can result from taking certain medications and is also a side effect of a number of diseases (see Symptom: Swelling).

BEST RESPONSE: The only way to counteract the weight gain that accompanies aging is to cut back on calories and begin a regular exercise program, says Dr. Norcross. A 20- to 30-minute aerobic workout at least three times a week, along with a sensible, well-balanced diet, will help get rid of the added poundage.

If this doesn't help, you should see your doctor. If an underactive thyroid is found to be your problem, medication can be prescribed that can help regulate the gland and bring your weight down.

Diuretics ("water pills") are sometimes prescribed for water retention, but most doctors do not recommend them for long-term use. Instead, a diet that is low in sodium—the mineral that enhances water retention—is the best solution.

ACCOMPANYING SYMPTOMS: If you're in your last three months of pregnancy and experience a sudden, unexplained weight gain and puffiness in the legs and feet, you should see your doctor. You could be suffering from toxemia, a potentially serious complication.

If your weight gain is most pronounced in the trunk, back and face, and you have acne, excessive hair growth, muscle wasting and bruising, you should see your doctor. You could be suffering from Cushing's disease, a rare disease of the pituitary and adrenal glands. Treatment involves surgery or radiation.

SYMPTOM: **Weight Loss, Unexplained**

COMMON CAUSES: Unexplained loss of weight is always a serious sign. It can be caused by a wide variety of ailments, including digestive disorders, pernicious anemia (see anemia under Whole Body Conditions), hyperthyroidism (see thyroid disease under Whole Body Conditions), Addison's disease and diabetes mellitus (see Common Whole Body Conditions), anorexia (see eating disorders under Common Whole Body

Conditions), tuberculosis and most forms of cancer.

Personal stress, anxiety and depression—emotional problems that can shrivel your appetite—are also factors that can make you lose weight.

BEST RESPONSE: You should see your doctor for a thorough examination if you have recently lost weight and haven't been consciously dieting or going through personal turmoil.

Treatment will depend on the doctor's findings. Pernicious anemia, for example, is treated with routine vitamin B_{12} injections, and the treatment for hyperthyroidism is surgical removal of most of the gland, radioactive iodine and medication. Addison's disease is treated with daily use of adrenal steroid hormones, such as cortisone and prednisone. Diabetes is treated with diet and, sometimes, insulin. Anorexia is treated with individual counseling and antidepressant drugs.

ACCOMPANYING SYMPTOMS: If your unexplained weight loss is accompanied by extreme fatigue, respiratory discomfort and lesions on the skin, you could have acquired immune deficiency syndrome, or AIDS (see Common Whole Body Conditions), and you should seek immediate medical attention.

Common Whole Body Conditions

Acquired immune deficiency syndrome. Commonly known as AIDS, this devastating disease is a total breakdown of the body's natural defenses, leaving the body completely vulnerable to a host of infections. Even the most innocuous virus—a cold, for example—can be troublesome to an AIDS victim.

AIDS is most commonly spread by sexual contact and most frequently strikes homosexual men. However, it's also contracted through transfusion of contaminated blood and use of contaminated needles or syringes, and it can be passed from an infected mother to her baby before birth and through breastfeeding.

Even though low concentrations of the AIDS virus are sometimes found in saliva, tears, urine, sweat and other body fluids of its victims, no one knows of anyone who has gotten AIDS through contact with these body fluids. Sex is the most common way of spreading the disease.

Exposure occurs when blood or semen that contains the infected cells is passed into an uninfected person's bloodstream.

When a person becomes infected with the virus, antibodies develop in about six weeks. A person can be infected and be contagious for many years without having any disease symptoms, but usually symptoms develop within 18 months. AIDS often goes undiagnosed until a life-threatening infection, cancer or tumor appears. The degree of symptoms varies greatly from patient to patient, however.

Symptoms at the time of diagnosis can include skin disease, respiratory problems, gastrointestinal infections or brain and neurological disorders. Weight loss, fatigue, fevers and loss of appetite are common.

Although the disease is considered fatal, a number of drugs that may be effective against AIDS are in various stages of investigation and testing.

Addison's disease. In this disease, the adrenal glands don't function properly, and thus slow down hormone production. And it's not just adrenalin that's affected. These glands are responsible for a number of regulatory processes, including the proper balance of water and salts in the body.

In most cases of Addison's disease, the adrenal glands just shrivel up, for reasons unknown to medical science. However, the disease can be brought on by injury due to bleeding, infection or a tumor. Failure of the pituitary gland, which regulates growth, can also result in adrenal insufficiency.

Addison's disease comes on slowly, with such symptoms as fatigue, fainting spells, loss of appetite and weight, nausea, vomiting and abdominal pain. Dark pigmentation somewhat resembling a suntan may appear on both exposed and unexposed areas of the body, especially on the skin over the knees, elbows and knuckles. Lips and gums also may be pigmented.

Diagnosis is made by measuring the amount of some of the adrenal hormones in the blood and urine. Those with Addison's disease—President John F Kennedy was one of its most noted victims—can live a normal life, with treatment that includes daily supplementation of adrenal steroid hormones such as cortisone and prednisone. The drug, however, may need to be adjusted in times of stress to avoid the major complication of the disease, adrenal crisis. If a victim goes into adrenal crisis, nausea, vomiting, dehydration, high temperature, severe drop in blood pressure and total collapse can result. Hospital treatment includes intravenous adrenal hormones and replacement of fluids and salts.

Alcoholism. Alcoholism is a chronic, debilitating disease brought on by long-term use and abuse of alcohol. Why some hard drinkers are vulnerable to the disease and others are not is unknown, although genetic or biochemical defects are suspected, since the problem often runs in families. Also considered as a possible cause is an allergy to either the alcohol itself or to the grains, corn, fruits, yeast or sugar from which alcoholic beverages are made.

The effects of alcoholism are far-reaching—from loss of job and spouse through neglect to loss of life through disease, such as cirrhosis of the liver. Gastrointestinal illnesses, neurological problems and heart disease also have been implicated in the disease.

"You know you're heading toward alcoholism when alcohol is causing a problem in any area of your life and yet you continue drinking," says Pat Mulcahy, R.N., nursing supervisor of the Sunrise Center at Pomerado Hospital Chemical Dependency Treatment Center in Poway, California. However, alcoholism very often is not a disease you recognize yourself. It usually requires others to show the alcoholic the error of his or her ways.

"If your loved one has an alcohol problem, you can use a technique called intervention to break through the denial and get the alcoholic to see the effect that alcohol is having and to admit the need for treatment," says Mulcahy. "This is best done with the assistance of a professional therapist."

Alcoholism is most effectively treated in a clinical setting. Counseling and close supervision are essential. Support groups, such as the highly successful Alcoholics Anonymous, are greatly encouraged.

Immediate withdrawal from alcohol is usually treated with increased fluids, vitamin therapy and medications when necessary. Depending on the degree of illness, withdrawal takes 24 to 72 hours.

Immediate withdrawal from alcohol abuse can cause minor symptoms such as tremors, sweating and weakness. A more serious backlash is delirium tremens—the d.t.'s—a syndrome characterized by hallucinations, tremors and fever. Because of the potentially serious nature of d.t.'s, withdrawal is best carried out in a hospital setting under medical supervision.

Anemia.   Anemia is a below-normal volume of red blood cells, which are responsible for carrying oxygen to the tissues.

Anemia is actually a syndrome of any number of disorders and comes in many forms, most of which carry the same, often vague symptoms—fatigue, pallor, breathlessness and palpitations. Its causes include poor diet, loss of blood, blood-related diseases or exposure to industrial chemicals. A few forms are hereditary.

The most common form of this syndrome is iron deficiency anemia, which develops most often because of blood loss. Women with heavy menstrual periods can have depleted blood iron reserves. So, too, can those with intestinal blood loss brought on by gastritis, peptic ulcer, hemorrhoids or cancer of the stomach or large intestine.

You can also come down with iron deficiency anemia if your body is unable to absorb iron or if your diet is deficient in iron. Infants kept too long on a milk diet, growing children with poor diets and pregnant women are most prone to this type of anemia. Treatment includes an iron-rich diet, iron tablets or iron injections.

Pernicious anemia is caused by the body's inability to absorb vitamin B_{12}, an essential factor in the production of red blood cells. If left untreated, the condition can lead to nerve damage.

Vitamin B_{12} absorption is interrupted when the stomach stops secreting a substance called intrinsic factor, which helps in the absorption process. That's why people who have had their stomach removed are the most common victims of B_{12} deficiency.

Since the body is able to store B_{12} efficiently, this form of anemia often takes years to develop. Treatment usually consists of a lifelong series of vitamin B_{12} injections.

Sickle cell anemia is an inherited disorder that attacks mostly blacks. What happens is that normally round blood cells take on the shape of a sickle. This makes the blood thicker and clogs the smallest vessels, reducing the blood supply to vital organs and causing periods of extreme pain.

There is no cure for this form of anemia, but serious symptoms are treated in the hospital with painkillers and sometimes transfusions.

Thalassemia major is another inherited form of anemia and is prevalent in persons from the Mediterranean area, the Middle East or the Far East. It reduces the blood's ability to release needed oxygen. Treatment includes regular, lifelong blood transfusions.

Hemolytic anemia occurs when the red blood cells are destroyed more rapidly than normal. The condition can be hereditary or can be caused by exposure to certain chemicals, taking medications or as part of a reaction to a blood transfusion.

One type of hemolytic anemia—hereditary spherocytosis—is treated by removing the spleen. Other causes may be treated by discontinuing the causative drugs or prescribing various medications.

Aplastic anemia occurs when the bone marrow's production of blood cells decreases either gradually or suddenly. As a result, the victim is more susceptible to infections, bruising and bleeding. The condition is caused by exposure to a number of toxic chemicals, radiation or x-rays.

Treatment involves removing the toxic agent, treating the anemia with blood transfusions and knocking out the infection with antibiotics. In severe cases, a bone marrow transplant may be necessary.

Diabetes insipidus.   This disease is characterized by passage of large amounts of fluids—up to several gallons a day—as a result of a deficiency of the antidiuretic hormone, also known as ADH or vasopressin.

When functioning properly, this hormone, which is produced in the hypothalamus and stored in the pituitary gland, helps regulate the balance of blood and fluids in the body. When deficiency occurs, output of fluid from the kidneys greatly exceeds normal, and the resulting fluid that is excreted is urine that is very dilute.

The disease can be brought on by damage to the pituitary gland as a result of injury, infection, tumor or aneurysm. Sometimes it's hereditary. The disease can also occur when the hormonal deficiency causes your kidneys to malfunction.

In addition to passing an unusual amount of fluid, another telling symptom is great thirst. It is important to drink plenty of liquids to prevent dehydration.

Treatment of the disease depends on the cause, although synthetic ADH injections or drops are often required. Sometimes surgery is necessary.

Diabetes mellitus.   Five percent of Americans—over 10 million people—suffer from diabetes mellitus, a chronic condition characterized by the body's inability to produce enough insulin to process food efficiently. The result is high levels of sugar in the blood.

Diabetes comes in two forms. Type I usually affects adolescents or young adults. It is the more severe but less common form, and always requires insulin injections. Type II, which usually occurs in adulthood, affects 90 percent of all diabetics. It's most common among overweight adults, and can often be controlled with weight loss, exercise and diet, although medication and insulin injections are sometimes necessary.

Symptoms of both types of diabetes include excessive thirst, frequent urination, fatigue, increased appetite and increased susceptibility to infections. Type I diabetics are usually thin; Type II diabetics are usually heavy. The disease tends to run in the family.

Definitive diagnosis of the disease is made with a fasting blood glucose test, in which a blood sample is taken after you've been without food for at least eight hours. If the level of sugar is borderline, a glucose tolerance test may also be necessary. This test, which also requires an eight-hour fast, measures the blood for sugar at specific levels after ingesting specific amounts of sugar.

Although diabetes can be controlled, it carries many risks, including heart disease, stroke, kidney failure, blindness, impotence in men and circulation problems which, if left untreated, can result in gangrene and amputation of legs or feet.

Clearly, diabetes requires constant supervision. If too much insulin is taken or a meal is missed, a diabetic can experience insulin shock or hypoglycemia (low blood sugar). Mild insulin shock causes weakness, confusion, nervousness, trembling, sweating and hunger and can be treated promptly by drinking a glass of milk or eating a piece of candy. More extreme symptoms of insulin shock, such as unconsciousness, may require hospitalization. A condition known as ketoacidosis (very high blood sugar) can occur when not enough insulin is available to the body. When this happens, breathing becomes heavy and the diabetic usually will have increased thirst and urination, fatigue, weakness and breath that has a sweet or fruity smell. The condition requires immediate hospital treatment.

With these kinds of complications, diabetics clearly need to watch sugar levels closely. Diet is important, and meals must never be missed. Blood testing is important, particularly for those who are insulin dependent.

Eating disorders. For a long time, gluttony—"pigging out," as it's otherwise known—was the only eating disorder people talked about. But a national poll recently determined that millions of American women (plus a handful of men) between the ages of 19 and 39 have suffered or are suffering from an altogether different, modern-day eating problem.

One is anorexia nervosa, a syndrome in which victims starve themselves to the point of emaciation. The other is bulimia, in which victims binge on vast quantities of food and then purge their system, either through vomiting or taking laxatives. Some suffer from both disorders. Teenage girls experiencing these disorders carry an extra burden of risk because excessive and unsupervised dieting can stunt growth and delay puberty.

Therapists say that anorexia nervosa and bulimia are an outgrowth of the current obsession with thinness. Although their cause is unknown, cultural, psychological and physiological factors play a part. Anorexics, in particular, are believed to have distorted self-images. Many victims starve themselves to the point of losing 25 percent of body weight. Some lose vital muscle mass and tissue to the point of death. In fact, studies show mortality rates to be between 2 and 5 percent.

Treatment for anorexia is difficult, because most victims deny their illness and are manipulative and isolated. Psychotherapy is often necessary, and antidepressant drugs are sometimes required. Because of the extreme weight loss that's prevalent with the condition, hospitalization is often necessary.

Bulimics are generally at normal weight or slightly underweight despite recurrent periods of secretive binge eating, in which large amounts of food—as much as 4,000 calories—are consumed in a short time. A typical binge could include a half-gallon of ice cream, two loaves of bread, two packages of cookies and 15 candy bars—all gobbled down in less than an hour. The bulimic, often because of feelings of depression or guilt, will then purge his or her body of the food.

Such a practice carries serious health implications because vomiting releases acids that can eat away at the teeth. Frequent vomiting can also cause loss of calcium, which may even result in osteoporosis. In addition, unhealthy purging practices can cause liver problems and other gastrointestinal difficulties, as well as heart troubles and metabolic disorders. Menstrual disorders are common in bulimics; anorexics frequently don't menstruate at all.

Treatment for bulimia varies according to the severity of the illness. In some cases, hospitalization is required to break the binge/purge cycle.

Self-help groups, along with individual psychotherapy, can be helpful. And even when depression is not present, antidepressant drugs help to curb the appetite of bulimics.

One reason that some of these drugs may be effective, researchers believe, is that they alter the levels of neurotransmitters, such as serotonin and epinephrine, the same way a carbohydrate binge does: by boosting brain serotonin levels until they relieve anxiety.

Heat exhaustion.   Also known as heat prostration, this is a condition brought on by exposure to high temperatures or the sun. It should not be confused with the more serious condition, heatstroke, which is life-threatening, carries a different set of symptoms and requires different treatment.

Heat exhaustion is due to excessive fluid loss and causes excessive sweating, nausea, anxiety and gradual weakness. The skin turns pale, grayish and clammy, and body temperature dips below normal. Because blood pressure is low and the pulse slow, fainting can occur.

Treatment of heat exhaustion includes lying down in a cool place with your head lower than your body and taking cool fluids by mouth every few minutes. Remove any excess clothing and, if possible, go to an air-conditioned area.

Heatstroke.   Sometimes known as sunstroke, heatstroke is a serious, life-threatening disorder caused by a failure of the body to regulate its own temperature. It occurs after exposure to high temperatures and is more common in older, debilitated people. It's also a threat to athletes.

Heatstroke, however, isn't only a result of the long, hot summer. Sitting too long in a hot tub or a too-hot bath (temperatures above 104°F) can cause it. People taking tranquilizers, antihistamines or medications for psychiatric disorders should not use hot tubs, because these medications make them more susceptible to heatstroke.

Early symptoms of heatstroke are headache, dizziness and fatigue. There is an absence of sweating, and the skin turns hot, red and dry. Body temperature can reach 106°F, and pulse rate increases rapidly to 150 beats per minute, resulting in convulsions, unconsciousness and even death. If the temperature is not brought down immediately, brain damage can result.

Heatstroke is a serious emergency that requires drastic measures.

Immediate hospital care is required. While waiting for transportation or medical treatment, the person should be placed in the coolest place possible—a shady area or an air-conditioned room. Remove any excess clothing. Cool the person by sponging with cool water or wrapping in a cool, wet sheet. Fan the person with your hand, an electric fan or a blow dryer on the cold setting.

In the hospital, the body temperature can be regulated more accurately and fluids and body salts replaced. Hospitalization for several days may be required.

Hypoglycemia.   Commonly known as low blood sugar, this is a condition in which the muscles and cells of the body are deprived of energy-providing glucose.

Hypoglycemia most frequently occurs in diabetics as a result of taking too much insulin or too much of an antidiabetic drug, or of missing meals. But hypoglycemia can also occur in nondiabetics as a result of abnormal functioning of the pancreas.

Symptoms include an insatiable appetite, weakness, nervousness, sweating and headache. In extreme cases, convulsions and unconsciousness can occur.

For the diabetic who takes insulin, hypoglycemia is a frequent complication. Most of the time a mild reaction—hunger, sweating, headache, nervousness—can be counteracted by drinking a glass of milk. For a moderate reaction—cold, clammy skin, memory loss, pounding heartbeat, difficulty in walking, numbness around the mouth or fingers—the same snack should be taken, followed by a complex carbohydrate such as bread, cereal or fruit. For a severe hypoglycemic reaction—muscle twitching, lack of urinary control, convulsions, unconsciousness—hospital care is required.

Hypothermia.   This is a sudden drop in body temperature—below 95°F—brought on by exposure to cold air or water. It's a condition that can affect anybody, especially alcoholics, although the elderly are more susceptible because the process of aging makes the body's built-in thermostat less reliable. Thin people are also more prone to hypothermia because they lack those layers of fat that can serve as a blanket against the cold.

Hypothermia is potentially dangerous because excessive exposure to cold temperatures can result in death. Symptoms include shivering, slow pulse and poor muscle coordination. In severe cases, body temperature can drop below 84°F, muscles become rigid, fingers, toes and nail beds become purple and loss of consciousness may occur. Complications include pneumonia, gangrene of the feet and legs, fluid around the heart, pancreatitis and kidney failure.

Treatment requires gradual rewarming of the body, preferably by a physician. If the body is warmed too fast, blood vessels can enlarge and create a loss of circulation to vital organs.

Infectious mononucleosis. Mono, as it is commonly called, also carries the moniker "the kissing disease" because it's often transferred by oral contact, and is most dominant among young people and during the spring. It's caused by the Epstein-Barr virus and can spread to almost every organ of the body.

Early symptoms are similar to those of influenza—fever, headache, sore throat and fatigue. In a day or two, glands in the neck, armpits and/or groin swell and become painful. Sometimes jaundice or a rash develops. These symptoms usually subside in two to three weeks, although weakness and fatigue can linger.

Diagnosis is made when a specific white blood cell is seen in a blood specimen under a microscope. There is little that can be done with this disease except wait it out. Treatment consists of rest—often for a month or more—plenty of fluids and aspirin or acetaminophen (Tylenol). Antibiotics, however, are not effective.

Influenza. Grandma may have called it "the grippe," but it is popularly known today as the flu, and it is one of the most contagious and perplexing diseases around. Epidemics usually occur in the wintertime, and new strains of the disease are constantly developing as others die out.

The flu is actually caused by a number of viruses that are spread easily from one person to another, usually through the respiratory tract. Symptoms are like those of a cold. Depending on the type of flu that happens to be going around at the time, other symptoms can include fever, chills, headache, muscular pain, sore throat, loss of appetite and extreme fatigue. The most severe complication is a lung infection, such as bronchitis or pneumonia, which is more likely to occur in the elderly and in smokers.

Inoculations are often given to prevent the flu, but a shot for one type will not prevent you from contracting a different strain. Efforts are made, however, to choose the most likely strain for inoculation. Inoculations are recommended for everyone of age 65 and older.

Antibiotics are usually not used in treating viral diseases. Bed rest for as long as fever is present—usually two or three days—will help prevent the virus from spreading through the body. Drinking lots of fluids and taking acetaminophen (Tylenol) are other self-help measures. It's especially important not to give aspirin to children who have the flu, since a number of studies have shown a link between aspirin and Reye's syndrome, a sudden, severe disease that affects the brain and liver.

Leukemia. Normally, the body processes only as many white blood cells as it needs to replace the ones that die off through natural processes. But sometimes the body's white blood cell production mechanisms go wild. Many more white cells are produced than the body can use—their purpose is to fight infection—and those that are produced tend to live longer than they normally should or would.

This is leukemia, a cancer of the white blood cells. And it's deadly because the "extra" white cells interfere with the function of various organs and wear down the body's defense systems. Leukemic cells, doctors explain, don't fight infections as effectively as normal cells.

There are two major types of leukemia—lymphocytic leukemia and myelocytic leukemia. The symptoms of lymphocytic leukemia include enlarged lymph glands in the neck, armpits or groin, or perhaps a feeling of fullness in the upper left part of the abdomen. Myelocytic leukemia is usually characterized by fatigue, infections (particularly of the mouth and throat), fever, lip and mouth sores and a tendency to bruise and bleed.

There is no cure for either form of adult leukemia, although treatments—antibiotics and anticancer drugs, for the most part—can prolong life and even send the disease into remission. A cure is possible, however, for the type of leukemia that affects children.

Lupus erythematosus. This chronic disease with the strange-sounding name actually has two forms. Discoid lupus erythematosus is a mild disorder affecting only the skin. Systemic lupus erythematosus is a serious disease affecting not only the skin but also any of a number of other vital organs, such as the muscular system, bones and joints, heart, lungs, intestinal tract, kidneys and bladder.

The characteristic symptom in both forms of the disease is the particular skin rash, which is red, scaly and appears on the cheeks and bridge of the nose in a butterfly pattern. Other skin eruptions may occur in light-exposed areas of the body. How serious lupus is varies greatly and depends on what parts of the body are affected.

Although the cause is not known, lupus is neither infectious nor contagious, nor is it a type of cancer. Treatment is individualized according to a patient's symptoms (no two patients are alike), but common therapy includes medication (aspirin, steroids, antimalarial drugs), rest and avoiding exposure to excessive sunlight.

Rheumatic fever. Rheumatic fever is a possible complication of a streptococcal (bacterial) infection that seems to play hide-and-seek throughout the body.

The infection starts out as a sore throat that goes away quickly and without any fuss. Then, one to six weeks later, you may notice that you feel tired and feverish. Soon after, your joints become swollen, tender, hot, red and painful. You may have red, ring-shaped rashes with white centers on your torso. As one ring fades, doctors say, another appears.

Fortunately, all of these symptoms will eventually disappear. It's when inflammation attacks your heart that you may be really headed for trouble. Inflammation around the heart, particularly around the valves (which control the flow of blood from one chamber in your heart to another), interferes with their work and can lead to heart failure.

The danger of rheumatic fever is the reason that no one should dismiss a sore throat as a minor aggravation. It is also why you should always check with your doctor if you have aching, swollen joints along with a feverish illness. You may need antibiotics to shoot down the bacterial infection. This would decrease your chances of getting rheumatic fever and the possibility of cardiac complications.

Thyroid disease. The thyroid is a butterfly-shaped gland, located in front of the neck, that produces hormones responsible for normal growth and metabolism.

When the thyroid is working properly, thyroxine, the hormone produced by the gland, affects a great number of the body's functions, including metabolic rate, metabolism of foods, growth and reproduction. In some people, however, the gland's activity goes awry, producing either too much or too little thyroxine.

Overactivity of the thyroid is known as hyperthyroidism and is more common in women than men. The cause of the condition is unknown—some believe it's a hereditary influence.

Symptoms include weight loss despite a healthy appetite, weakness, insomnia, rapid heartbeat, protruding eyes, sensitivity to heat and hand tremors. The victim may also experience emotional upsets, such as excessive crying or depression. There may also be a swelling of the neck due to an enlarged thyroid, known as a goiter. The condition can be corrected with surgical removal of part of the thyroid, radioactive iodine treatment and/or drug therapy.

When the thyroid is producing too little thyroxine, the condition is called hypothyroidism. Because the chemical processes in the body slow down, the victim may become obese despite a depressed appetite and feel mentally and physically weak. A deepened voice, thickened skin, sensitivity to cold and loss of hair are other symptoms.

The disease can come on for no apparent reason, although sometimes the surgical removal of part of the thyroid to treat hyperthyroidism can result in hypothyroidism. In newborns, the disease causes cretinism, or arrested mental and physical development. Treatment is lifelong medication with artificial thyroid hormones.

Index

Puberty, nipple problems and, 99, 100
Pulse
    rapid, 307, 336, 360, 386, 472, 483
    slow, 485
Purine, 82–83, 90
Pus, 14, 193. *See also specific body areas*
Pyelonephritis, 364, 439, 442, 444, 445–46
Pyorrhea, 405, *See also* Gum disease

Q

Quinidine, bruising from, 348
Quinine, bruising from, 348
Quinsy, 185–86, 197–98, 432

R

Rabies, 340, 341
Radiation therapy, 191, 228
Rash(es), 378–80
    on cheek and nose, 363, 487
    from chickenpox, 392
    in colicky baby, 6
    from dermatitis/eczema, 393–94
    on extremities after tick bite, 336
    with fever, 380–81, 463
    from German measles, 395
    heat, 349
    from infectious mononucleosis, 485
    with itching, 363
    from measles, 396
    in pregnancy, 365
    red or purple, 202, 277
    from roseola, 397
    from shingles, 398
    from toxic shock syndrome, 335
    with white centers, 487
Raynaud's disease, 124, 353
Rectocele, 7
Rectum
    bleeding from, 1, 30, 44, 48, 55
    burning in, 9
    discharge from, 1, 55
    pain in, 42
    prolapse of, 26, 27, 37
    warm, 42
Regurgitation, 32–33
Reproductive system. *See also* Penis; Vagina
    common disorders of, 327
    female, 296–316, 457

    male, 316–35
    urgent symptoms with, 296
Reserpine, nose stuffiness from, 291
Respiratory infection, 139, 247
Respiratory problems, 146, 360, 476, 477
Restlessness, 269
Retinal problems, 170, 172, 174
Reye's syndrome, 247, 463, 486
Rheumatic fever, 380, 474, 487
    lumps from, 367
    pallor from, 374
    strep throat in, 428, 429
    swelling around joint from, 79
Rheumatism, 84
Rheumatoid arthritis, 74, 87, 89, 157, 168, 191
Riboflavin deficiency, 185, 349
Ribs, pain at end of, 65–66
Ringworm, 381, 397
    blisters from, 345
    nail problems from, 235
    of scalp, 225, 226, 231
Rocky Mountain spotted fever, 340, 341, 381
Rosacea, 285, 376
Roseola, 380, 381, 397
Roundworms, 36
Rubella. *See* German measles
Running, breast pain from, 101

S

Sacroiliac pain, 62
St. Anthony's fire, 380
St. Vitus' dance, 474
Saliva, dry mouth and, 190–91, 192, 193
Salivary duct stones, 203, 204
Salivary glands, 203–4, 205
Salmonella poisoning, 46
Salt, 9, 143, 146
Saturated fats, 116, 117, 122
Scabies, 346, 377, 397–98
Scalp, **222–31**
    bleeding wound on, 222
    blisters on, 346
    brown or yellow lesions on, 367
    flaking from, 222
    inflammation of, 231
    itching, 225–27, 231
    lump on, 222